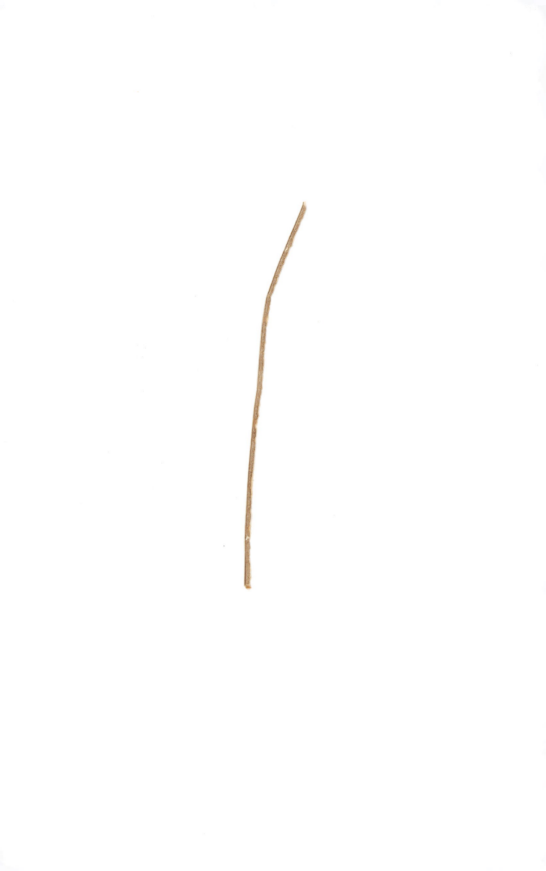

Nutrition and Bariatric Surgery

Nutrition and Bariatric Surgery

Edited by
Robert F. Kushner
Christopher D. Still

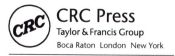

CRC Press
Taylor & Francis Group
Boca Raton London New York

CRC Press is an imprint of the
Taylor & Francis Group, an **informa** business

CRC Press
Taylor & Francis Group
6000 Broken Sound Parkway NW, Suite 300
Boca Raton, FL 33487-2742

© 2015 by Taylor & Francis Group, LLC
CRC Press is an imprint of Taylor & Francis Group, an Informa business

No claim to original U.S. Government works

Printed on acid-free paper
Version Date: 20140612

International Standard Book Number-13: 978-1-4665-5769-7 (Hardback)

Library of Congress Cataloging-in-Publication Data

Nutrition and bariatric surgery / editors, Robert F. Kushner, Christopher D. Still.
    p. ; cm.
    Includes bibliographical references and index.
    Summary: "While bariatric surgery can lead to positive effects, it can also result in increased risk for nutrient malabsorption, deficiency, and clinical complications. This book addresses the dietary and nutritional care of the bariatric surgery patient. It explores the physiological changes that underlie selective nutrient malabsorption, preoperative nutritional assessment and dietary care of the patient through the surgery process, and nutritional clinical complications manifesting in anemia, neurological disorders, metabolic bone disease, and protein-calorie malnutrition. It also covers special populations, including adolescents and pregnant and lactating patients"--Provided by publisher.
    ISBN 978-1-4665-5769-7 (hardcover : alk. paper)
    I. Kushner, Robert F., 1953- editor. II. Still, Christopher D., editor.
    [DNLM: 1. Bariatric Surgery--rehabilitation. 2. Nutrition Disorders--prevention & control.
3. Feeding Behavior--physiology. 4. Postoperative Complications--prevention & control. WD 100]

RA645.N87
616.3'9--dc23
                                            2014022608

Visit the Taylor & Francis Web site at
http://www.taylorandfrancis.com

and the CRC Press Web site at
http://www.crcpress.com

This book is dedicated to the patients and families we have cared for who have enriched our lives.

RFK
CDS

Contents

Preface

Bariatric surgery has been shown to be an effective weight loss option for patients with moderate or severe obesity, leading to significant weight loss and improvement of multiple comorbid conditions. It is estimated that approximately 220,000 operations are performed annually in the United States and Canada. Exponential growth in procedures over the past 20 years is due to several factors, including improved surgical techniques (particularly laparoscopic exposure), reduction in the postoperative mortality rate, significant improvement in multiple obesity-related comorbid conditions, and increased media attention. Although greater weight loss and improvement in obesity-related comorbid conditions are commonly seen compared with nonsurgical treatments, these procedures place patients at high risk for development of both macro- and micronutrient deficiencies unless patients are routinely monitored, counseled, and provided with proper supplementation. Since most of the deficiencies can be identified early at a preclinical stage, early treatment will prevent or reduce symptoms and deficiency syndromes.

Perioperative nutritional and metabolic care is especially important since bariatric surgical patients pose a particular nutritional challenge due to risk of preoperative deficiency, reduced dietary intake, malabsorption, and inadequate supplementation. Multiple guidelines recommend that all patients who are considering weight loss surgery should undergo a comprehensive assessment by a multidisciplinary team of healthcare providers. During the preoperative process, patients are typically instructed on healthy eating and physical activity patterns, behavioral strategies to implement the lifestyle changes, and the importance of stress reduction and social support for long-term success. The primary focus of nutritional care after bariatric surgical procedures is to facilitate weight loss while ensuring adequate provision of nutrients and reducing the risk for nutritional deficiencies. Bariatric surgery necessitates dietary modification of food texture, consistency, volume (of both solids and liquids), frequency and duration of meals, and adjustments for food intolerances and potential nutrient deficiencies. In order to maximize successful outcomes, healthcare providers responsible for care of bariatric surgical patients must be knowledgeable in the special dietary and nutritional needs of this population.

Nutrition and Bariatric Surgery is the first comprehensive book that uniquely addresses the dietary and nutritional care of the bariatric surgery patient. The book is intended as an authoritative practical guide for all healthcare professionals who are responsible for the perioperative nutritional care of the bariatric surgical patient. Chapter authors are senior professionals who provide a thorough review of the literature as well as share their extensive clinical experience in patient care.

The first three chapters address overarching nutritional considerations for assessment and management. Chapter 1 reviews the nutritional and physiological changes imposed by surgical revision of the gastrointestinal tract. Chapters 2 and 3 provide an overview of the nutritional assessment process and pre- and postoperative dietary management recommendations. In Chapters 4 through 9, we turn our attention to disease states and individual nutrient deficiencies, including nutritional anemias, metabolic bone disease, neurological disorders, protein–calorie malnutrition, and selected less common micronutrient deficiencies. The important topic of pharmacology of nutritional supplementation and drugs is thoroughly covered in Chapter 8. In the remaining six chapters we delve into unique topics that are pertinent to special patient populations undergoing bariatric surgery. The particular nutritional needs of adolescents, women who are pregnant or lactating, and patients in the intensive care unit are each addressed in a separate chapter. In Chapter 12 we review the psychology of eating and associated issues related to undergoing surgery, and in Chapter 13 we address nutritional concerns of body contouring procedures. The final chapter considers dietary and nutritional concerns associated with weight regain.

It is our intention to improve the dietary and nutritional management of patients who undergo bariatric surgery. We hope that you will find *Nutrition and Bariatric Surgery* a valuable resource that supports this goal.

Robert F. Kushner

Christopher D. Still

About the Editors

Robert F. Kushner, MD, MS, is professor of medicine at Northwestern University Feinberg School of Medicine, clinical director of the Northwestern Comprehensive Center on Obesity, and medical director of the Center for Lifestyle Medicine in Chicago. He earned his medical degree from the University of Illinois. After finishing a residency in internal medicine at Northwestern University, he went on to complete a postgraduate fellowship in clinical nutrition and earned a master's degree in clinical nutrition and nutritional biology from the University of Chicago. Dr. Kushner is past president of The Obesity Society (TOS), past president of the American Society for Parenteral and Enteral Nutrition (ASPEN), past president of the American Board of Physician Nutrition Specialists (ABPNS), and fellow of the American College of Physicians (FACP) and TOS. He currently serves as the first chair of the American Board of Obesity Medicine (ABOM). Dr. Kushner has authored over 190 original articles, reviews, books, and book chapters covering medical nutrition, medical nutrition education, and obesity, and is an internationally recognized expert on the care of overweight and obese patients.

Christopher D. Still, DO, MS, is medical director of the Center for Nutrition and Weight Management and director of the Geisinger Obesity Research Institute at Geisinger Heath System in Danville, Pennsylvania. He earned his master of science at Columbia University Institute of Human Nutrition and his osteopathic medical degree from the Philadelphia College of Osteopathic Medicine. He completed his residency in internal medicine and fellowship in obesity medicine/nutrition support at Geisinger Medical Center. Dr. Still is past president of the American Board of Physician Nutrition Specialists and founding board member of the Obesity Action Coalition. He is a fellow of the American College of Physicians (FACP) and is board certified in internal medicine with the American Board of Physician Nutrition Specialists and the American Board of Obesity Medicine. In addition to his strong interest in obesity research, Dr. Still has authored numerous clinical- and research-oriented publications in the field of obesity and obesity-related comorbid medical problems. He has been featured on CNN and the Discovery Channel as well as other national and local media outlets.

List of Contributors

Siamak Agha-Mohammadi
Plastic Surgery Body Contouring
  Center
Newport Beach, California

Hira Ahmad
Department of General Surgery
Bariatric and Metabolic Institute
Cleveland Clinic Florida
Weston, Florida

Caroline M. Apovian
Boston University School of Medicine
and
Center for Nutrition and Weight
  Management
Boston Medical Center
Boston, Massachusetts

Maria L. Collazo-Clavell
Division of Endocrinology, Diabetes,
  Metabolism, and Nutrition
Mayo Clinic
Rochester, Minnesota

Yaniv Cozacov
Department of General Surgery
Bariatric and Metabolic Institute
Cleveland Clinic Florida
Weston, Florida

Sue Cummings
MGH Weight Center
Massachusetts General Hospital
Boston, Massachusetts

Stephanie F. Deivert
Geisinger Health System
Danville, Pennsylvania

Rebecca J. Dilks
Perelman School of Medicine
University of Pennsylvania
Philadelphia, Pennsylvania

Thomas H. Frazier
Department of Medicine
University of Louisville School of
  Medicine
Louisville, Kentucky

Holly Herrington
Center for Lifestyle Medicine
Northwestern Medicine
Chicago, Illinois

Kathleen B. Hrovat
Surgical Weight Loss Program for
  Teens
Cincinnati Children's Hospital Medical
  Center
Cincinnati, Ohio

Ryan T. Hurt
Department of Medicine
University of Louisville School of
  Medicine
Louisville, Kentucky

and

Division of General Internal Medicine
Mayo Clinic
Rochester, Minnesota

Thomas H. Inge
Surgical Weight Loss Program for
  Teens
Cincinnati Children's Hospital Medical
  Center
Cincinnati, Ohio

Linda M. Kollar
Surgical Weight Loss Program for
   Teens
Cincinnati Children's Hospital Medical
   Center
Cincinnati, Ohio

Michelle A. Kominiarek
Obstetrics and Gynecology
University of Illinois at Chicago
Chicago, Illinois

Neeraj Kumar
College of Medicine and Department of
   Neurology
Mayo Clinic
Rochester, Minnesota

Robert F. Kushner
Feinberg School of Medicine
Northwestern University
Chicago, Illinois

Margaret Malone
Department of Pharmacy Practice
Albany College of Pharmacy and
   Health Sciences
Albany, New York

Mark A. Marinella
Dayton Physicians, LLC
Wright State University School of
   Medicine
Dayton, Ohio

Stephen A. McClave
Department of Medicine
University of Louisville School of
   Medicine
Louisville, Kentucky

Jeffrey I. Mechanick
Division of Endocrinology, Diabetes
   and Bone Disease
Icahn School of Medicine at Mount
   Sinai
New York, New York

Pornpoj Pramyothin
Faculty of Medicine Siriraj Hospital
Mahidol University
Bangkok, Thailand

Raul J. Rosenthal
Department of General Surgery
Bariatric and Metabolic Institute
Cleveland Clinic Florida
Weston, Florida

David B. Sarwer
Perelman School of Medicine
University of Pennsylvania
Philadelphia, Pennsylvania

Kirsten Webb Sorensen
Center for Lifestyle Medicine
Northwestern Medicine
Chicago, Illinois

Christopher D. Still
Geisinger Health System
Danville, Pennsylvania

Samir D. Vermani
Department of Medicine
George Washington University School
   of Medicine
Washington, DC

Michael A. Via
Beth Israel Medical Center
Albert Einstein College of Medicine
New York, New York

1 Review of Nutritional Gastrointestinal Physiology Imposed by Bariatric Surgical Procedures

Michael A. Via and Jeffrey I. Mechanick

CONTENTS

The human gastrointestinal (GI) tract has evolved into a complex physiological system that is responsible for not only the consumption, digestion, and absorption of nutrients, but also the integration of neurohumoral metabolic signals from the brain, visceral organs (liver, gallbladder, and pancreas), and substrate reservoirs (muscle, bone, and fat). Bariatric surgical procedures can exploit nearly all elements of GI physiology to reduce cardiometabolic risks, such as overweight/obesity, dysglycemia, dyslipidemia, hypertension, and vascular inflammation. Two broad therapeutic interventional modalities include restriction, leading to decreased nutrient intake, and malabsorption, leading to impaired nutrient digestion and entry into the portal circulation. Strategic surgical planning based on an individual's metabolic profile can involve one, the other, or both modalities. This chapter addresses the question: What are the specific GI physiological targets of bariatric surgery that confer a safe and effective metabolic intervention?

1.1 GASTRIC PHYSIOLOGY

GI physiology begins with mastication within the oral cavity, where there is a small degree of protein and carbohydrate hydrolysis via salivary proteases and glucosidases (Bader 2011). The proximal GI tract is essentially unaltered following bariatric surgery. In one study, no changes in salivary flow or dental disease were noted in patients that underwent bariatric surgery (Marsicano et al. 2012). After swallowing, food boluses propagate through the esophagus to the stomach where an acid environment continues the digestion process. The stomach acts to store ingested food boluses for prolonged acid exposure and can expand in volume to a maximum of 1 to 1.5 L to accommodate the ingestion of large meals (Ramsay and Carr 2011).

The stomach is divided anatomically into four main sections: the fundus, body, antrum, and pylorus. Gastric acid is produced by parietal cells that are located mainly in the body and to a lesser extent in the antrum and fundus (Ramsay and Carr 2011). Acid production is stimulated by gastrin, histamine, prostaglandins, and vagal nerve signaling, and it is inhibited by somatostatin (Ramsay and Carr 2011). The acid environment of the stomach facilitates protein degradation, allowing for the release and dissolution of calcium, magnesium, iron, and other trace elements for eventual absorption (Ramsay and Carr 2011). The acid environment also activates the protease pepsin from its proenzyme form, pepsinogen. Activated pepsin serves to hydrolyze ingested protein that is amenable to peptide bond cleavage in an acid environment. Chief cells, located throughout the stomach, are responsible for the production and release of pepsinogen (Ramsay and Carr 2011).

1.1.1 ANATOMIC MANIPULATION

Restrictive bariatric surgical procedures reduce the capacity of the stomach, and consequently the amount of ingested calories. Contemporary restrictive procedures, including laparoscopic adjustable gastric banding (LAGB) and laparoscopic sleeve gastrectomy (LSG), induce early satiety, leading to a reduction in oral intake and weight loss. Some authors argue that the severe reduction on postoperative stomach pouch size must exert some effect other than simple physical restriction (Burton and

Brown 2011), though no hormonal or other physiologic mechanism has been shown to explain the weight loss following LGB surgery (Dixon et al. 2005). The pattern of weight loss and changes in metabolism that mirrors the weight loss following LAGB suggests that physical restriction serves as the main underlying mechanism to the success of this bariatric procedure (Dixon et al. 2005).

The LAGB procedure is a purely restrictive procedure. A band is inserted that surrounds the stomach, reducing its overall capacity. Tension in the band can be adjusted by infusion of saline for optimal effect on early satiety and weight loss. The vertical gastric banding operation, commonly known as stomach stapling, has fallen out of favor as a bariatric procedure due to high rates of morbidity (Trenkner 2012). The hybridized Roux-en-Y gastric bypass (RYGB) and biliopancreatic diversion with duodenal switch (BPD-DS) procedures combine restriction of stomach size with malabsorption by bypassing large portions of the intestine.

Gastric emptying studies show no difference in gastric motility in patients that undergo LAGB surgery (de Jong et al. 2009). As expected, following restriction of stomach volume, these patients exhibit increased gastroesophageal reflux. Distal esophagus retention of the oral contrast agent for a median of 10 min has been observed in patients following LAGB (de Jong et al. 2009). Metabolic improvements in cholesterol profile, blood pressure, and diabetes control are associated with weight loss in LAGB, supporting the premise that these effects are secondary (Strohmayer et al. 2010). In contrast, many of these improvements in metabolic function are observed directly postoperative in RYGB surgery, prior to any weight loss. This immediate improvement following RYGB is due to considerable increases in circulating levels of incretin hormones that occur immediately following RYGB, driving many of these metabolic phenomena as described further below (Harvey et al. 2010).

The restrictive component of the RYGB procedure involves creation of a gastric pouch, approximately 200 ml in size. This pouch is anastamosed to the distal ileum approximately 150–200 cm from the ileocecal valve. The remaining portion of the stomach is left in place and creates a blind loop of bowel that is anastamosed in a Y configuration with the distal ileum for drainage (Lynch and Belgaumkar 2012). RYGB induces weight loss by both restriction of stomach capacity and malabsorption through intestinal bypass.

The BPD-DS procedure is a malabsorptive bariatric procedure in which a distal gastrectomy is performed, creating a small gastric pouch of approximately 250–300 ml. This conduit is anastamosed to the distal ileum, approximately 50–100 cm from the ileocecal valve. These surgical manipulations bypass a significant portion of the intestine, leading to decreased nutrient absorption and substantial weight loss (Totte et al. 1999). The high degree of malabsorption that is induced by BPD-DS or in biliopancreatic diversion without duodendal switch yields high rates of micronutrient deficiencies and macronutrient malnutrition. Consequently, these surgeries have fallen out of favor, and presently, they are rarely performed (Totte et al. 1999).

The LSG procedure is performed by resecting a portion of the gastric antrum, body, and fundus, thereby creating a smaller "sleeve" to act as a stomach (Updated Position Statement 2010). Patients that undergo LSG surgery develop less gastric wall tension following a meal. The restrictive component of LSG plays only a minor role for overall weight loss (Harvey et al. 2010).

1.1.2 MECHANISMS OF WEIGHT LOSS

The main mechanistic effect leading to weight loss in both LSG and RYGB surgery is via surgically induced changes in metabolic hormone secretion: reduction in gastric ghrelin secretion in the case of LSG, and altered intestinal secretion of incretin hormones in RYGB (Harvey et al. 2010).

The P/D1 cells located in the stomach fundus are responsible for the vast majority of ghrelin production and release, which is stimulated by fasting and suppressed after food consumption, physical exercise, and acute illness or surgery (Stengel and Tache 2012). Ghrelin functions via activation of agouti-related peptide and neuropeptide Y positive cells within the arcuate nucleus of the hypothalamus (Stengel and Tache 2012). These pathways have a profound effect that enhances appetite and food consumption. Ghrelin also exhibits several important peripheral effects. Long-term administration of ghrelin increases body weight, stimulates increased lipid uptake by visceral fat tissue, and inhibits catabolism of lipids (Stengel and Tache 2012). Considerable reduction in ghrelin levels following LSG surgery leads to the weight loss and improved metabolism, which may be seen even in the immediate postoperative period following this procedure, prior to weight loss (Dimitriadis et al. 2012).

The incretin hormones include glucagon-like peptide-1 (GLP-1) and glucose-dependent insulinotropic polypeptide (GIP) that are secreted by the L-cells and K-cells of the small intestine, respectively. Both function to enhance insulin secretion, decrease glucagon secretion, inhibit gastric emptying, and exert trophic effects on pancreatic beta cells in response to meals (Peterli et al. 2009; Thaler and Cummings 2009; Salinari et al. 2009). All of these mechanisms improve glucose metabolism. Meal-stimulated peptide YY (PYY) is also secreted by the intestinal L-cells and acts centrally to increase satiety and peripherally to delay gastric emptying. GLP-1 and, to a lesser extent, GIP also bind receptors within the hypothalamus and reduce appetite.

Due to the transposition of distal ileum to a more proximal position in RYGB and BPD-DS, levels of GLP-1, GIP, and PYY increase substantially. This effect starts in the immediate postoperative period (Thaler and Cummings 2009).

Similar to the immediate postoperative results for LSG, patients that undergo RYBG or BPD-DS experience improvement in markers of metabolism that include reduced blood pressure reduction and improved glycemic control, which may be seen prior to significant weight loss in both of these procedures, often within days to weeks postoperatively (Strohmayer et al. 2010). As with LSG, this phenomenon of immediate improvement in metabolism after surgery results from the surgically induced elevations in GI hormone signaling—elevated incretin hormones and PYY in RYGB and BPD-DS (Harvey et al. 2010).

Still, a significant portion of the observed weight loss in both RYGB and LSG procedures is believed to be due to stomach volume restriction (Updated Position Statement 2010). Restriction also plays a small role in BPD-DS, although most of the weight loss is achieved through surgically induced malabsorption in this procedure. Following the restrictive procedures, patients can reduce the weight loss effect of RYGB, LSG, or LABG surgery by consuming multiple small meals and high-calorie liquids, demonstrating the importance of restriction in these procedures (Ribeiro et al. 2009).

1.1.3 GASTRIC ABSORPTION

1.1.3.1 Alcohol Absorption

Restrictive procedures have little effect on gastric water and alcohol absorption. No differences in breath alcohol concentration or in subjective measures of sobriety were noted after alcohol ingestion in individuals both before and at 3 and 6 months after either LAGB or LSG procedures (Changchien et al. 2012). In contrast, RYGB patients demonstrate a 24 and 80% increased time to sobriety and an approximate two- and threefold increased peak breath alcohol concentration after consumption of 5 oz red wine at both postoperative months 3 and 6, respectively, compared to preoperative levels (Woodard et al. 2011). The mechanism for this change is not clear, but may contribute to the increased risk of alcohol use disorders in this group of patients. In one recent study, the prevalence of alcohol use disorders increases by approximately 50% for RYGB patients during the second postoperative year (King et al. 2012). Patients undergoing bariatric surgery are typically counseled on alcohol consumption in moderation (Ertelt et al. 2008; Mechanick et al. 2008).

1.1.3.2 Cobalamin Absorption

The stomach also contributes an important role in vitamin B_{12} (cobalamin) absorption (Allen 2010). B_{12} is bound to haptocorrin, a salivary protein that serves to insulate the B_{12} moiety from gastric acid. Parietal cells located in the body, fundus, and antrum of the stomach secrete an intrinsic factor, which binds and protects vitamin B_{12} that is released after hydrolysis of haptocorrin-B_{12} complexes by pancreatic proteases in the duodenum. As chyme migrates distally through the intestine, intrinsic factor–B_{12} complexes are absorbed in the distal ileum via receptor-mediated endocytosis. Thus, procedures that reduce gastric acid production, parietal cell mass, and parietal cell exposure to ingested materials, such as RYGB, BPD-DS, and LSG, can lead to B_{12} deficiency (Strohmayer et al. 2010). Intestinal malabsorption following RYBG and BPD-DS also contributes to B_{12} deficiency.

Direct measurement of serum B_{12} levels as well as markers of B_{12} activity that include measurement of homocysteine and methylmalonic acid may aid in the diagnosis of B_{12} deficiency. Because body stores can last for over 1 year, B_{12} deficiencies may not develop in the immediate postoperative phase.

1.2 SMALL INTESTINE PATHOPHYSIOLOGY

1.2.1 FUNCTIONAL ANATOMY

Gastric chyme enters the intestine through the pylorus. The majority of macronutrient digestion and absorption occurs in the small intestine (Thomson and Wild 1997). Pancreatic enzymes, secreted into the duodenum, via the sphincter of Oddi, catalyze peptide and polysaccharide hydrolysis. Liberated amino acids, di- and tripeptides, and mono- and disaccharides are absorbed by the intestinal epithelium throughout the jejunum and ileum. Dietary fats are emulsified by bile salts secreted by the liver and gallbladder through the common bile duct that also passes through the sphincter of Oddi. Triglycerides and other lipophilic esters are hydrolyzed by pancreatic lipase. Micelles form within the intestinal lumen that contain dietary phospholipids, free fatty acids, monoglycerols, cholesterol, and lipid-soluble vitamins (Borel 2003). Intestinal enterocytes absorb micelles via specific carrier proteins and process the lipid contents. Within intestinal enterocytes, triglycerides are synthesized from the free fatty acids and glycerol and packaged into chylomicrons that are transferred into the lymphatic system (Reboul and Borel 2011).

1.2.2 MACRONUTRIENT MALABSORPTION

Macronutrient malabsorption contributes significantly to the degree of observed weight loss following either RYGB or BPD-DS. In both types of procedures, a large portion of bowel is bypassed, leaving only a short segment of distal ileum for macronutrient absorption. By design, all patients that undergo these procedures experience protein-calorie malabsorption to some degree. In some cases, the amount of malabsorption leads to clinical malnutrition that may necessitate supplementation or nutrition support, including parenteral nutrition (Faintuch et al. 2004). In patients with severe malnutrition, surgical revision or reversal of the bariatric procedure may be performed (Faintuch et al. 2004).

Severe protein malabsorption has been reported in 22–30% of patients that have undergone BPD-DS (Fox 1991). Moreover, high rates of fat malabsorption following BPD-DS procedures may contribute to weight loss, protein-calorie malnutrition, and deficiencies of lipid-soluble vitamins. Consequently, the use of this procedure is declining (Mechanick et al. 2008).

Uncommonly, patients that undergo RYGB may also experience severe protein-calorie malabsorption necessitating nutritional support (Skroubis et al. 2002). Approximately 1% of RYGB patients are hospitalized annually for severe protein-calorie malnutrition (Bock 2003). Long-term studies demonstrate a 5% lifetime risk of severe protein-calorie malabsorption, necessitating nutritional support and parenteral nutrition (Skroubis et al. 2002; Bock 2003). In addition to malabsorption, patients that undergo RYGB and BPD-DS surgery commonly display an aversion to protein rich foods, which may exacerbate malnutrition (Bloomberg et al. 2005). Postoperatively, these patients must be monitored regularly for clinical signs of protein-calorie malnutrition (Mechanick et al. 2008).

1.2.3 WATER-SOLUBLE VITAMIN PHYSIOLOGY AND MALABSORPTION

Water-soluble vitamins are structurally dissimilar substances that are required in small amounts and are generally absorbed via the intestinal epithelium (see Tables 1.1 and 1.2). These compounds serve as important cofactors at enzyme active sites and provide unique chemical properties that are necessary to drive nearly all metabolic pathways. While the exact physiological mechanisms and regulation of micronutrient absorption are not fully understood for many water-soluble vitamins, these essential compounds must be consumed in the diet and then chemically processed and absorbed in the small

TABLE 1.1

Anatomy and Physiology of Micronutrient Absorption

Anatomic Site	Micronutrient	Key Physiologic Digestion and Absorption Processes
Stomach	Cobalamin (B_{12})	Requires haptocorrin and intrinsic factor
Duodenum	Copper	Competes with zinc for absorption and secretion
Jejunum/ileum	Thiamin (B_1)	Requires hydrolysis by phosphatase secreted in the proximal small intestine
	Riboflavin (B_2)	Absorbed throughout the intestine and colon, intestinal phosphatase required for absorption; also synthesized by GI microflora
	Niacin (B_3)	Absorbed throughout the intestine and colon, synthesized by GI microflora
	Pantothenic acid (B_5)	Absorbed throughout the intestine and colon, synthesized by GI microflora
	Pyridoxine (B_6)	Absorbed throughout the intestine and colon, synthesized by GI microflora
	Biotin	Absorbed throughout the intestine and colon, synthesized by GI microflora
	Folate	Synthesized only in small amounts by GI mircoflora
	Vitamin C	Absorbed via sodium cotransport and glucose transport channels
	Vitamin A	Ester hydrolysis within the duodenum
	Vitamin D	Ester hydrolysis within the duodenum
	Vitamin E	Ester hydrolysis within the duodenum
	Vitamin K	Ester hydrolysis within the duodenum
	Calcium	Absorption depends on gastric acid and adequate vitamin D
	Iron	Requires gastric acid for release and intestinal ferroreductase activity for absorption
	Zinc	May be lost by conditions that cause diarrhea
	Selenium	Best absorbed in organic forms such as selenomethionine or selenocysteine

intestine through specific channels (Said 2011). Some water-soluble vitamins, including biotin, niacin, folate, pantothenic acid, pyridoxine, riboflavin, and thiamin, are derived from both dietary consumption and enterocolonic bacterial synthesis (Said 2011). This subset of vitamins is absorbed in the small intestine and colon. Since the colon is left intact in malabsorptive procedures, deficiency of many of these individual water-soluble vitamins is less common. However, as in the case of folate absorption, dietary sources provide the majority of the required amount, and significant intestinal malabsorption can lead to deficiency (Said 2011).

Thiamin is one such vitamin that is obtained from dietary sources and colonic microflora. As with folate, the former process appears to be more important for thiamin. Patients with small bowel malabsorption of various etiologies, including those with celiac disease or inflammatory bowel disease, commonly have thiamin

TABLE 1.2

Summary of Nutrient Absorption and Deficiencies before and after Bariatric Surgery

Nutrient	Functional Anatomy Absorption	Nutrient Deficiencies				
		Preoperative	LAGB	LSG	RYGB	BPD-DS
Protein	Jejunum/ileum	−	−	−	+	++
Fat/lipids	Jejunum/ileum	−	−	−	+	++
Carbohydrates	Jejunum/ileum, colon	−	−	−	+	+
Thiamine (B$_1$)	Jejunum/ileum, colon	+	−	+	+	+
Riboflavin (B$_2$)	Jejunum/ileum, colon	−	−	−	−	−
Niacin (B$_3$)	Jejunum/ileum, colon	−	−	−	−	−
Pantothenic acid (B$_5$)	Jejunum/ileum, colon	−	−	−	−	−
Pyridoxine (B$_6$)	Jejunum/ileum, colon	+	+	−	+	+
Cobalamin (B$_{12}$)	Stomach, distal ileum	+	+	+	++	+
Ascorbic acid	Jejunum/ileum	++	+	+	+	++
Biotin	Jejunum/ileum, colon	+	−	−	−	−
Folate	Jejunum/ileum, colon	−	+	++	+	−
Vitamin A	Jejunum/ileum	−	−	NA	+	+
Vitamin D	Jejunum/ileum	+++	++	++	++	+++
Vitamin E	Jejunum/ileum	−	−	NA	+	+
Vitamin K	Jejunum/ileum	−	−	NA	−	++
Calcium	Duodenum/proximal jejunum	−	+	+	++	++
Iron	Jejunum/ileum	+	+	+	+	+
Zinc	Jejunum/ileum	+	NA	+	+	+
Copper	Duodenum	NA	NA	NA	NA	++
Selenium	Jejunum/ileum	++	NA	NA	−	+++

deficiency (Thomson 1966). Dietary thiamin exists in a phosphorylated form that is hydrolyzed by phosphatases in the proximal small intestine and absorbed throughout the small intestine (Said 2011; Sklan and Trostler 1977). Surgery that bypasses the proximal intestine reduces thiamine phosphate hydrolysis and overall thiamin absorption. Thiamin deficiency is commonly observed following malabsorptive bariatric surgery (Said 2011). Severe cases of Wernicke's encephalopathy as well as both wet and dry beriberi have been reported in RYGB patients (Bhardwaj et al. 2008; Matrana et al. 2008). More commonly, mild deficiency of thiamin may present as chronic unexplained nausea and vomiting or neuropathy. Patients that undergo malabsorptive procedures should be monitored for thiamin deficiency (Mechanick et al. 2008). Since thiamin deficiency has also be described acutely following gastrectomy, patients that undergo LSG procedures should also be monitored for thiamin deficiency, especially if symptoms of neuropathy develop. LAGB patients with persistent vomiting may also develop thiamin deficiency (Gascon-Bayarri et al. 2011).

Ascorbic acid is absorbed by sodium-dependent vitamin C transporter proteins (SVCT-1 and SVCT-2) that are expressed in intestinal epithelial cells (Said 2004). Dehydro-L-ascorbic acid, an oxidized form of vitamin C, is absorbed through hexose transporter proteins (GLUT-1, GLUT-3, and GLUT-4) (Liang et al. 2001). Intestinal absorption of ascorbic acid is regulated by its own dietary intake. Abundant dietary vitamin C suppresses the transcription of intestinal SVCT-1 (Maulen et al. 2003). High rates of vitamin C deficiency are reported, both before and after malabsorptive bariatric surgery procedures (Coupaye et al. 2009; Kaidar-Person et al. 2008a, 2008b). The deficiency of vitamin C in the preoperative obese population may result from poor dietary intake of foods rich in vitamin C, and by intake of foods containing high amounts of carbohydrates that compete with vitamin C absorption at the GLUT-1, GLUT-3, and GLUT-4 channels (Kaidar-Person et al. 2008a). Postoperatively, a prevalence of 10–50% has been noted for vitamin C deficiency in malabsorptivie surgery patients (Bloomberg et al. 2005). Screening may include regular measurement of serum vitamin C levels (Mechanick et al. 2008).

Pantothenic acid and lipoic acid, an intracellular antioxidant, are also both absorbed via the same sodium multivitamin transport protein as biotin and may also be absorbed by colonic epithelial cells (Said 2011). Niacin is acquired through exogenous sources and endogenous synthesis using tryptophan as a substrate. Niacin is absorbed in the jejunum, ileum, and throughout the colon via a carrier-medicated pathway (Nabokina et al. 2005; Gopal et al. 2007). Deficiencies of these vitamins are uncommon following malabsorptive bariatric surgery (Strohmayer et al. 2010). Synthesis of pantothenic acid and niacin by enterocolonic microflora can attenuate deficiency states.

Absorption of pyridoxine has been demonstrated in enterocolonocytes, and the colonic microflora produce sufficient quantities for most individuals (Said et al. 2003). Nevertheless, pyridoxine deficiency has been described in malabsorptive bariatric surgery patients (Strohmayer et al. 2010; Hallert et al. 2009). Riboflavin is also absorbed by epithelial cells in both the colon and the small intestine. Intestinal phosphatases play an important role in hydrolysis of dietary sources, which include flavin mononucleotide phosphate and flavin adenine dinucleotide phosphate (Daniel et al. 1983). Only the native nonphosphorylated form of these compounds is absorbed (Daniel et al. 1983). Deficiency states of riboflavin are rare due to the combination of synthesis by enterocolonic microflora and the highly efficient absorption of riboflavin in both the colon and small intestine (Kasper 1970). Riboflavin deficiency has been reported in inflammatory bowel disease and chronic alcoholism (Said 2011); however, it is not commonly observed in malabsorptive bariatric procedures.

1.2.4 LIPID-SOLUBLE VITAMIN MALABSORPTION

Lipid- (or fat-) soluble vitamins (LSVs) are absorbed through transport proteins in the small intestine (see Tables 1.1 and 1.2). Only the free vitamin compounds are absorbed; ingested ester forms must be hydrolyzed for absorption to occur (Borel et al. 2001). Under normal physiologic conditions, hydrolysis primarily occurs in the duodenum, catalyzed by pancreatic lipase, while a small portion of LSV-ester hydrolysis occurs in the stomach (Borel et al. 2001; Carriere et al. 1993). Subsequent to intestinal LSV-ester hydrolysis, LSVs are transferred to the lipid phase of digested materials in a process that depends on bile salt concentration (Tyssandier et al. 2001; Borel et al. 1994). Although LSVs are absorbed throughout the intestine, they are most efficiently absorbed in the distal ileum via carrier protein-mediated micelle absorption (Reboul and Borel 2011). Under normal physiologic conditions, the efficiency of LSV absorption is variable, and thought to depend on individual patient factors and on the contents of the meal (Reboul and Borel 2011). Absorption of LSVs has been measured to be approximately 75–100% for ingested vitamin A (Sivakumar and Reddy 1972), 99% for vitamin D (Thompson et al. 1966), 10–33% for vitamin E (Bruno et al. 2006), and 13–20% for vitamin K (Shearer et al. 1974).

LSV deficiency has been observed in obese individuals who are planning on a bariatric surgical procedure, prior to surgery (Kaidar-Person et al. 2008a). This is thought to be due to poor nutritional choices that lead to obesity as well as a higher volume of LSV distribution in obese individuals (Via 2012). Prevalence of frank deficiency of vitamin D has been reported as high as 60%, while the prevalence of other LSV deficiencies ranges from 15 to 30% in the preoperative obese population (Kaidar-Person et al. 2008a).

After RYGB, vitamin D absorption declines by approximately 25–30% (Thompson et al. 1966; Aarts et al. 2011). Absorption of other LSVs also declines following RYGB, leading to a reported prevalence of vitamin A deficiency in 10–52% and vitamin D insufficiency (less than 30 ng/dl) in 30–50% (Coupaye et al. 2009). Synthesis of vitamin K by enterocolonic bacteria may help to reduce rates of deficiency after RYGB (Kasper 1970). Reported prevalence of LSV deficiency ranges from 60 to 70% for each vitamin A, D, E, and K following BPD-DS (Marinari et al. 2004; Marceau et al. 1995).

1.2.5 CALCIUM MALABSORPTION

Dietary calcium absorption is affected in both restrictive and malabsorptive bariatric procedures. Most patients that undergo bariatric surgery develop some degree of secondary hyperparathyroidism due to the reduced calcium absorption that predictably results from these procedures (Jin et al. 2007; Youssef et al. 2007). Under normal physiological conditions, calcium ions are liberated from dietary sources in the acid environment of the stomach for later absorption. Therefore, reduced stomach acid production resulting from restrictive procedures leads to poor calcium absorption (DiGiorgi et al. 2008).

Additionally, the majority of ingested calcium is absorbed through vitamin D-dependent transcellular transport in the duodenum and proximal jejunum (Johnson et al. 2006). Because the duodenum is bypassed in malabsorptive procedures, these patients demonstrate significantly diminished calcium absorption (Johnson et al. 2005).

A high rate of vitamin D insufficiency is noted in obese individuals prior to bariatric surgery, which also contributes to poor calcium absorption (Kaidar-Person et al. 2008). This is especially true in patients that undergo malabsorptive procedures and typically require relatively high-dose vitamin D supplementation to improve calcium absorption (Aarts et al. 2011).

As with calcium from dietary sources, most forms of calcium supplements also require acid for dissolution and adequate absorption. Calcium citrate dissolves at higher pH levels than other calcium supplements and is recommended for all patients that undergo bariatric surgery (Mechanick et al. 2008).

Bone loss is commonly observed following bariatric surgical procedures due to vitamin D insufficiency, calcium malabsorption, and secondary hyperparathyroidism that develop. Weight loss itself can lead to reduction in bone density simply from reduced mechanical loads (Strohmayer et al. 2010). Another important pathway in the regulation of bone metabolism is through serotonin release from the GI tract. Serotonin has an inhibitory effect on osteoblast function and proliferation by reducing cyclin D activity within osteoblasts (Karsenty and Yadav 2011). Circulating serotonin levels increase following RYGB, which also contributes to the bone loss in these patients (Kellum et al. 1990). Bone metabolism following bariatric surgery is described in greater detail in Chapter 6.

1.2.6 TRACE METALS

Copper is an important cofactor for enzymes involved in oxidative phosphorylation, iron absorption and transport, neurotransmitter synthesis, and in the genesis of superoxides (van den Berghe and Klomp 2009). The majority of ingested copper is absorbed in the duodenum (van den Berghe and Klomp 2009). Approximately 1–2 mg copper is required daily, and excess copper is secreted in bile and pancreatic juice under tight regulation (van den Berghe and Klomp 2009). Due to the bypassed proximal intestine, which represents the major site of copper absorption, patients that undergo RYGB and BPD-DS are at risk for copper deficiency. Since zinc competes with copper ions for intestinal absorption and can induce biliary excretion of copper, overly aggressive supplementation with zinc, as may occur following bariatric surgery, can lead to a copper deficiency.

Dietary iron exists in two distinct forms: heme and nonheme iron (Han 2011). Heme iron is complexed tightly within a porphyrin ring and is derived from animal myoglobin and hemoglobin sources that undergo proteolysis within the stomach and duodenum (Conrad et al. 1966). Nonheme iron must also be liberated from chelated forms that exist in dietary sources so that iron absorption may occur (Han 2011).

During the early stages of digestion, the acid environment of the stomach maintains the solubility of ingested iron in both the heme and nonheme forms. At this point, iron mainly exists in the oxidized ferric state. In the intestine, dietary iron is reduced to the ferrous state by ferroreductase. Only iron in the ferrous state can be absorbed (Han 2011). Bariatric procedures that reduce gastric acid production, including RYGB, BPD-DS, and LSG, impair dietary iron processing for absorption and may increase the risk of iron deficiency (Coupaye et al. 2009).

The majority of iron absorption occurs within the duodenum at the apical surface of enterocytes. Since copper moieties are present in iron transport proteins, efficient iron absorption is dependent on sufficient copper levels (Shi et al. 2008). Copper deficiency may lead to recalcitrant iron deficiency that only improves after copper levels are restored. Important regulation of iron absorption is based on total body iron stores and on the iron load of a meal (Han 2011). Since there is minimal capacity to excrete excess iron, iron absorption is tightly regulated and limited (King 2010).

Both RYGB and BPD-DS bypass the duodenum and proximal intestine. This reduces ferroreductase activity and diminishes the absorptive surface area for iron, leading to iron deficiency in many patients that undergo RYGB or BPD-DS (Han 2011).

Zinc is an essential trace element that serves as an important cofactor for enzymes that control DNA regulation, growth, brain development, and wound healing, among other functions (Barceloux 1999). Total body zinc levels are primarily regulated by enhancing or repressing zinc excretion in the urine or feces, rather than changing absorption (King 2010). Intestinal absorption of zinc remains relatively constant in both states of zinc deficiency or excess (Hambidge et al. 2010), although administration of oral zinc supplements may acutely reduce absorption via transporter protein downregulation (Cragg et al. 2005). Malabsorptive bariatric procedures, as well as simply the presence of diarrhea or dumping syndrome, can increase the risk for zinc deficiency (King 2010).

The essential trace metal selenium is substituted for sulfur moieties in cysteine and methionine to form the seleno-amino acids selenocysteine and selenomethionine. These specialized seleno-amino acids are incorporated into 25 known enzymes that participate in important oxidation-reduction reactions such as thyroid peroxidase, iodothyronine deiodonases, and glutathione peroxidases (Fairweather-Tait et al. 2010). Dietary selenium may be obtained as selenocysteine and selenomethionine, often from cereals and animal skeletal muscle sources, or selenium may be acquired as selenate and selenite salts (Fairweather-Tait et al. 2010). The different forms of dietary selenium are efficiently absorbed, but seleno-amino acids are more readily retained. In contrast, selenate and selenite salts must be converted to organic forms before they are used and can be excreted before these species are fully processed or utilized (Rayman et al. 2008; Steen et al. 2008). Intestinal absorption and processing of selenium may be impaired following malabsorptive bariatric surgery. A substantial portion of patients have low circulating levels of selenium, and some develop frank deficiency states following baritric surgery (Coupaye et al. 2009). This is especially evident in patients following BPD-DS due to the extreme malabsorption that results from this surgery, in which approximately 15% of patients develop deficiency noted by low blood levels of selenium. Individuals with severe selenium deficiency may develop congestive heart failure and impaired immune function. Measurement of selenium should be included in periodic malnutrition screening following BPD-DS (Mechanick et al. 2008).

The absorption and metabolism of other trace metals, including manganese, molybdenum, vanadium, and nickel, in both health and disease are less well characterized and therefore relegated to an academic discussion. In general, these elements are acquired via small intestinal absorption, although the exact location for absorption within the intestine, as well as the mechanism and regulation of absorption, is not fully understood for these elements. Moreover, clinical deficiency states may exist for these micronutrients, but the manifestations of such deficiencies have not been well described. The means for suitable measurement of body stores are not currently available. Further study of patients that have undergone malabsorptive surgery may demonstrate deficiencies in these important cofactors (Coupaye et al. 2009; Miller and Smith 2006).

1.2.7 OXALATE ABSORPTION

A number of observational studies demonstrate increased frequency of nephrolithiasis following RYGB surgery due to calcium oxalate stone formation (Lieske et al. 2008; Nelson et al. 2005; Matlaga et al. 2009). The largest study to date demonstrates a 7.6% incidence of nephrolithiasis in 4,636 subjects that were monitored for 5 years following RYGB compared to a 4.5% incidence in matched obese controls (Matlaga et al. 2009). This phenomenon has not been described following LABG or LSG (Semins et al. 2009, 2010; Penniston et al. 2009). Increased plasma and urine oxalate levels are observed in patients that have undergone RYGB and BPD-DS (Kumar et al. 2011). Although the exact mechanism is yet to be worked out, increased intestinal absorption of oxalate is believed to result indirectly from fat malabsorption. The excess of unconjugated fatty acids in the intestinal lumen leads to increased luminal calcium–fatty acid salt formation. This diminishes the sequestration of luminal oxalate by ingested calcium, leading to greater oxalate absorption (Kumar et al. 2011).

Increases in urinary oxalate and in the prevalence of nephrolithiasis are noted in patients with other medical conditions that lead to fat malabsorption, including inflammatory bowel disease and mesenteric ischemia (Pardi et al. 1998; Canos et al. 1981). Oral calcium administration can help to reduce oxalate absorption in patients that have undergone RYGB or BPD-DS and is currently recommended in these patients (Mechanick et al. 2008).

1.2.8 PHARMACEUTICAL ABSORPTION

The pharmacokinetic profile of many medicines may be potentially altered following malabsorptive procedures due to reduced intestinal absorption surface as well as the higher pH that results from gastric bypass in both RYGB and BPD-DS procedures (Edwards and Ensom 2012). In these conditions, absorption of weakly acidic drugs is reduced, while absorption of weakly basic drugs is enhanced (Miller and Smith 2006; Skottheim et al. 2009). Extended release drugs and drugs that depend on intestinal enzyme activity for activation may have diminished bioavailability (Edwards and Ensom 2012). If available, immediate release medications are preferred over extended release forms in restricted procedures (Edwards and Ensom 2012).

Intestinal CYP3A activity is reduced in RYGB and BPD-DS procedures (Edwards and Ensom 2012). This first-pass intestinal metabolism serves as an important step that contributes to the circulating concentrations of some pharmaceutical agents. For example, atorvastatin concentration increases following RYGB surgery, which is thought to be due to decreased intestinal CYP3A activity in these patients (Skottheim et al. 2009, 2010). Sertraline is also partially metabolized via the intestinal CYP3A system; however, pharmacokinetic studies demonstrate a lower absorption of sertraline following RYGB, suggesting that decreased absorptive surface area is the predominant factor for the bioavailability of this medication (Roerig et al. 2010). Metformin demonstrated higher bioavailability following RYGB, though this finding is thought to be due to delayed gastric emptying and enhanced expression of the intestinal monoamine transport proteins that are responsible for the absorption of metformin (Padwal et al. 2011). The bioavailability of levothyroxine is reduced by approximately 30% following RYGB, owing to decreased stomach acid production and intestinal malabsorption (Rubio et al. 2012).

Following RYGB, patients given orally administered morphine demonstrated a higher circulating concentration and a decreased time to maximum concentration compared to preoperative evaluation. This is thought to be related to faster drug delivery to the distal ileum that rapidly absorbs opiate class medications (Edwards and Ensom 2012). Circulating levels of acetaminophen after a test dose are unchanged in the immediate postoperative phase, but are increased when administered orally 1 year following RYGB (Edwards and Ensom 2012). Intestinal adaptation over time may explain this finding, as discussed below.

1.2.9   INTESTINAL ADAPTATION

After prolonged periods of malabsorption, the small intestine is capable of an adaptation process that leads to both increased surface area and improved efficiency of nutrient absorptive capacity, which can lessen the severity of malabsorption (Norholk et al. 2012). This is driven by a series of complex physiological mechanisms that stimulate intestinal enterocyte proliferation. This process is dependent on nutrients as well as pancreatic and biliary secretions present within the intestinal lumen (Cisler and Buchman 2005). A number of humoral factors stimulate the proliferation of intestinal enterocytes that include insulin-like growth factors 1 and 2 (IGF-1 and IGF-2), hepatocyte growth factor (HGF), transforming growth factor-α (TGF-α), growth hormone, gastrin, GIP, PYY, and neurotensin (Cisler and Buchman 2005). Of these, IGF-1, IGF-2, HGF, and TGF-α exert their effects directly on intestinal enterocytes, while GIP and PYY function to slow intestinal transit, thereby increasing the exposure of epithelial cells to intraluminal nutrients. As a result, proliferation of the intestinal epithelium leads to increased surface area for increased absorption.

This adaptive phenomenon is commonly noted in individuals with short bowel syndrome due to inflammatory bowel disease or in individuals that have undergone extensive bowel resection for ischemia or other causes (Norholk et al. 2012). Intestinal adaptation has also been demonstrated in animal models of malapsorptive bariatric surgery, and may contribute to the diminishing weight loss over time that is typically observed in patients that undergo malabsorptive procedures (Borg et al. 2007; Taqi et al. 2010).

1.3   COLON

1.3.1   WATER AND ELECTROLYTES

The colon serves to absorb dietary and secreted water, electrolytes, and some vitamins. Approximately 90% of the electrolyte content that propagates through the proximal colon is absorbed by epithelial cells that line the colonic crypts and villae (Bachmann et al. 2011). In disease states, electrolytes such as Na^+, Cl^-, and HCO_3^- are actively secreted. Highly efficient transport proteins at the apical and basolateral surfaces of colonic epithelial cells minimize electrolyte loss and maintain low fecal electrolyte concentrations that are generally less than 5 mM for Na^+, 2 mM for Cl^-,

9 mM for K^+, and 5 mM for HCO_3^- (Bachmann et al. 2011). Presently, little data exist regarding changes in electrolyte and water absorption with bariatric surgical procedures. One animal model of RYGB demonstrated increased water intake and increased urinary sodium excretion, suggesting an improvement in sodium balance following RYGB (Bueter et al. 2011).

1.3.2 ENTEROCOLONIC MICROFLORA

The colon also functions in the storage and elimination of undigestable waste. Dietary nonstarch polysaccharides that include cellulose, pectin, and β-glucan, among other plant-derived polysaccharides, are not easily hydrolyzed by endogenous enzymes of the human GI tract. These substances are classified as soluble and insoluble dietary fiber, and generally represent approximately 5–10% of ingested carbohydrates. Microflora that reside within the colon ferment much of the dietary fiber, which leads to the production of short-chain fatty acids (SCFAs) (Kumar et al. 2012). Epithelial cells of the colon absorb SCFAs, and either metabolize these compounds as an energy source or release them for systemic use. SCFAs represent approximately 7–10% of caloric intake (Kumar et al. 2012; Tilg and Kaser 2011).

In individuals with macronutrient malabsorption, such as following RYGB or BPD-DS, an increased carbohydrate load reaches the lumen of the colon. This increased substrate allows the microflora to produce greater amounts of SCFAs in this setting, thereby providing increased SCFAs as an energy source by the human host (Cisler and Buchman 2005). This process is known as carbohydrate salvage, and may be partly responsible, along with intestinal adaptation, for the diminished amount of weight loss over the long term following malabsorptive bariatric procedures (Cisler and Buchman 2005).

Ingested dietary fiber also leads to the proliferation of colonic microflora that contributes a significant amount of bulk to the fecal matter and allows easier passage of fecal material (Kumar et al. 2012). Incompletely fermented fiber forms a water-avid gel matrix that adds to the viscosity and overall structure of fecal material (Tilg and Kaser 2011).

Over 1,100 species of bacteria and yeasts inhabit the human colon, though an individual human may harbor approximately 160 separate species (Qin et al. 2010). The bacterial species are members of four bacterial phyla: Firmicutes, Bacteroidetes, Proteobacteria, and Actinobacteria. The interaction of enterocolonic microbiota and the human host is complex and involves hormonal signal pathways, usable energy in the form of SCFAs, production of micronutrients and essential amino acids, and immune modulation, among other functions that remain under investigation.

A number of studies demonstrate that obese individuals tend to have an increase in the ratio of Firmicutes/Bacteroidetes compared to nonobese controls (Ley et al. 2006; Zhang et al. 2009; Armougom et al. 2009; Santacruz et al. 2010), though several studies fail to demonstrate this phenomenon (Schwiertz et al. 2010; Duncan et al. 2008). Studies in animal models of obesity also demonstrate differences in prevalence of microflora phyla compared to lean controls (Ley et al. 2005; Turnbaugh et al. 2008; Fleissner et al. 2010). Mice in a germ-free environment gained less weight than control mice, suggesting the importance of the energy contribution and metabolic regulation of colonic microflora (Turnbaugh et al. 2006).

One study demonstrated that specific gene expression within the enterocolonic microflora correlated more closely with host obesity than differences in phyla prevalence (Turnbaugh et al. 2006). In this study, obese individuals were found to harbor microflora that decreased adenosine monophosphate-activated protein kinase activity, an important regulator of metabolism in both bacteria and humans that affects hepatic glycogen storage and insulin resistance. These findings suggest that specific microflora-host interactions involving energy metabolism are more important than the phyla prevalence of Firmicutes and Bacteroidetes (Tilg and Kaser 2011).

Regardless of the exact mechanism, weight loss in the host is associated with a change in the enterocolonic microbiota profile. RYGB leads to changes in the microbiota profile that more closely represent that of lean individuals (Zhang et al. 2009). Similar changes are expected to occur with weight loss that accompanies the other bariatric procedures, though this has not been investigated to date (Tilg and Kaser 2011). The physiologic importance of enterocolonic microbiota with regard to the overall health and energy metabolism of the host remains an important area of study within the field of obesity.

1.4 SUMMARY

Bariatric surgery alters the functional anatomy of the GI tract. While this can adversely affect nutritional status and GI symptomatology, this phenomenon enables surgically targeted metabolic interventions and strategies that optimize risk-benefit ratios. Specific features of postoperative assessment of the bariatric surgery patient should include protein–energy malnutrition, micronutrient status, risk for oxalosis, disruption of intestinal microflora, absorption of medications, supplements, and alcohol, and in severe and recalcitrant instances, the need for nutrition support, surgery revision, and surgical reversal. These details should be familiar to all members of the bariatric surgery care team.

REFERENCES

Aarts, E., L. van Groningen, R. Horst, D. Telting, A. van Sorge, I. Janssen, and H. de Boer. 2011. Vitamin D absorption: consequences of gastric bypass surgery. *Eur J Endocrinol* 164(5):827–32.

Allen, L. H. 2010. Bioavailability of vitamin B₁₂. *Int J Vitam Nutr Res* 80(4–5):330–35.

Armougom, F., M. Henry, B. Vialettes, D. Raccah, and D. Raoult. 2009. Monitoring bacterial community of human gut microbiota reveals an increase in *Lactobacillus* in obese patients and *Methanogens* in anorexic patients. *PLoS One* 4(9):e7125.

Bachmann, O., M. Juric, U. Seidler, M. P. Manns, and H. Yu. 2011. Basolateral ion transporters involved in colonic epithelial electrolyte absorption, anion secretion and cellular homeostasis. *Acta Physiol (Oxf)* 201(1):33–46.

Bader, H. I. 2011. Salivary diagnostics in medicine and dentistry: a review. *Dent Today* 30(8):46, 48, 50–51; quiz 52–53.

Barceloux, D. G. 1999. Zinc. *J Toxicol Clin Toxicol* 37(2):279–92.

Bhardwaj, A., M. Watanabe, and J. R. Shah. 2008. A 46-yr-old woman with ataxia and blurred vision 3 months after bariatric surgery. *Am J Gastroenterol* 103(6):1575–77.

Bloomberg, R. D., A. Fleishman, J. E. Nalle, D. M. Herron, and S. Kini. 2005. Nutritional deficiencies following bariatric surgery: what have we learned? *Obes Surg* 15(2):145–54.

Bock, M. A. 2003. Roux-en-Y gastric bypass: the dietitian's and patient's perspectives. *Nutr Clin Pract* 18(2):141–44.

Borel, P. 2003. Factors affecting intestinal absorption of highly lipophilic food microconstituents (fat-soluble vitamins, carotenoids and phytosterols). *Clin Chem Lab Med* 41(8):979–94.

Borel, P., M. Armand, B. Pasquier, M. Senft, G. Dutot, C. Melin, H. Lafont, and D. Lairon. 1994. Digestion and absorption of tube-feeding emulsions with different droplet sizes and compositions in the rat. *JPEN J Parenter Enteral Nutr* 18(6):534–43.

Borel, P., B. Pasquier, M. Armand, V. Tyssandier, P. Grolier, M. C. Alexandre-Gouabau, M. Andre, M. Senft, J. Peyrot, V. Jaussan, D. Lairon, and V. Azais-Braesco. 2001. Processing of vitamin A and E in the human gastrointestinal tract. *Am J Physiol Gastrointest Liver Physiol* 280(1):G95–103.

Borg, C. M., C. W. le Roux, M. A. Ghatei, S. R. Bloom, and A. G. Patel. 2007. Biliopancreatic diversion in rats is associated with intestinal hypertrophy and with increased GLP-1, GLP-2 and PYY levels. *Obes Surg* 17(9):1193–98.

Bruno, R. S., S. W. Leonard, S. I. Park, Y. Zhao, and M. G. Traber. 2006. Human vitamin E requirements assessed with the use of apples fortified with deuterium-labeled alpha-tocopheryl acetate. *Am J Clin Nutr* 83(2):299–304.

Bueter, M., H. Ashrafian, A. H. Frankel, F. W. Tam, R. J. Unwin, and C. W. le Roux. 2011. Sodium and water handling after gastric bypass surgery in a rat model. *Surg Obes Relat Dis* 7(1):68–73.

Burton, P. R., and W. A. Brown. 2011. The mechanism of weight loss with laparoscopic adjustable gastric banding: induction of satiety not restriction. *Int J Obes (Lond)* 35(Suppl 3):S26–30.

Canos, H. J., G. A. Hogg, and J. R. Jeffery. 1981. Oxalate nephropathy due to gastrointestinal disorders. *Can Med Assoc J* 124(6):729–33.

Carriere, F., J. A. Barrowman, R. Verger, and R. Laugier. 1993. Secretion and contribution to lipolysis of gastric and pancreatic lipases during a test meal in humans. *Gastroenterology* 105(3):876–88.

Changchien, E. M., G. A. Woodard, T. Hernandez-Boussard, and J. M. Morton. 2012. Normal alcohol metabolism after gastric banding and sleeve gastrectomy: a case-cross-over trial. *J Am Coll Surg* 215(4):475–9.

Cisler, J. J., and A. L. Buchman. 2005. Intestinal adaptation in short bowel syndrome. *J Investig Med* 53(8):402–13.

Conrad, M. E., S. Cortell, H. L. Williams, and A. L. Foy. 1966. Polymerization and intraluminal factors in the absorption of hemoglobin-iron. *J Lab Clin Med* 68(4):659–68.

Coupaye, M., K. Puchaux, C. Bogard, S. Msika, P. Jouet, C. Clerici, E. Larger, and S. Ledoux. 2009. Nutritional consequences of adjustable gastric banding and gastric bypass: a 1-year prospective study. *Obes Surg* 19(1):56–65.

Cragg, R. A., S. R. Phillips, J. M. Piper, J. S. Varma, F. C. Campbell, J. C. Mathers, and D. Ford. 2005. Homeostatic regulation of zinc transporters in the human small intestine by dietary zinc supplementation. *Gut* 54(4):469–78.

Daniel, H., E. Binninger, and G. Rehner. 1983. Hydrolysis of FMN and FAD by alkaline phosphatase of the intestinal brush-border membrane. *Int J Vitam Nutr Res* 53(1):109–14.

de Jong, J. R., B. van Ramshorst, H. G. Gooszen, A. J. Smout, and M. M. Tiel-Van Buul. 2009. Weight loss after laparoscopic adjustable gastric banding is not caused by altered gastric emptying. *Obes Surg* 19(3):287–92.

DiGiorgi, M., A. Daud, W. B. Inabnet, B. Schrope, M. Urban-Skuro, N. Restuccia, and M. Bessler. 2008. Markers of bone and calcium metabolism following gastric bypass and laparoscopic adjustable gastric banding. *Obes Surg* 18(9):1144–48.

Dimitriadis, E., M. Daskalakis, M. Kampa, A. Peppe, J. A. Papadakis, and J. Melissas. 2013. Alterations in gut hormones after laparoscopic sleeve gastrectomy: prospective clinical and laboratory investigational study. *Ann Surg* 257(4):647–54.

Dixon, A. F., J. B. Dixon, and P. E. O'Brien. 2005. Laparoscopic adjustable gastric banding induces prolonged satiety: a randomized blind crossover study. *J Clin Endocrinol Metab* 90(2):813–19.

Duncan, S. H., G. E. Lobley, G. Holtrop, J. Ince, A. M. Johnstone, P. Louis, and H. J. Flint. 2008. Human colonic microbiota associated with diet, obesity and weight loss. *Int J Obes (Lond)* 32(11):1720–24.

Edwards, A., and M. H. Ensom. 2012. Pharmacokinetic effects of bariatric surgery. *Ann Pharmacother* 46(1):130–36.

Ertelt, T. W., J. E. Mitchell, K. Lancaster, R. D. Crosby, K. J. Steffen, and J. M. Marino. 2008. Alcohol abuse and dependence before and after bariatric surgery: a review of the literature and report of a new data set. *Surg Obes Relat Dis* 4(5):647–50.

Faintuch, J., M. Matsuda, M. E. Cruz, M. M. Silva, M. P. Teivelis, A. B. Garrido Jr., and J. J. Gama-Rodrigues. 2004. Severe protein-calorie malnutrition after bariatric procedures. *Obes Surg* 14(2):175–81.

Fairweather-Tait, S. J., R. Collings, and R. Hurst. 2010. Selenium bioavailability: current knowledge and future research requirements. *Am J Clin Nutr* 91(5):1484S–91S.

Fleissner, C. K., N. Huebel, M. M. Abd El-Bary, G. Loh, S. Klaus, and M. Blaut. 2010. Absence of intestinal microbiota does not protect mice from diet-induced obesity. *Br J Nutr* 104(6):919–29.

Fox, S. R. 1991. The use of the biliopancreatic diversion as a treatment for failed gastric partitioning in the morbidly obese. *Obes Surg* 1(1):89–93.

Gascon-Bayarri, J., J. Campdelacreu, M. C. Garcia-Carreira, J. Estela, S. Martinez-Yelamos, A. Palasi, T. Delgado, and R. Rene. 2011. [Wernicke's encephalopathy in non-alcoholic patients: a series of 8 cases]. *Neurologia* 26(9):540–47.

Gopal, E., S. Miyauchi, P. M. Martin, S. Ananth, P. Roon, S. B. Smith, and V. Ganapathy. 2007. Transport of nicotinate and structurally related compounds by human SMCT1 (SLC5A8) and its relevance to drug transport in the mammalian intestinal tract. *Pharm Res* 24(3):575–84.

Hallert, C., M. Svensson, J. Tholstrup, and B. Hultberg. 2009. Clinical trial: B vitamins improve health in patients with coeliac disease living on a gluten-free diet. *Aliment Pharmacol Ther* 29(8):811–16.

Hambidge, K. M., L. V. Miller, J. E. Westcott, X. Sheng, and N. F. Krebs. 2010. Zinc bioavailability and homeostasis. *Am J Clin Nutr* 91(5):1478S–83S.

Han, O. 2011. Molecular mechanism of intestinal iron absorption. *Metallomics* 3(2):103–9.

Harvey, E. J., K. Arroyo, J. Korner, and W. B. Inabnet. 2010. Hormone changes affecting energy homeostasis after metabolic surgery. *Mt Sinai J Med* 77(5):446–65.

Jin, J., A. V. Robinson, P. T. Hallowell, J. J. Jasper, T. A. Stellato, and S. M. Wilhem. 2007. Increases in parathyroid hormone (PTH) after gastric bypass surgery appear to be of a secondary nature. *Surgery* 142(6):914–20.

Johnson, J. M., J. W. Maher, E. J. DeMaria, R. W. Downs, L. G. Wolfe, and J. M. Kellum. 2006. The long-term effects of gastric bypass on vitamin D metabolism. *Ann Surg* 243(5):701–4; discussion 704–5.

Johnson, J. M., J. W. Maher, I. Samuel, D. Heitshusen, C. Doherty, and R. W. Downs. 2005. Effects of gastric bypass procedures on bone mineral density, calcium, parathyroid hormone, and vitamin D. *J Gastrointest Surg* 9(8):1106–10; discussion 1110–1.

Kaidar-Person, O., B. Person, S. Szomstein, and R. J. Rosenthal. 2008a. Nutritional deficiencies in morbidly obese patients: a new form of malnutrition? Part A: vitamins. *Obes Surg*
18(7):870–76.

Kaidar-Person, O., B. Person, S. Szomstein, and R. J. Rosenthal. 2008b. Nutritional deficiencies in morbidly obese patients: a new form of malnutrition? Part B: minerals. *Obes Surg*
18(8):1028–34.

Karsenty, G., and V. K. Yadav. 2011. Regulation of bone mass by serotonin: molecular biology
and therapeutic implications. *Annu Rev Med* 62:323–31.

Kasper, H. 1970. Vitamin absorption in the colon. *Am J Proctol* 21(5):341–45.

Kellum, J. M., J. F. Kuemmerle, T. M. O'Dorisio, P. Rayford, D. Martin, K. Engle, L. Wolf, and
H. J. Sugerman. 1990. Gastrointestinal hormone responses to meals before and after gastric bypass and vertical banded gastroplasty. *Ann Surg* 211(6):763–70; discussion 770–71.

King, J. C. 2010. Does zinc absorption reflect zinc status? *Int J Vitam Nutr Res* 80(4–5):300–6.

King, W. C., J. Y. Chen, J. E. Mitchell, M. A. Kalarchian, K. J. Steffen, S. G. Engel, A. P.
Courcoulas, W. J. Pories, and S. Z. Yanovski. 2012. Prevalence of alcohol use disorders
before and after bariatric surgery. *JAMA* 307(23):2516–25.

Kumar, R., J. C. Lieske, M. L. Collazo-Clavell, M. G. Sarr, E. R. Olson, T. J. Vrtiska, E. J.
Bergstralh, and X. Li. 2011. Fat malabsorption and increased intestinal oxalate absorption are common after Roux-en-Y gastric bypass surgery. *Surgery* 149(5):654–61.

Kumar, V., A. K. Sinha, H. P. Makkar, G. de Boeck, and K. Becker. 2012. Dietary roles
of non-starch polysaccharides in human nutrition: a review. *Crit Rev Food Sci Nutr*
52(10):899–935.

Ley, R. E., F. Backhed, P. Turnbaugh, C. A. Lozupone, R. D. Knight, and J. I. Gordon. 2005.
Obesity alters gut microbial ecology. *Proc Natl Acad Sci USA* 102(31):11070–75.

Ley, R. E., P. J. Turnbaugh, S. Klein, and J. I. Gordon. 2006. Microbial ecology: human gut
microbes associated with obesity. *Nature* 444(7122):1022–23.

Liang, W. J., D. Johnson, and S. M. Jarvis. 2001. Vitamin C transport systems of mammalian
cells. *Mol Membr Biol* 18(1):87–95.

Lieske, J. C., R. Kumar, and M. L. Collazo-Clavell. 2008. Nephrolithiasis after bariatric surgery for obesity. *Semin Nephrol* 28(2):163–73.

Lynch, J., and A. Belgaumkar. 2012. Bariatric surgery is effective and safe in patients over 55:
a systematic review and meta-analysis. *Obes Surg* 22(9):1507–16.

Marceau, S., S. Biron, M. Lagace, F. S. Hould, M. Potvin, R. A. Bourque, and P. Marceau.
1995. Biliopancreatic diversion, with distal gastrectomy, 250 cm and 50 cm limbs: long-
term results. *Obes Surg* 5(3):302–7.

Marinari, G. M., F. Murelli, G. Camerini, F. Papadia, F. Carlini, C. Stabilini, G. F. Adami,
and N. Scopinaro. 2004. A 15-year evaluation of biliopancreatic diversion according to
the Bariatric Analysis Reporting Outcome System (BAROS). *Obes Surg* 14(3):325–28.

Marsicano, J. A., A. Sales-Peres, R. Ceneviva, and S. H. de C. Sales-Peres. 2012. Evaluation
of oral health status and salivary flow rate in obese patients after bariatric surgery. *Eur
J Dent* 6(2):191–97.

Matlaga, B. R., A. D. Shore, T. Magnuson, J. M. Clark, R. Johns, and M. A. Makary. 2009.
Effect of gastric bypass surgery on kidney stone disease. *J Urol* 181(6):2573–77.

Matrana, M. R., S. Vasireddy, and W. E. Davis. 2008. The skinny on a growing problem: dry
beriberi after bariatric surgery. *Ann Intern Med* 149(11):842–44.

Maulen, N. P., E. A. Henriquez, S. Kempe, J. G. Carcamo, A. Schmid-Kotsas, M. Bachem, A.
Grunert, M. E. Bustamante, F. Nualart, and J. C. Vera. 2003. Up-regulation and polar-
ized expression of the sodium-ascorbic acid transporter SVCT1 in post-confluent dif-
ferentiated CaCo-2 cells. *J Biol Chem* 278(11):9035–41.

Mechanick, J. I., R. F. Kushner, H. J. Sugerman, J. M. Gonzalez-Campoy, M. L. Collazo-
Clavell, S. Guven, A. F. Spitz, C. M. Apovian, E. H. Livingston, R. Brolin, D. B. Sarwer,
W. A. Anderson, and J. Dixon. 2008. American Association of Clinical Endocrinologists,

The Obesity Society, and American Society for Metabolic and Bariatric Surgery Medical guidelines for clinical practice for the perioperative nutritional, metabolic, and nonsurgical support of the bariatric surgery patient. *Endocr Pract* 14(Suppl 1):1–83.

Miller, A. D., and K. M. Smith. 2006. Medication and nutrient administration considerations after bariatric surgery. *Am J Health Syst Pharm* 63(19):1852–57.

Nabokina, S. M., M. L. Kashyap, and H. M. Said. 2005. Mechanism and regulation of human intestinal niacin uptake. *Am J Physiol Cell Physiol* 289(1):C97–103.

Nelson, W. K., S. G. Houghton, D. S. Milliner, J. C. Lieske, and M. G. Sarr. 2005. Enteric hyperoxaluria, nephrolithiasis, and oxalate nephropathy: potentially serious and unappreciated complications of Roux-en-Y gastric bypass. *Surg Obes Relat Dis* 1(5):481–85.

Norholk, L. M., J. J. Holst, and P. B. Jeppesen. 2012. Treatment of adult short bowel syndrome patients with teduglutide. *Expert Opin Pharmacother* 13(2):235–43.

Padwal, R. S., R. Q. Gabr, A. M. Sharma, L. A. Langkaas, D. W. Birch, S. Karmali, and D. R. Brocks. 2011. Effect of gastric bypass surgery on the absorption and bioavailability of metformin. *Diabetes Care* 34(6):1295–300.

Pardi, D. S., W. J. Tremaine, W. J. Sandborn, and J. T. McCarthy. 1998. Renal and urologic complications of inflammatory bowel disease. *Am J Gastroenterol* 93(4):504–14.

Penniston, K. L., D. M. Kaplon, J. C. Gould, and S. Y. Nakada. 2009. Gastric band placement for obesity is not associated with increased urinary risk of urolithiasis compared to bypass. *J Urol* 182(5):2340–46.

Peterli, R., B. Wolnerhanssen, T. Peters, N. Devaux, B. Kern, C. Christoffel-Courtin, J. Drewe, M. von Flue, and C. Beglinger. 2009. Improvement in glucose metabolism after bariatric surgery: comparison of laparoscopic Roux-en-Y gastric bypass and laparoscopic sleeve gastrectomy: a prospective randomized trial. *Ann Surg* 250(2):234–41.

Qin, J., R. Li, J. Raes, M. Arumugam, K. S. Burgdorf, C. Manichanh, T. Nielsen, N. Pons, F. Levenez, T. Yamada, D. R. Mende, J. Li, J. Xu, S. Li, D. Li, J. Cao, B. Wang, H. Liang, H. Zheng, Y. Xie, J. Tap, P. Lepage, M. Bertalan, J. M. Batto, T. Hansen, D. Le Paslier, A. Linneberg, H. B. Nielsen, E. Pelletier, P. Renault, T. Sicheritz-Ponten, K. Turner, H. Zhu, C. Yu, M. Jian, Y. Zhou, Y. Li, X. Zhang, N. Qin, H. Yang, J. Wang, S. Brunak, J. Dore, F. Guarner, K. Kristiansen, O. Pedersen, J. Parkhill, J. Weissenbach, P. Bork, and S. D. Ehrlich. 2010. A human gut microbial gene catalogue established by metagenomic sequencing. *Nature* 464(7285):59–65.

Ramsay, P. T., and A. Carr. 2011. Gastric acid and digestive physiology. *Surg Clin North Am* 91(5):977–82.

Rayman, M. P., H. G. Infante, and M. Sargent. 2008. Food-chain selenium and human health: spotlight on speciation. *Br J Nutr* 100(2):238–53.

Reboul, E., and P. Borel. 2011. Proteins involved in uptake, intracellular transport and basolateral secretion of fat-soluble vitamins and carotenoids by mammalian enterocytes. *Prog Lipid Res* 50(4):388–402.

Ribeiro, A. G., M. J. Costa, J. Faintuch, and M. C. Dias. 2009. A higher meal frequency may be associated with diminished weight loss after bariatric surgery. *Clinics (Sao Paulo)* 64(11):1053–58.

Roerig, J. L., K. Steffen, C. Zimmerman, J. E. Mitchell, R. D. Crosby, and L. Cao. 2010. Preliminary comparison of sertraline levels in postbariatric surgery patients versus matched nonsurgical cohort. *Surg Obes Relat Dis* 8(1):62–66.

Rubio, I. G., A. L. Galrao, M. A. Santo, A. C. Zanini, and G. Medeiros-Neto. 2012. Levothyroxine absorption in morbidly obese patients before and after Roux-En-Y gastric bypass (RYGB) surgery. *Obes Surg* 22(2):253–58.

Said, H. M. 2004. Recent advances in carrier-mediated intestinal absorption of water-soluble vitamins. *Annu Rev Physiol* 66:419–46.

Said, H. M. 2011. Intestinal absorption of water-soluble vitamins in health and disease. *Biochem J* 437(3):357–72.

Said, H. M., A. Ortiz, and T. Y. Ma. 2003. A carrier-mediated mechanism for pyridoxine uptake by human intestinal epithelial Caco-2 cells: regulation by a PKA-mediated pathway. *Am J Physiol Cell Physiol* 285(5):C1219–25.

Salinari, S., A. Bertuzzi, S. Asnaghi, C. Guidone, M. Manco, and G. Mingrone. 2009. First-phase insulin secretion restoration and differential response to glucose load depending on the route of administration in type 2 diabetic subjects after bariatric surgery. *Diabetes Care* 32(3):375–80.

Santacruz, A., M. C. Collado, L. Garcia-Valdes, M. T. Segura, J. A. Martin-Lagos, T. Anjos, M. Marti-Romero, R. M. Lopez, J. Florido, C. Campoy, and Y. Sanz. 2010. Gut microbiota composition is associated with body weight, weight gain and biochemical parameters in pregnant women. *Br J Nutr* 104(1):83–92.

Schwiertz, A., D. Taras, K. Schafer, S. Beijer, N. A. Bos, C. Donus, and P. D. Hardt. 2010. Microbiota and SCFA in lean and overweight healthy subjects. *Obesity (Silver Spring)* 18(1):190–95.

Semins, M. J., J. R. Asplin, K. Steele, D. G. Assimos, J. E. Lingeman, S. Donahue, T. Magnuson, M. Schweitzer, and B. R. Matlaga. 2010. The effect of restrictive bariatric surgery on urinary stone risk factors. *Urology* 76(4):826–29.

Semins, M. J., B. R. Matlaga, A. D. Shore, K. Steele, T. Magnuson, R. Johns, and M. A. Makary. 2009. The effect of gastric banding on kidney stone disease. *Urology* 74(4):746–49.

Shearer, M. J., A. McBurney, and P. Barkhan. 1974. Studies on the absorption and metabolism of phylloquinone (vitamin K1) in man. *Vitam Horm* 32:513–42.

Shi, H., K. Z. Bencze, T. L. Stemmler, and C. C. Philpott. 2008. A cytosolic iron chaperone that delivers iron to ferritin. *Science* 320(5880):1207–10.

Sivakumar, B., and V. Reddy. 1972. Absorption of labelled vitamin A in children during infection. *Br J Nutr* 27(2):299–304.

Sklan, D., and N. Trostler. 1977. Site and extent of thiamin absorption in the rat. *J Nutr* 107(3):353–56.

Skottheim, I. B., G. S. Jakobsen, K. Stormark, H. Christensen, J. Hjelmesaeth, T. Jenssen, A. Asberg, and R. Sandbu. 2010. Significant increase in systemic exposure of atorvastatin after biliopancreatic diversion with duodenal switch. *Clin Pharmacol Ther* 87(6):699–705.

Skottheim, I. B., K. Stormark, H. Christensen, G. S. Jakobsen, J. Hjelmesaeth, T. Jenssen, J. L. Reubsaet, R. Sandbu, and A. Asberg. 2009. Significantly altered systemic exposure to atorvastatin acid following gastric bypass surgery in morbidly obese patients. *Clin Pharmacol Ther* 86(3):311–18.

Skroubis, G., G. Sakellaropoulos, K. Pouggouras, N. Mead, G. Nikiforidis, and F. Kalfarentzos. 2002. Comparison of nutritional deficiencies after Roux-en-Y gastric bypass and after biliopancreatic diversion with Roux-en-Y gastric bypass. *Obes Surg* 12(4):551–58.

Steen, A., T. Strom, and A. Bernhoft. 2008. Organic selenium supplementation increased selenium concentrations in ewe and newborn lamb blood and in slaughter lamb meat compared to inorganic selenium supplementation. *Acta Vet Scand* 50:7.

Stengel, A., and Y. Tache. 2012. Ghrelin—a pleiotropic hormone secreted from endocrine x/a-like cells of the stomach. *Front Neurosci* 6:24.

Strohmayer, E., M. A. Via, and R. Yanagisawa. 2010. Metabolic management following bariatric surgery. *Mt Sinai J Med* 77(5):431–45.

Taqi, E., L. E. Wallace, P. de Heuvel, P. K. Chelikani, H. Zheng, H. R. Berthoud, J. J. Holst, and D. L. Sigalet. 2010. The influence of nutrients, biliary-pancreatic secretions, and systemic trophic hormones on intestinal adaptation in a Roux-en-Y bypass model. *J Pediatr Surg* 45(5):987–95.

Thaler, J. P., and D. E. Cummings. 2009. Minireview: hormonal and metabolic mechanisms of diabetes remission after gastrointestinal surgery. *Endocrinology* 150(6):2518–25.

Thompson, G. R., B. Lewis, and C. C. Booth. 1966. Absorption of vitamin D3-3H in control subjects and patients with intestinal malabsorption. *J Clin Invest* 45(1):94–102.

Thomson, A. B., and G. Wild. 1997. Small bowel review: part I. *Can J Gastroenterol* 11(6):515–31.

Thomson, A. D. 1966. The absorption of radioactive sulphur-labelled thiamine hydrochloride in control subjects and in patients with intestinal malabsorption. *Clin Sci* 31(2):167–79.

Tilg, H., and A. Kaser. 2011. Gut microbiome, obesity, and metabolic dysfunction. *J Clin Invest* 121(6):2126–32.

Totte, E., L. Hendrickx, and R. van Hee. 1999. Biliopancreatic diversion for treatment of morbid obesity: experience in 180 consecutive cases. *Obes Surg* 9(2):161–65.

Trenkner, S. W. 2012. Historical perspectives of bariatric surgery: the jejunoileal bypass and vertical banded gastroplasty. *Abdom Imaging* 37(5):683–6.

Turnbaugh, P. J., F. Backhed, L. Fulton, and J. I. Gordon. 2008. Diet-induced obesity is linked to marked but reversible alterations in the mouse distal gut microbiome. *Cell Host Microbe* 3(4):213–23.

Turnbaugh, P. J., R. E. Ley, M. A. Mahowald, V. Magrini, E. R. Mardis, and J. I. Gordon. 2006. An obesity-associated gut microbiome with increased capacity for energy harvest. *Nature* 444(7122):1027–31.

Tyssandier, V., B. Lyan, and P. Borel. 2001. Main factors governing the transfer of carotenoids from emulsion lipid droplets to micelles. *Biochim Biophys Acta* 1533(3):285–92.

Updated position statement on sleeve gastrectomy as a bariatric procedure. 2010. *Surg Obes Relat Dis* 6(1):1–5.

van den Berghe, P. V., and L. W. Klomp. 2009. New developments in the regulation of intestinal copper absorption. *Nutr Rev* 67(11):658–72.

Via, M. 2012. The malnutrition of obesity: micronutrient deficiencies that promote diabetes. *ISRN Endocrinol* 2012:103472.

Woodard, G. A., J. Downey, T. Hernandez-Boussard, and J. M. Morton. 2011. Impaired alcohol metabolism after gastric bypass surgery: a case-crossover trial. *J Am Coll Surg* 212(2):209–14.

Youssef, Y., W. O. Richards, N. Sekhar, J. Kaiser, A. Spagnoli, N. Abumrad, and A. Torquati. 2007. Risk of secondary hyperparathyroidism after laparoscopic gastric bypass surgery in obese women. *Surg Endosc* 21(8):1393–96.

Zhang, H., J. K. DiBaise, A. Zuccolo, D. Kudrna, M. Braidotti, Y. Yu, P. Parameswaran, M. D. Crowell, R. Wing, B. E. Rittmann, and R. Krajmalnik-Brown. 2009. Human gut microbiota in obesity and after gastric bypass. *Proc Natl Acad Sci USA* 106(7):2365–70.

2 Nutritional Assessment of the Bariatric Surgery Patient

Maria L. Collazo-Clavell

CONTENTS

Nutritional assessment is an important component of the preoperative evaluation of the patient pursuing bariatric surgery. It is a requirement by most third-party payers to fulfill the prior authorization criteria in order to deem bariatric surgery medically necessary. More importantly, a careful nutritional assessment offers relevant information regarding a patient's medical and emotional health, health risks, eating habits, weight history, and weight loss efforts that can help both the patient and clinician assess the role of bariatric surgery on a patient's health and his or her lifelong efforts at weight management.

2.1 WHO COMPLETES THE NUTRITION ASSESSMENT?

The evaluation of the patient interested in bariatric surgery involves several disciplines.[1,2] The nutritional assessment is the responsibility of the medical clinician guiding the medical evaluation (surgeon or obesity specialist) and an experienced registered dietitian (RD).[1–3]

2.2   WHAT ARE THE GOALS OF THE MEDICAL NUTRITIONAL ASSESSMENT?

One of the goals of the medical evaluation is to determine whether the patient fulfills the currently accepted criteria for consideration of bariatric surgery.[1,2,4] It requires assessment of the patient's health risk based on body mass index (BMI),[2,4] and the identification of existing weight-related medical complications and risk factors that can lead to higher perioperative morbidity and mortality[1–3] (Figure 2.1). Individuals with a BMI value greater than 40 kg/m^2 or those with BMI values between 35 and 40 kg/m^2 with obesity-related comorbidities are potential candidates.[1,2,4] However, many bariatric programs and third-party payers have additional criteria that must be fulfilled before bariatric surgery is recommended and approved as a covered benefit.[2,5] The role of bariatric surgery in patients with lower BMI values (30–35 kg/m^2) is a topic of active investigation and discussion.[6,7] Laparoscopic adjustable gastric banding (LAGB) was approved by the Food and Drug Administration for use in this patient population in 2011.[8] However, most third-party payers will not cover bariatric surgery for patients in this BMI range.[5] Often, the patient considered for bariatric surgery within this BMI range has significant obesity-related morbidity such as diabetes and is willing to participate in a clinical trial.[6]

The medical history, in addition to clarifying weight trends and previous weight loss effort, should focus on identifying weight-related medical comorbidities that may improve with weight loss. Another important component is to identify medical conditions and behaviors that may increase perioperative risk and threaten long-term success[1–4] (Figure 2.1). The number of individuals with metabolic complications of obesity seeking bariatric surgery is increasing as a result of favorable remission rates reported for diabetes, hypertension, and hyperlipidemia.[9,10] Additional comorbidities that can potentially improve after bariatric surgery include joint pain from degenerative joint disease (DJD), obstructive sleep apnea (OSA), gastroesophageal reflux disease (GERD), nonalcoholic fatty liver disease (NAFLD), hypoventilation syndromes, and asthma, among others.[1,2] The clinician should also recognize existing medical conditions and therapies that might impact the decision to proceed with bariatric surgery, the operation offered, and potential risks. For example, a preexisting diagnosis of autoimmune diseases is a contraindication to LAGB.[8] Celiac sprue or inflammatory bowel disease can introduce intricacies that impact recommendations and management.[5] Deep venous thrombosis (DVT) and subsequent pulmonary embolism (PE) are the most common causes for mortality in this population.[1] Hence, assessing the individual's risk and perioperative management to lower the risk for thromboembolism is critical. This is particularly true for the patient with a preexisting diagnosis of DVT/PE or coagulopathy.[11,12]

Accurate medication reconciliation and review is an important aspect of any medical evaluation. Metformin therapy is a first-line agent for the management of type 2 diabetes in the overweight/obese patient. Metformin has been associated with vitamin B$_{12}$ deficiency as a result of impaired absorption. Although not all patients will develop vitamin B$_{12}$ deficiency, it is important to recognize the patient at risk, especially when considering a bariatric operation that can further impair vitamin B$_{12}$ metabolism and increase the risk for deficiency.[13] In addition to metformin, other medications can impact nutrition. Proton pump inhibitors and any medication/condition decreasing gastric acid can impair absorption of nutrients, particularly vitamin B$_{12}$.[14] Other medications can present challenges for

BMI calculation (kg/m^2)	30–35**	35–40*	>40
IDENTIFY			
Obesity related comorbidities **Currently under investigation *With established comorbidities		DM2/HTN/hyperlipidemia OSA/hypoventilation syndrome/asthma DJD NAFLD GERD	
Risk factors for perioperative morbidity/mortality			BMI >50 Kg/m^2 In activity Smoking Untreated OSA H/O thromboembolism DM2
Nutritional risk factors		Medications H/O ETOH/substance abuse Diet H/O GI disease/surgeries	
Suggested laboratory testing	CBC Ferritin Vitamin B12 25 OH vitamin D Thiamine	FBG, HgbA1c Lipid profile Serum creatinine Liver transaminases TSH	Polysomnography
Dietary assessment		Weight history/weight loss efforts Diet recall/monitoring tools Cultural preferences/dietary restrictions	
Interventions		Dietary modification Regular physical activity Smoking cessation Optimal management of comorbidities	

FIGURE 2.1 Nutritional assessment of the patient during bariatric surgery. (DM2, type 2 diabetes mellitus; HTN, hypertension; OSA, obstructive sleep apnea; DJD, degenerative joint disease; NAFLD, nonalcoholic fatty liver disease; GERD, gastroesophageal reflux disease; H/O, history of; ETOH, alcohol; CBC, complete blood count; FBG, fasting blood glucose; TSH, thyroid-stimulating hormone; BMI, body mass index.)

long-term weight management, as can be the case with many medications used for the management of psychiatric and neurologic disorders known to promote weight gain.[15,16] There is a scarcity of studies looking at absorption of commonly used medications after bariatric operations. However, recognizing which medications will be required after bariatric surgery should be taken into consideration when deciding on the bariatric operation to be performed. The use of nonsteroidal anti-inflammatory drugs (NSAIDs) is often discouraged after bariatric surgery as a result of increased risk for anastomotic ulcerations observed after Roux-en-Y gastric bypass (RYGB).[1] Accurate documentation of vitamin and other nutritional supplements should be completed in order to have an informed discussion with the patient regarding their use/discontinuation after surgery.[3]

A social history review should identify behaviors that increase the risk for nutritional deficiencies, perioperative complications, or may represent obstacles to long-term success. Smoking has been recognized as a risk factor for higher morbidity and mortality after bariatric surgery. Frank discussion regarding smoking cessation in preparation for surgery should be completed.[17] Unfortunately, smoking cessation can be associated with weight gain.[18] As a result, strategies to minimize weight gain should be discussed. Prior history of alcohol or substance abuse can be associated with higher risk for nutritional deficiencies and must be carefully monitored during, before, and after bariatric surgery to minimize the risk for relapse.[3,19]

Both the review of systems and physical examination should be aimed at identifying the presence of undiagnosed weight-related comorbidities such as obstructive sleep apnea (OSA) and screen for potential secondary causes for obesity; albeit, these are rare. Accurate measurement of height (cm), weight (kg), and BMI (kg/m^2) is a critical component of the physical examination. A large neck circumference raises the suspicion for obstructive sleep apnea, or suspicious physical stigmata may prompt screening for Cushing's syndrome.[1]

Laboratory testing recommended is aimed at screening for suspected medical conditions, assessing the management of established comorbidities or screening for suspected nutritional deficiencies[1] (Figure 2.1).

Several investigators have reported that commonly recognized nutritional deficiencies after bariatric surgery can be identified in the obese patients seeking bariatric surgery. The most commonly identified deficiencies include vitamin D, iron, and thiamine. Hence, it is often recommended to screen for these most common deficiencies, especially in high-risk patients and when contemplating a bariatric operation that introduces maldigestion or malabsorption as a mechanism for weight loss.[20–22] Although recommendations vary, commonly recommended tests are 25-OH vitamin D in individuals with limited sun exposure, complete blood count (CBC), and serum ferritin in actively menstruating women and thiamine in patients with other nutritional risks, such as prior or current alcohol intake or persistent vomiting.[1,3]

2.3   WHAT ARE THE GOALS OF DIETITIAN ASSESSMENT?

The importance of the dietitian's role in the nutritional assessment of the patient seeking bariatric surgery cannot be understated. The goal is to establish a foundation from which patients can develop a path toward successful weight management and improved health.[1–3,23] Most patients contemplating bariatric surgery, especially those with metabolic complications of obesity (e.g., diabetes, hyperlipidemia) have had prior experience consulting a dietitian with variable success at instituting recommendations provided.[24] The dietitian is responsible for learning about the patient's eating habits, general nutrition knowledge, weight history, and weight loss efforts. He or she can identify potential obstacles to sustained dietary change and assess an individual's readiness for change. This information can guide the dietitian in helping patients recognize potential areas for change and providing support as patients try to implement changes in preparation for the operation contemplated.[23] This is not an easy process, since dietitians often have to navigate patients' preexisting biases, help them overcome ingrained obstacles (behavioral, cultural, psychosocial, and financial), and support positive changes in order to improve the patients' chances of managing their weight successfully long term.[3,23]

Most assessments by a dietitian will include a dietary intake. This is a diet recall from the patient of his or her food intake for the previous few days. Although often plagued with inaccuracies, it can help the dietitian learn about the patient's dietary patterns: frequency of preparing meals at home or meals consumed at restaurants, food and dietary preferences, disordered eating patterns (irregular meals, snacking, grazing, binge eating behaviors), and attitudes toward food. It can be the basis for nutrition education, including helping the patient recognize the importance of personal responsibility in his or her lifestyle choices, practice realistic goal setting, and suggest techniques/tools available for self-monitoring of eating and activity habits.[3,23]

Not uncommonly, this preoperative assessment and counseling can help patients identify aspects of their eating habits that are difficult to change and may impact the success of the surgery contemplated. Although debated, consumption of high-calorie sweets can limit the success of mainly restrictive bariatric operations such as the vertical banded gastroplasty (VBG), the LAGB, and sleeve gastrectomy (SG). These patients may do better with a Roux-en-Y gastric bypass due to the dumping physiology that is introduced.[25,26] For the patient with diabetes or hyperlipidemia, dietary changes implemented, such as restriction of calories and dietary fat, can lead to better control of metabolic parameters.[1] For some, modifications to glucose-lowering therapy to avoid hypoglycemia may be necessary.

Upon completion of the medial nutritional assessment, the clinician should be able to determine if the patient meets the currently accepted criteria for consideration of bariatric surgery, based on BMI and obesity-related comorbidities with acceptable perioperative risks. Uncontrolled medical or psychiatric conditions associated with unacceptable perioperative risks or limited long-term success represent contraindications to proceeding with bariatric surgery.[1,2] The patient should be well informed regarding benefits and risks of the bariatric operation being offered and the importance of lifestyle changes for long-term success.

2.4 WHAT MEDICAL INTERVENTIONS ARE CONSIDERED IN PREPARATION FOR BARIATRIC SURGERY?

Helping our patients institute lifestyle changes in preparation for surgery provides benefits in controlling perioperative risk for morbidity and mortality. Higher BMI, especially for those with values greater than 50 kg/m², and inactivity are well-recognized risk factors for higher morbidity and mortality after bariatric surgery.[12] This fact highlights the importance of the dietitian's efforts in helping patients institute dietary changes to control weight in preparation for surgery.[23] A large percentage of patients interested in bariatric surgery will report limited mobility. For many, obstacles to regular physical activity are related to comorbidities such as joint pain, pulmonary complications, deconditioning, etc.[28] It is important to recognize these obstacles and establish a management plan seeking the assistance of specialists when necessary. Often, we need to introduce novel options for physical activity to our patients with the goal of gradually improving their physical fitness in order to minimize their perioperative risks.[12,29] Levels of preoperative physical activity have also been shown to correlate with improved weight loss outcomes and greater physical activity levels after surgery.[30,31]

Newly diagnosed and established medical comorbidities should be optimally managed.[1,2] Untreated OSA is a risk factor for higher perioperative morbidity and mortality, and its management important in controlling perioperative risk.[12] Optimizing the management of type 2 diabetes, hypertension, and dyslipidemia is recommended.[1–3]

Type 2 diabetes has been recognized as a risk factor for increased risk for anastomotic leaks, another cause for significant morbidity and mortality after bariatric surgery.[32] For those patients hoping to achieve remission of their type 2 diabetes, higher remission rates are reported for those with preoperative HgbA1c values of <8%.[33] Strong consideration should be given to glucose-lowering medications and their impact in our patients' efforts at managing their weight in preparation for surgery.

A diagnosis of nonalcoholic fatty liver disease (NAFLD) can often present a challenge since it represents a broad spectrum of disease.[34] The strongest risk factors for NAFLD are obesity and type 2 diabetes, with the prevalence of hepatic steatosis reaching 90% depending on the modality of diagnosis.[35] The challenge is to identify the patient with more advanced disease with either fibrosis or cirrhosis noninvasively.[36] Patients with more advanced fibrosis and cirrhosis, especially if uncompensated, have been reported to have higher morbidity and mortality.[37] In less advanced disease, several bariatric operations have been studied, and which bariatric operation offers the most benefit with limited risks remains under active investigation.[38] Consultation with a hepatologist, and potentially a liver biopsy, may be required for clarification.[34]

A cardiac assessment should be considered in the patient with established coronary heart disease (CHD) or its equivalents, and in those with significant risk factors for CHD, especially if they are unable to achieve the accepted level of physical activity to assess for the presence of ischemia.[1]

2.5   ARE THERE ANY DIETARY INTERVENTIONS CONSIDERED IN PREPARATION FOR BARIATRIC SURGERY?

Although general principles are similar, there are variations in the manner bariatric programs institute preoperative dietary interventions. Some are guided by third-party payers, often requiring monthly dietitian visits for anywhere from 6–18 months to fulfill their prior authorization criteria.[3,24]

A common source of controversy is whether patients should achieve weight loss in preparation for surgery. Many third-party payers and, as a result, bariatric programs may require a weight loss of 5–10% of initial body weight before proceeding with surgery. To date, there is no consistent data supporting a beneficial impact of preoperative weight loss on long-term weight loss outcomes.[24] However, weight loss in preparation for bariatric surgery has been shown to have short-term benefits on perioperative risks. Patients who have achieved weight loss in preparation for bariatric surgery compared to those who have not have shorter operative times and decreased liver size and visceral adipose tissue, facilitating the laparoscopic approach. These benefits have been associated with shorter hospital length of stay, but no differences in postoperative complication rates.[39,40]

The role of empiric preoperative vitamin supplementation has not been formally studied. Iron deficiency is the most common, particularly among women of childbearing years, which represent the majority of the patients seeking bariatric surgery (78%). Among all patients seeking bariatric surgery, the prevalence of iron deficiency is reported at 44%. The most common vitamin and mineral deficiencies identified are vitamin D and calcium, with prevalence rates of up to 62%. In decreasing order of reported prevalence, the next is folate deficiency (56%), vitamin B_{12} (10–30%), and thiamine (15%). However, thiamine deficiency is particularly common among patients of Hispanic heritage, representing 47% of the cases reported. African Americans represent 30% of the cases reported and Caucasians <7%.[3,20,21] As a result, many bariatric programs empirically advise their patients to start a mineral-containing multivitamin, vitamin D, and calcium supplement, but only screen for vitamin deficiencies when suspected from medical history or clinical findings.[1,3]

The patient contemplating a revision of a previous bariatric surgery can be at significant risk for existing vitamin and mineral deficiencies. Although the minority of patients undergoing revision operations are doing so for malnutrition (<10%),[41] subclinical vitamin and mineral deficiencies can exist with the potential to worsen when more restriction to eating, and especially malabsorption of nutrients, is introduced.[42,43]

2.6 SUMMARY

The nutritional assessment is an important component of the evaluation of the patient interested in bariatric surgery. It assures that the patient meets the currently accepted criteria for bariatric surgery, but more importantly, educates the patient regarding the potential health benefits and risks of the operation being contemplated. It allows the clinician to identify and manage medical comorbidities and behaviors that can impact perioperative risk and long-term success at weight management. With the expertise provided by a dietitian, patients can institute lifestyle changes that can lower perioperative risks and establish a foundation for successful weight management.

REFERENCES

1. Mechanik JI, Youdim A, Jones DB, et al. 2013. Clinical practice guidelines for the perioperative nutritional, metabolic and non-surgical support of the bariatric surgery patient—2013 update: cosponsored by American Association for Clinical Endocrinologist, The Obesity Society and American Society for Metabolic and Bariatric Surgery. *Obesity* 21:S1–27.
2. Collazo-Clavell ML, Clark MM, McAlpine DE, et al. 2006. Assessment and preparation of patients for bariatric surgery. *Mayo Clin Proc* 81(10, Suppl):S11–17.
3. Aills L, Blankenship J, Buffington C, et al. 2008. ASMBS Allied Health nutritional guidelines for the surgical weight loss patient. *Surg Obes Relat Dis* 4:S73–108.
4. The practical guide: identification, evaluation, and treatment of overweight and obesity in adults. http://www.nhlbi.nih.gov/guidelines/obesity/prctgd_c.pdf.
5. Sadhasi vam S, Larson CJ, Lambert PJ, et al. 2007. Refusals, denials and patient choice: reasons prospective patients do not undergo bariatric surgery. *Surg Obes Relat Dis* 3:531–536.
6. Schauer PR, Kashyap SR, Wolski K, et al. 2012. Bariatric surgery versus intensive medical therapy in obese patients with diabetes. *N Engl J Med* 366(17):1567–1576.
7. ASMBS Clinical Issues Committee. 2013. Bariatric surgery in class I obesity (body mass index 30–35 kg/m²). *Surg Obes Relat Dis* 9:e1–10.
8. U.S. Food and Drug Administration. Lap-Band adjustable gastric banding system P000008/S017. http://www.accessdata.fda.gov/cdrh_docs/pdf/p000008s017a.pdf.

9. Sjostrom L, Lindroos AK, Peltonen M, et al. 2004. Swedish Obese Subjects Study Scientific Group. Lifestyle, diabetes and cardiovascular risk factor 10 years after bariatric surgery. *N Engl J Med* 351(26):2683–93.

10. Buchwald H, Avidor Y, Braunwald E, et al. 2004. Bariatric surgery: a systematic review and meta-analysis. *JAMA* 292(14):1724.

11. DeMaria EJ, Portenier D, Wolfe L. 2007. Obesity surgery mortality risk score: proposal for a clinically useful score to predict mortality risk in patients undergoing gastric bypass. *Surg Obes Relat Dis* 3(2):134–40.

12. The Longitudinal Assessment of Bariatric Surgery (LABS) Consortium. 2009. Perioperative safety in the longitudinal assessment of bariatric surgery. *N Engl J Med* 361(5):445–54.

13. de Jager J, Kooy A, Lehert P, et al. 2010. Long term treatment with metformin in patients with type 2 diabetes and risk of vitamin B_{12} deficiency: randomized placebo controlled trial. *BMJ* 340:c2181.

14. Sheen E, Triadafilopoulos G. 2011. Adverse effects of long-term proton pump inhibitor therapy [Review]. *Dig Dis Sci* 56(4):931–50.

15. McCloughen A, Foster K. 2011. Weight gain associated with taking psychotropic medication: an integrative review. *Int J Ment Health Nurs* 20(3):202–22.

16. Patten SB, Williams JV, Lavorato DH, Khaled S, Bulloch AG. 2011. Weight gain in relation to major depression and antidepressant medication use. *J Affect Disord* 134(1–3):288–93.

17. Livingston EH, Arterburn D, Schifftner TL, Henderson WG, DePalma RG. 2006. National Surgical Quality Improvement Program analysis of bariatric operations: modifiable risk factors contribute to bariatric surgical adverse outcomes. *J Am Coll Surg* 203(5):625–33.

18. Levine MD, Kalarchian MA, Courcoulas AP, Wisinski MS, Marcus MD. 2007. History of smoking and postcessation weight gain among weight loss surgery candidates. *Addict Behav* 32(10):2365–71.

19. Iverzaj V, Saules KK, Wiedemann AA. 2012. "I didn't see this coming": why are post bariatric patients in substance abuse treatment? Patients' perceptions of etiology and future recommendations. *Obes Surg* 22(8):1308–14.

20. Flancbaum L, Belsley S, Drake V, Colarusso T, Tayler E. 2006. Preoperative nutritional status of patients undergoing Roux-en-Y gastric bypass for morbid obesity. *J Gastrointest Surg* 10:1033–37.

21. Snyder-Marlow G, Tayor D, Lenhard J. 2010. Nutrition care for patients undergoing laparoscopic sleeve gastrectomy for weight loss. *J Am Diet Assoc* 110:600–7.

22. Nocca D, Krawczykowsky D, Bomas B, Noel P, Picot MC, Blanc PM, de Sequin de Hons C, Millat B, Gagner M, Monnier L, Fabre JM. 2008. A prospective multicenter study of 163 sleeve gastrectomies: results at 1 and 2 years. *Obes Surg* 18:560–65.

23. Kulick D, Hark L, Deen D. 2010. The bariatric surgery patient: a growing role for registered dietitians. *J Am Diet Assoc* 110:593–99.

24. Brethauer S. 2011. ASMBS position statement on preoperative supervised weight loss requirements. *Surg Obes Relat Dis* 7:257–60.

25. Goergen M, Arapis K, Limgba H, Lens V, Azagra JS. 2007. Laparoscopic Roux-en-Y gastric bypass versus laparoscopic vertical banded gastroplasty: results of 2 year follow up study. *Surg Endosc* 21(4):659–64.

26. Hudson SM, Dixon JB, O'Brien PE. 2002. Sweet eating is not a predictor of outcome after Lap-Band placement. Can we finally bury the myth? *Obes Surg* 12(6):789–94.

27. Lindroos AK, Lissner L, Sjostrom L. 1996. Weight change in relation to intake of sugar and sweet foods before and after weight reducing gastric surgery. *Int J Obes Relat Metab Disord* 20(7):634–43.

28. King WC, Engel SG, Elder KA, Chapman WH, Eid GM, Wolfe BM, Belle SH. 2012. Walking capacity of bariatric surgery candidates. *Surg Obes Relat Dis* 8(1):48–59.
29. McCullough PA, Gallagher MJ, Dejong AT, et al. 2006. Cardiorespiratory fitness and short-term complications after bariatric surgery. *Chest* 130:517–25.
30. Livhits M, Mercado C, Yermilov I, et al. 2010. Exercise following bariatric surgery: systematic review. *Obes Surg* 20:657–65.
31. Bond DS, Phelan S, Wolfe LG, et al. 2009. Becoming physically active after bariatric surgery is associated with improved weight loss and health-related quality of life. *Obes Silver Spring* 17:78–83.
32. Fernandez AZ Jr, DeMaria EJ, Tichansky DS, et al. 2004. Experience with over 3,000 open and laparoscopic bariatric procedures: multivariate analysis of factors related to leak and resultant mortality. *Surg Endosc* 18:193–97.
33. Schernthaner G, Kopp HP, Brix JM, Schernthaner GH. 2011. Cure of type 2 diabetes by metabolic surgery: a critical analysis of the evidence in 2010. *Diabetes Care* 34(2):S355–60.
34. Chalasani N, Younossi Z, Lavine J, et al. 2012. The diagnosis and management of non-alcoholic fatty liver disease: practice guideline by the American Association for the Study of Liver Diseases, American College of Gastroenterology, and the American Gastroenterological Association. *Hepatology* 55:2005–23.
35. Leite NC, Salles GF, Araujo AI, Villela-Nogueira CA, Cardoso CR. 2009. Prevalence and associated factors of non-alcoholic fatty liver disease in patients with type-2 diabetes mellitus. *Liver Int* 29:113–19.
36. Gambino G, Cassader M, Pagano G. 2011. Meta-analysis: natural history of non-alcoholic fatty liver disease (NAFLD) and diagnostic accuracy of non-invasive tests for liver disease severity. *Ann Med* 43(8):617–49.
37. Mosko JD, Nguyen GC. 2011. Increased perioperative mortality following bariatric surgery among patients with cirrhosis. *Clin Gastroenterol Hepatol* 9(10):897–901.
38. Mathurin P, Hollebecque AK, Arnalsteen BD, et al. 2009. Prospective study of the long-term effects of bariatric surgery on liver injury in patients without advanced liver disease. *Gastroenterology* 137:532–40.
39. Alami RS, Morton JM, Schuster R, et al. 2007. Is there a benefit to preoperative weight loss in gastric bypass patients? A prospective randomized trial. *Surg Obes Relat Dis* 3:141–46.
40. Liu RC, Sabnis AA, Forsyth C, Chand B. 2005. The effects of acute preoperative weight loss on laparoscopic Roux en Y gastric bypass surgery. *Obes Surg* 15:1396–402.
41. Patel S, Szomstein S, Rosenthal RJ. 2011. Reasons and outcomes of reoperative bariatric surgery for failed and complicated procedures (excluding adjustable gastric banding). *Obes Surg* 21:1209–19.
42. Rawlins ML, Teel D 2nd, Hedgcroth K, Maguire JP. 2011. Revision of Roux-en-Y gastric bypass for failed weight loss. *Surg Obes Relat Dis* 7(1):45–49.
43. Hamoui N, Chock B, Anthone GJ, Crookes PF. 2007. Revision of the duodenal switch: indications, technique and outcomes. *J Am Col Surg* 204(4):603–8.

3 Nutrition Management, Pre- and Postsurgery

Sue Cummings

CONTENTS

3.1   INTRODUCTION

The decision to recommend weight loss surgery (WLS) for patients with obesity requires a multidisciplinary team to evaluate the indications for an operation, to define and manage comorbidities, and to provide short- and long-term post-WLS monitoring, support, and education. Most current recommendations for the nutritional care of WLS patients are based on case reports, nonrandomized, small samples, retrospective studies, and expert opinion. Although there are some published guidelines, to date, there has been no standardization of the nutrition management of the pre- or post-WLS patient.[1–3] All WLS procedures have nutritional implications, and this chapter will provide guidance for the nutritional evaluation and care for pre- and post-WLS patients.

3.2   PRESURGERY NUTRITION

3.2.1   NUTRITION EVALUATION

Since we have limited capacity to predict success or failure of a given procedure in a given patient, the choice of which procedure to perform is often influenced by the local or regional expertise of surgeons and patient preference. However, strong consideration should be given to risk stratification, patient comorbidities, as well as weight loss expectations. Although risk will never be reduced to zero, it is important that we make every attempt to do so through careful and thorough medical, psychological, nutritional, and surgical evaluation. Registered dietitians (RDs) play an important role in the nutrition care of the bariatric patient.[3,4] The components of a thorough nutrition evaluation are outlined in Table 3.1 and include laboratory assessment of patients' current nutrition status. Table 3.2 provides a list of pre- and postsurgical nutritional labs. Weight and dieting history and triggers to weight gain, including environmental challenges to following a healthy diet, should also be assessed and documented. The medical letter of necessity sent to insurance providers for approval of bariatric surgery will require documentation of previous failed weight loss attempts. For patients prescribed specialized diets and medications for nutrition-related comorbidities such as diabetes mellitus (DM), hypertension (HTN), hyperlipidemia, chronic kidney disease (CKD), and end-stage renal disease (ESRD), an assessment of adherence and barriers to adherence should also be performed. Assessment of patients' expectations, knowledge, and self-efficacy regarding post-WLS diet recommendations and supplementation is an important component of the initial evaluation. The presurgery nutrition assessment also provides baseline data used to assess postsurgery outcomes. By synthesizing and classifying patient assessment information, a presurgery *nutrition prescription* can be formulated and presurgery nutrition goals can be set.[5]

3.2.1.1   Presurgery Nutritional Labs

Obesity itself is a risk factor for a number of nutrition deficiencies.[7] Since combination procedures put patients at additional risk, an important component of the nutrition evaluation is laboratory assessment of nutritional status. Deficiencies should

TABLE 3.1
Pre-WLS Nutrition Evaluation

1. Reason for referral
2. Anthropometric measurements:
   a. Weight:
   b. Height:
   c. Body mass index (BMI):
3. Patient goals and expectations:
   a. Patient-stated weight goal
   b. Reason patient wants to lose weight
   c. Patient's expectations regarding treatment
4. Nutrition-related medical diagnosis/problems
5. Medications
6. Abnormal nutrition-related labs (if available); see Table 3.2
7. Weight history (inquire about triggers to weight gain):
   a. Onset of obesity (circle one):   Childhood   Adolescent   Adult
   b. Chronology of weight gain:
      i. Lowest adult weight:
      ii. Highest adult weight:
   c. Family history of obesity:
   Possible triggers to weight gain:
   d. Life events that may have led to weight gain
   e. Weight-promoting medications
   f. Postpartum weight retention
   g. Menopause
   h. Smoking cessation
   i. Hours of sleep per night
   j. Work schedule: Shift worker?
8. Prior weight loss effort: (The letter of medical necessity required by all insurance providers must include patient's previous, failed attempts at weight loss and maintenance)
   a. Prior weight loss surgery: Y/N
   b. Commercial programs
   c. Has worked with a registered dietitian on weight loss
   d. Medical programs (including weight loss medications)
   e. Self-directed diets
9. Current intake:
   a. Who shops and prepares food at home?
   b. Diet recall:
      i. Wakes:
      ii. Breakfast:
      iii. Snack:
      iv. Lunch:
      v. Snack:
      vi. Dinner:

(Continued)

TABLE 3.1 (CONTINUED)
Pre-WLS Nutrition Evaluation

      vii.   Snack:

    c.   Food allergies/intolerance:

    d.   Vitamin/mineral supplements:

10.   Patterns/habits:

    a.   Feeling after meals: Comfortable   Stuffed   Can eat more

    b.   Skips meals: Y/N

    c.   Unplanned snacking: If yes, what times of day?

    d.   Wakes during the night to eat: Y/N

    e.   Is there a time of feeling "out of control" when eating: Y/N

    f.   Nutrition quality: Do you think you eat healthfully (follow guidelines below):

        i.   Poor:

            1.   Does not eat fruits or vegetables on a daily basis

            2.   Never eats fruits

            3.   Never eats vegetables

            4.   Consumes high amounts of processed fruits

            5.   High daily intake of empty-calorie foods: Sweets fatty/salty foods

        ii.   Good:

            1.   Eats some fruits and/or vegetables daily

            2.   "Tries" to eat healthy—whole wheat bread, moderate to high intake of noncalorie foods (sweets/salty/fatty foods)

        iii.   Excellent:

            1.   Daily intake of fruits and vegetables

            2.   Eats whole grains, lean meats, low-fat meals

    g.   Consumption of high-calorie beverages: Y/N

        i.   If yes, what kind; how much per day: Juice, soda, whole or 2% milk, alcohol

    h.   Eating out: (Note how often per: Day? Week? Month?)

        i.   Fast food restaurants:

        ii.   Order out or delivery:

        iii.   Restaurants:

11.   Physical activity pattern

    a.   Work-related activity: Sedentary   Moderate   Heavy

    b.   Time spent in sedentary activities per day (computer, TV, etc.):

    c.   Planned exercise (type):

        i.   Time spent in planned exercise:

    d.   If patient does not exercise, are there specific barriers to exercise? List:

12.   Assess:

    a.   Motivation for healthy eating

    b.   Weight loss expectations

    c.   Understanding of post-WLS diet changes, supplementation

    d.   Ability and willingness to commit to all pre- and post-WLS appointments

    e.   Need for additional nutrition education, support, counseling prior to WLS

    f.   Ability to financially afford post-operative vitamin and mineral supplements.

TABLE 3.2 Pre- and Post-WLS Nutrition Biochemical Surveillances, Sleeve Gastrectomy, and Rous-en-Y Gastric Bypass

	Presurgery	2 Months Postsurgery	Post Month 6	Post Yearly
Iron status	√	√	√	√
Serum folate				
Ferritin				
TIBC				
Thiamin (B$_1$)	√	√	√	√
B$_{12}$ cobalamin Methylmalonic acid (optional)	√	√	√	√
Vitamin D, 25-OH	√	√	√	√
Serum calcium				
PTH				
Alkaline phosphatase				
Hemoglobin A1c	√	√	√	√
Phosphorus	√	√	√	√
Magnesium	√	X	√	√
Vitamin A	X	X	X	Optional
Zinc	√	X	√	√
Copper[a]	X	X	RYGB	RYGB
Selenium[a]	X	X	RYGB	RYGB

Source: Adapted from Mechanick, J. I. et al., *SOARD,* 9, 159–191, 2013; Moize, V. et al., *JAND,* 113, 400–410, 2013.

Note: Shaded areas indicate that it is not necessary unless indicated by physical assessment/specific findings; there are no data regarding copper or selenium post-SG.

[a] With specific findings.

be replete prior to WLS. Special considerations should be given to the following micronutrients:[3,6]

- *Vitamin D*: The primary source of vitamin D is the sun. In addition to inadequate sun exposure, the uses of sunscreens block the absorption of vitamin D. Since vitamin D deficiency is common in the U.S. population and obesity is also a risk factor for deficiency, vitamin D status, measured as 25 (OH) vitamin D, should be assessed and deficiencies corrected prior to WLS.
- *Calcium*: Adequate calcium consumption and weight-bearing physical activity build strong bones, optimize bone mass, and may reduce the risk of osteoporosis later in life. Since calcium absorption after the Roux-en-Y gastric bypass (RYGB) and possibly the sleeve gastrectomy (SG) may be compromised, patients, especially women who are peri- or postmenopausal, should be monitored closely and instructed to have a baseline bone density test that is repeated every 2 to 5 years post-WLS.

- *Thiamin (vitamin B_1)*: Thiamin deficiency is seen more commonly in African American and Hispanic patients with obesity. Thiamin should be tested and low levels replete prior to WLS.
- *Folate (folic acid)*: Folate should be tested and replete, especially in women of childbearing age. Pregnancy is discouraged until 18–24 months post-WLS, and women should be advised to use appropriate contraception until that time. Female patients who may be planning a pregnancy any time after WLS should be educated regarding the importance of folic acid in the prevention of spina bifida in the fetus.
- *Iron*: All patients should be screened for iron deficiency. Iron deficiency may be a particular problem for women who are menstruating, and they should be screened and replete if deficient prior to surgery. It would be prudent to recommend all women who are menstruating to start a multivitamin with iron prior to surgery.
- *Vitamin B_{12}*: Although not common, there are reports of patients presenting for WLS who have preoperative low levels of vitamin B_{12}.[7,8] Since vitamin B_{12} absorption from dietary sources post-RYGB and SG may be compromised, vitamin B_{12} should be assessed prior to surgery and deficiencies corrected. Varying levels of B_{12} storage among individuals will affect post-surgical status; therefore, patients need to be educated prior to surgery of the increased risk of deficiency occurring late, >2 years, post-WLS, and as with all nutritional laboratory studies, monitored on a yearly basis.

3.2.1.2 Presurgery Medical Nutrition Therapy: Education and Counseling

All patients considering WLS should have access to preoperative nutrition education and counseling, in either group or individual sessions. These sessions can be burdensome to patients both financially and in terms of time commitment, and delays before surgery can be an obstacle for patients in the most need of effective obesity treatment. Providers can help patients through this process by (1) establishing cost-effective programs, (2) motivating patients by emphasizing the benefits of presurgical preparation, both physically and psychologically, and (3) using this time to shape patient expectations regarding the early postsurgical challenges and the lifestyle changes required for long-term success. Once patients make a decision to have weight loss surgery, the process of preparation should begin immediately.

Fearing food restriction and deprivation, which is often experienced by patients when "dieting," many patients may be tempted to prepare for surgery as they are going to be starting a diet. They may want to engage in food-centered activities such as planning gatherings with friends and family to their favorite restaurants, consuming more of their favorite foods, etc. This may lead to presurgery weight gain or poor control of nutrition-related comorbidities. Patients should be advised not to prepare for surgery as if they are going to be going on a diet, but prepare for surgery as if their life depends on it. Surgical risks and complications should be made clear, and the patient's role in reducing perioperative risks emphasized. Getting physically ready for surgery by focusing on stabilizing blood glucose, blood pressure, and other nutrition-related comorbidities is an important aspect of pre-WLS preparation.

Counseling patients to engage in behaviors that may help them to walk into the hospital on the day of their surgery as healthy as they can be may potentially lower peri- and postoperative complications. In addition, although hunger, satiety, food tolerance, and amount of foods eaten, especially early post-WLS, will change dramatically, the environmental challenges will not. Presurgery nutrition education and care include assisting patients with an understanding of how the procedures influence nutritional status, food choices, and eating behaviors both short- and long-term postsurgery.

Additional nutritional changes to encourage prior to WLS include the following:

- *Eliminating caffeine*: Caffeine acts like a diuretic and may potentially contribute to dehydration. For many, abrupt caffeine withdrawal can lead to uncomfortable side effects, including headaches and extreme fatigue. Gradually weaning off of caffeine prior to surgery will help to avoid these effects.
- *Physical activity*: Encourage all patients to schedule mini-walks throughout the day. This will assist in setting the expectation and habit prior to surgery and may help patients to develop strength and stamina for post-WLS activity. Patients should be educated about postsurgical risks for venous thrombosis and the important role of activity in prevention.
- *Hydration:* Encourage patients to get in the habit of drinking 48 to 64 oz of noncalorie, noncarbonated, noncaffeinated beverages each day. Patients are at risk for early postoperative dehydration. Patients will need to start early and sip all day long to get in adequate amounts of fluids. Provide patients with lists of appropriate post-WLS liquids.
- *Structuring meals and snacks*: Many patients skip meals, which tends to lead to large meals and snacks consumed at one time, often later in the day. Patients should be educated about the importance of planning and preparing meals and snacks and setting up a routine meal pattern. Setting a schedule of when and what to drink will be essential for meeting nutrition needs.
- *Mindful eating*: Since the new pouch/sleeve will not grind food or secrete acid or digestive enzymes and the volume is significantly diminished, patients need to learn to chew food thoroughly, to breathe between bites, and to check in with their body to assess fullness. Teaching patients techniques of mindful eating and encouraging them to start practicing this presurgery will prepare them for the dramatic change in eating style required postsurgery.

3.2.2 PRESURGERY WEIGHT LOSS

A 10% preoperative weight loss has been associated with decreased complications after gastric bypass surgery.[9] Preoperative weight loss has also been shown to exert a favorable effect on hospital length of stay for bariatric surgery.[10] Some surgeons require a preoperative weight loss ranging from 5 to 10% of current weight. The pre-WLS diet can be individually tailored based on patients' medical or nutritional status. Diets that incorporate meal replacement products and very low-calorie diets are commonly used. The length of time a patient follows the presurgery diet is variable and commonly based on amount of weight loss required.

3.2.3 Presurgery Insurance Provider Requirements

Some federal and private insurers may require that patients participate in a 3- to 6-month medically supervised nutrition program. For most insurance companies, proper documentation is critical and must consist of date of visit, current weight, and specific goals relating to three categories: nutrition, exercise, and behavior modification. These visits can be provided by a registered dietitian; some insurance providers also require monthly psychology visits. Patients should be advised to contact their individual insurance provider to learn what is required to get insurance authorization for WLS.

3.2.4 Summary of Presurgery Nutrition Preparation

Goals of presurgery nutrition intervention:

- Education regarding nutritional implications of WLS
- Guiding patients toward starting the process of meal and snack planning and healthy eating and activity
- Achieving better control of nutrition-related comorbidities
- Repletion of nutrition deficiencies
- Presurgery weight loss (5–10% of current weight)

3.3 DISCHARGE DIET AND NUTRITION GUIDELINES

Once a patient has been approved for surgery and has been given a surgery date, he or she should be scheduled to meet with a dietitian to begin the pre-WLS nutrition education that focuses on the discharge diet and vitamin and mineral supplementation. All patients should be provided with educational material and access to educational sessions at the prospective surgery center.[2] A shopping list of liquids and appropriate WLS supplements in chewable or liquid form should be provided. See Table 3.3 for the standard supplementation recommendations for all RYGB and SG patients. Since not all multivitamins are formulated the same, Table 3.4 lists the vitamins and minerals that need to be in the multivitamins for patients post-WLS. Patients should purchase their postop liquids and supplements prior to going into the hospital so that they are prepared and can begin diet stage 2 at discharge (see Tables 3.5 and 3.6 for diet stage 2 after RYGB, SG, and LAGB).

3.4 POSTOP NUTRITIONAL CARE

It is imperative that ongoing nutritional assessment and follow-up occur at regular intervals to maintain a healthy nutritional status. Nutritional management after bariatric surgery has been determined to be a significant factor in postoperative patients maintaining weight loss.[4] Suggestions regarding important areas of pre-and postoperative nutritional monitoring, evaluation, and education have been outlined in the American Society for Metabolic and Bariatric Surgery (ASMBS) nutritional guidelines for the surgical weight loss patient.[2,3]

TABLE 3.3 Standard Post-RYGB and SG Supplementation[a]

Supplement	Dosage
Multivitamin	1–2 daily, should contain RDA for all nutrients listed in Table 3.5; early postop recommend 2/day; >3 months may switch to 1 daily
Calcium citrate divided dose[b]	1,200–1,500 mg/day
Vitamin D	3,000 IU of D titrate to >30 ng/ml
Folic acid	400 µg/day in multivitamin
Elemental iron	18–27 mg/day elemental
Not to be taken with calcium; taken with vitamin C will increase iron absorption	40–65 mg/day menstruating females
Vitamin B$_{12}$	350–500 µg/day orally/sublingual, nasal, or 1,000 µg/month intramuscularly

Source: Mechanick, J. I. et al., *Endocrine Practice*, 14(1), July/August 2008; Aills, L. et al., SOARD, 4, S73–S108, 2008.

[a] Patients with preoperative or postoperative biochemical deficiency states are treated beyond these recommendations.

[b] Calcium citrate is the preferable form of calcium supplementation for absorption in a hypochlorhydric stomach such as the RYGB pouch; however, attention should be paid to cost, availability, and feasibility when recommending calcium supplements, as calcium carbonate may lead to better patient adherence.

TABLE 3.4
Dietary Reference Intakes (DRIs): All Post-WLS Multivitamins Should Contain 100% of the Nutrients Listed Below

DRI	Vitamin K (µg)	Biotin (µg)	Zinc (mg)	Thiamin (mg)	B$_{12}$ (µg)	Folic Acid (µg)	Iron (mg)	Copper (mg)
Adult males	120	30	11	1.2	2.4	400	8	0.7
Adult females	90	30	8	1.1	2.4	400	18	0.7

Source: Dietary Reference Intakes (DRIs). These reports may be accessed via www.nap.edu.

3.4.1 POST-WLS DIET STAGES

The post-WLS diet progression is a staged approach based on *nutritional needs* during each phase of weight loss and the *texture* of foods that can be tolerated during each phase; see Table 3.5 for diet stages post-RYGB and SG. The general guidelines for diet stages post-RYGB and SG are the same. The diet progression post-LAGB varies from these procedures and is outlined in Table 3.6. Progression of the liquid diet to a full solid food diet is as tolerated, and food tolerance varies widely among post-WLS patients, even those that have the same procedure; therefore, it is important for all patients to be followed frequently early post-WLS. Table 3.7 provides a guideline for frequency of dietitian follow-up appointments. Much of the postoperative nutrition sessions can be provided in a group format, which offers patients the added support of their peers.

TABLE 3.5
Diet Stages RYGB/SG[d]

Diet Stage[b]	Begin	Fluids/Food	Guidelines
Stage 1	Postop days 1 and 2	GBP clear liquids; noncarbonated; no calories, no sugar, no caffeine	Postop day 1 patients may undergo a gastrogaffin swallow test for leak; once tested, begin sips of water

Stage 2
Begin supplementation:
• Chewable multivitamin with minerals (2/day); see list of standard post-WLS supplementation
• Chewable or liquid calcium citrate with vitamin D
• Sublingual, liquid, or nasal 350–500 μg vitamin B$_{12}$
• Vitamin D$_3$, 3,000 IU total per day
	Postop day 3 (discharge diet)	GBP clear liquids:
		• Variety of no sugar liquids or artificially sweetened liquids
		• Encourage patients to have salty fluids at home and solid liquids: Sugar-free ice pops/gelatin
		Plus full liquids:
		• Less than 25 g sugar per serving in full liquids
		• Protein-rich liquids
			Patients should consume a minimum of 48–60 oz of total fluids per day; 24–32 oz or more clear liquids; plus 24–32 oz of any combination of full liquids; examples of full liquids listed below:
			• 1% or skim milk
			• Smooth tomato soup, no chunks, mixed with 1% or skim milk
			• Whey, whey isolate, or soy protein powder (limit 25–30 g protein per serving) mixed with
			  • Lactaid milk, soy milk, or almond milk
			• Light yogurt or Greek yogurt:
			  • Less than 25 g of sugar per serving listed on label; no chunks of fruit
			• Plain yogurt

(Continued)

TABLE 3.5 (CONTINUED)
Diet Stages RYGB/SG[d]

Diet Stage[b]	Begin	Fluids/Food	Guidelines
Stage 3	Postop days 10–14[b]	Increase clear liquids (total liquids 48–64 oz or more per day) and replace full liquids with soft, moist, diced, ground, or pureed protein sources as tolerated Stage 3 protein sources: Eggs, ground meats, ground or pureed poultry, soft, moist fish, added gravy, bouillon, light mayo to moisten, cooked beans, hearty bean soups, cottage cheese, low-fat cheese, yogurt	• Protein food choices are encouraged for 3–6 small meals per day; patients may only be able to tolerate a couple of tablespoons at each meal/snack • Encourage patients not to drink with meals and to wait ~30 min after each meal before resuming fluids • Patients can supplement small amounts of soft protein intake with one full liquid as listed in stage 2
Stage 3: Week 2	4 weeks postop	Advance diet as tolerated; if protein foods well tolerated, add well-cooked soft vegetables and soft or peeled fruit	• Adequate hydration is essential and a priority for all patients during the rapid weight loss phase • Patient should be encouraged to add fruits/vegetables in a texture that is tolerated; added fruits and vegetables and adequate hydration will help prevent constipation • Full liquids may be used for meal or snack replacement

(Continued)

TABLE 3.5 (CONTINUED)
Diet Stages RYGB/SG[d]

Diet Stage[b]	Begin	Fluids/Food	Guidelines
Stage 3: Week 3 May switch to pill form supplementation if liquid or chewable not tolerated; encourage liquid or chewable forms of supplements for at least 3 months	5 weeks postop	Continue to consume protein with some fruit or vegetable at each meal; some people tolerate salads 1 month postop	Avoid rice, bread, and pasta until patient is comfortably consuming adequate protein per day and fruits/vegetables Consider diet a "prescription" to meet nutritional needs during rapid weight loss and healing phase Diet prescription: 1. Adequate hydration 2. Some protein sources 3–5 times a day with fruits and vegetables 3. Post-WLS supplementation; as hunger increases and patients are meeting the DRI for protein and consuming fruits and vegetables, whole grains can be introduced
Stage 4 Vitamin and mineral supplementation daily[c]	As hunger increases and more food is tolerated	Healthy solid food diet	Healthy, balanced diet consisting of adequate protein (plant or animal sources), fruits, vegetables, and whole grains; calorie needs based on individual needs

Source: Adapted from Mechanick, J. I. et al., *Endocr Pract,* 14(Suppl 1), 2008; Aills, L. et al., *SOARD,* 4:S73–S108, 2008.

Note: When diet advanced to soft solids, special attention to mindful eating and chewing until liquid is key, since more restriction may increase risk for food getting stuck above stoma of band if not properly chewed (e.g., if not chewed until liquid).

[a] RYGBP, Roux-en-Y gastric bypass.

[b] There is no standardization of diet stages. There are a wide variety of diet protocols varying from how long patients stay on each stage and what types of fluids/foods are recommended.

[c] Nutritional labs should be drawn 2, 6, and 12 months and yearly indefinitely. Bone density test at baseline and every 2 years.

[d] The same nutritional guidelines and diet advancements for post-RYGBP are also recommended post-SG.

TABLE 3.6
LAGB

Diet Stages[b]	Begin	Fluids/Food	Guidelines
Stage 1	Postop days 1 and 2	LAGB clear liquids; noncarbonated; no calories, no sugar, no caffeine	Postop LAGB day 1, patients may begin sips of water, ice chips, and avoid carbonation

Stage 2 Begin supplementation: Chewable multivitamin with minerals Chewable or liquid calcium citrate with vitamin D	Postop days 2–3 (discharge diet)	LAGB clear liquids:
		• 0-calorie liquids; avoid caffeine, carbonation, alcohol
		Plus LAGB full liquids:
		• Less than 25 g sugar per serving, and no more than 3 g fat per serving protein-rich liquids
			Patients should consume a minimum of 48–60 oz of total fluids per day; 24–32 oz or more clear liquids; plus 24–32 oz of any combination of full liquids; examples of full liquids listed below:
			• 1% or skim milk
			• Smooth tomato soup, no chunks, mixed with 1% or skim milk
			• Whey, whey isolate, or soy protein powder (limit 25–30 g protein per serving) mixed with
			  • Lactaid milk, soy milk, or almond milk
			• Light yogurt or Greek yogurt:
			  • Less than 25 g of sugar per serving listed on label; no chunks of fruit
			• Plain yogurt

(Continued)

TABLE 3.6 (CONTINUED)
LAGB

Diet Stages[b]	Begin	Fluids/Food	Guidelines
Stage 3: Week 1	Postop days 10–14[b]	Increase LAGB clear liquids (total liquids 48–64 oz or more per day) and replace full liquids with soft, moist, diced, ground, or pureed protein sources as tolerated Stage 3, week 1: Very well-chewed, soft eggs, ground meats, or poultry, soft, moist fish, added gravy, bouillon, light mayo to moisten, cooked beans, hearty bean soups, cottage cheese, low-fat cheese, yogurt	Note: Patients should be reassured that hunger is common and normal after AGB • Protein food (moist, ground) choices are encouraged for 3–6 small meals per day, to help with satiety • Mindful, slow eating is essential • Encourage patients not to drink with meals and to wait ~30 min after each meal before resuming fluids
Stage 3: Week 2	4 weeks postop	Advance diet as tolerated; if protein foods well tolerated in week 1, add well-cooked, soft vegetables and soft or peeled fruit	• Adequate hydration is essential and a priority for all patients during the rapid weight loss phase • Protein at every meal and snack, especially if increased hunger noted prior to initial fill or adjustment • Very well-cooked vegetables may also help to increase satiety
Stage 3: Week 3	5 weeks postop	Continue to consume protein with some fruit or vegetable at each meal; some people tolerate salads 1 month postop	If patient is tolerating soft, moist, ground, diced, or pureed proteins with small amounts of fruits and vegetables, may add crackers (use with protein) Avoid rice, bread, and pasta

(Continued)

TABLE 3.6 (CONTINUED)
LAGB

Diet Stages[b]	Begin	Fluids/Food	Guidelines
Stage 4 Vitamin and mineral supplementation daily	As hunger increases and more food is tolerated	Healthy solid food diet	Healthy, balanced diet consisting of adequate protein, fruits, vegetables, and whole grains; calorie needs based on height, weight, age
Post-LAGB fill/ adjustment	~6 weeks postop LAGB, and possibly every 6 weeks until satiety reached	Full liquids × 2 days postfill; advance to stage 3, week 1 guidelines above, as tolerated; × 4–5 days, then advance as above	Same as stage 2 liquids above × 48 h (or as otherwise advised by surgeon) Note: When diet advanced to soft solids, special attention to mindful eating and chewing until liquid key, since more restriction may increase risk for food getting stuck above stoma of band if not properly chewed (e.g., if not chewed until liquid)

Source: Diet stage tables provided with permission by Sue Cummings, MS, RD, MGH Weight Center, Boston, Massachusetts, ACS.org (accessed September 2011).

[a] RYGBP, Roux-en-Y gastric bypass.

[b] There is no standardization of diet stages. There are a wide variety of diet protocols varying from how long patients stay on each stage and what types of fluids/foods are recommended.

[c] Nutritional labs should be drawn 2, 6, and 12 months and yearly indefinitely. Bone density test at baseline and every 2 years.

[d] The same nutritional guidelines and diet advancements for post-RYGBP are also recommended post-SG.

3.4.1.1 Early Post-WLS Nutritional Priorities

- *Hydration*: Some patients may find it difficult to reach the recommended goal of 48–60 oz of fluid per day. Although uncommon, patients who continue diuretic medications post-WLS need to be monitored very closely for hydration status and medications adjusted accordingly. Patients should be taught signs and symptoms of dehydration, which include dark urine, hypotension upon standing, and in some cases, extreme fatigue and nausea. Suggestions for how to increase fluids through solid liquids (sugar-free ice pops, diet gelatin, etc.) and a list of salty liquids such as broth should be provided to all patients prior to discharge and included in the preoperative nutrition education materials. Since IV hydration contains a

TABLE 3.7

Postsurgery: Center of Excellence Recommended Follow-Up Postop Visits

1. Two weeks postoperatively (**advance diet to stage 3**)
2. Several weeks later as indicated (**nutrition groups, 6 weeks and 9 weeks postop**)
3. Three months (**individual RD to assess progress**)
4. Six months (**months 4–9, nutrition groups to address behavioral issues, nutrition, building healthy habits, physical activity**)
5. Six to nine months (**individual RD to assess progress**)
6. One year (**medical, biochemical surveillance, RD visit to assess progress**)
7. Every year thereafter (**medical, biochemical surveillance, RD**)

Monthly surgical support and education groups—open to all postsurgery patients.

Since most patients experience increased hunger and some see weight regain in years 2–5 postsurgery, this is a good time for RDs to offer groups or individual sessions for support and education and to reinforce healthy behaviors and review weight loss expectations; focus on what has been achieved versus what hasn't.

Source: American Chemical Society, http://www.acs.org.

Note: Chapter author suggestions for medical nutrition therapy visits with the registered dietitian (RD) in bold. (All patients should have access to a bariatric dietitian as needed; the above visits are the author's suggestions for standardizing MNT visits with the bariatric RD specialist across surgical centers.)

glucose-dextrose solution, administration of 100 mg of thiamin (vitamin B_1) should be included in the IV to avoid precipitation of thiamin deficiency in patients receiving IV rehydration.

- *Dietary protein*: Randomized studies among bariatric surgery patient populations are necessary to establish the exact quantity of protein that should be prescribed during the rapid weight loss phase. It is useful for dietitians to provide patients with specific products and guidelines for purchasing recommended protein supplements. Sample meal patterns outlining meal times, type and amount of fluids, and when to take supplements should be provided to all patients. Because of the limited volume capacity of the sleeve and pouch, patients do better with small, frequent feedings, especially if there are numerous comorbidities and complications. According to Soeters et al.,[11] empiric and theoretic evidence suggests bolus feeding is ineffective for patients with compromised gut function, stomach capacity, or liver function; they advise continuous feeding or frequent but small meals. Balanced daily distribution of protein intake at each meal protects metabolically active tissues, including skeletal muscle, during weight loss.[12]

The first 2 weeks following WLS patients are instructed to follow a liquid diet consisting of *full* liquids, which are liquids that contain protein and carbohydrate, and *clear* liquids (noncalorie, noncaffeine, noncarbonated, decaffeinated). Although individual hydration needs vary, general recommendations suggest starting with 60 oz of total fluids a day for men, with a minimum of 30 oz from protein-containing full liquids and 30 oz of clear liquids. For women a general guideline of 48 total fluid ounces or more a day, with a minimum of 24 oz of protein-containing full liquids and 24 oz of clear liquids. Caution should be given regarding the amount of protein contained in protein supplements, and patients should avoid protein shakes or powders that provide zero amounts of carbohydrates and excessive amounts of protein (general guidelines no more than 30 g of protein per serving). Several studies indicate that healthy adults are able to tolerate higher protein intakes without changes in hydration status. However, adequate fluid intake following WLS is vital to processing renal solute load, especially if patients are consuming large amounts of protein and minimal amounts of total fluids.[13] Individuals with compromised kidney and liver function may not be able to process high protein intakes, and recommendations in this population should be made with caution.[14]

Protein deficiency in post-WLS patients who do not have surgical complications is not common. If serum albumin, historically used as a measure of protein status, is low, it is more likely an indication of hydration status or inflammation than protein malnutrition.[15]

3.4.2 Macronutrients

3.4.2.1 Protein Supplements

Body protein is composed of 9 indispensable, also called essential (meaning that they must be consumed in the diet), amino acids and 11 dispensable (nonessential) amino acids. Whey, casein, milk, soy, and egg white protein sources contain all of the essential amino acids.[16] Although taste, cost, and availability of protein supplements are all important factors, it's vital that the quality of a protein supplement be deemed the most important variable in order to allow for optimal protein absorption and repletion in the postoperative bariatric patient.[17]

An objective measurement of protein supplement quality, called the protein digestibility corrected amino acid score (PDCAAS), compares indispensable amino acids (IAAs) of a protein to the dispensable amino acid content. The PDCAAS allows even the new bariatric practitioner or non-RD team member to objectively assess the quality of a particular protein supplement. The score is indicative of the ability of the human body to utilize a particular protein source for protein synthesis. A perfect PDCAAS of 100 is found among protein sources, including whey, casein, milk, soy, and egg whites.[16,18] Overall, the highest-quality protein supplements contain whey protein, due to the high amounts of branched-chain amino acids, vital in periods of physiological stress, such as found in the bariatric surgery perioperative period. Whey concentrates are also of high quality, but unlike whey isolates, they may contain significant amounts of lactose. Since many patients have some degree of lactose intolerance and some gastric bypass surgery patients may encounter lactose intolerance issues postoperatively, suggesting lactose-free protein products, such as soy, egg whites, and whey protein isolates, may be preferable for many bariatric patients.

After 2 weeks on a liquid diet, patients are advanced to a soft food diet. Hydration continues to be a priority, and as patients switch to soft food sources of protein, they need to be advised to maintain adequate hydration, with a minimum of 48–60 oz of total fluids, which may be met by substituting full liquids for clear liquids. Protein shakes can be used to supplement food intake; however, it is also important that patients incorporate some sources of carbohydrate in their diet.

3.4.2.2   Dietary Carbohydrates

Exact carbohydrate goals after bariatric procedures have not been defined, and there are limited published papers regarding carbohydrate needs post-WLS.[19] The Food and Agriculture Organization (FAO) and World Health Organization (WHO) recommend a minimum consumption of 50 g of carbohydrate per day to maintain normal brain activity.[20] Great caution should be taken when designing a postoperative diet. Patients should be encouraged to eliminate the more processed forms of carbohydrates in the diet and consume complex forms, especially in the form of fruits and vegetables. As external caloric needs increase and protein, fruits, and vegetables are being consumed in adequate amounts, patients can be counseled to incorporate whole grains.

3.4.3   Calorie Goals

It is not unusual for bariatric patients to become concerned regarding caloric intake in the perioperative period and beyond. Another goal of post-WLS counseling is to help patients to change the focus from emphasis on caloric intake, which many bariatric patients struggle with preoperatively, to incorporating a healthy diet and obtaining adequate amounts of macronutrients, including protein and healthy carbohydrates. Emphasis should be shifted from calories to adequate nutrition.

Early postoperative nutrition recommendations are very prescriptive. Whether hungry or not, patients need to meet nutrient needs, and the diet can be thought of as a "nutrition prescription," meaning he or she has to get in certain nutrition (e.g., adequate amount of fluids to prevent dehydration, protein, carbohydrates, essential fats, vitamin and mineral supplements) that body fat stores do not provide.

3.4.4   Early Postoperative Nutrition Prescription

1. *Hydration*: Minimum total of 60 oz for men, 48–60 oz for women. These amounts are only guidelines; amounts may need to be increased based on an individual's needs. Hydration is the first and foremost nutrition priority.
2. *Protein source*: Three to five times a day. This may be limited initially to only a few bites per meal, as the amount is specifically determined by patients' tolerance and fullness. It is essential to reassure patients that as the weeks and months pass, they will be able to tolerate increased portion sizes. Adding a liquid protein source (a full liquid protein shake) once a day will help to ensure adequate protein intake. Listening to their body through mindful eating is the key to learning when to stop eating.
3. *Fruits and vegetables*: A small amount of fruits and vegetables should be consumed with their protein and at least three times a day.

4. *Vitamin and mineral supplements*: Standard supplementation includes a daily multivitamin with minimum of 100% of DRI for B vitamins, including B_1, biotin, B_{12}, and folate; vitamin K, vitamin D and iron; a sublingual B_{12}; and calcium citrate with vitamin D in divided doses, vitamin D up to 3,000 IU (titrate to >30 ng/ml).

3.4.5 DIETARY PROGRESSION

Diet progression post-WLS, as discussed earlier in this chapter, is based on nutritional needs and texture of the foods. The use of a clear liquid diet is usually short term (1–2 days), which is then advanced to a full liquid diet (liquids that contain dietary nutrients, specifically protein and carbohydrate), starting at days 3–4 postop and lasting ~10–14 days, at which time patients are advanced to soft solid foods (pureed, diced, ground, or moist protein sources). Protein supplements are often included within all phases of dietary progression, depending on the individual patient's intake. Food tolerances and the pace and rate of the diet progression vary widely among patients, which is why close and frequent postop nutritional support and counseling is recommended.

3.4.6 EARLY POST-WLS NUTRITION CONCERNS THAT ARE SPECIFIC TO THE TYPE OF SURGERY PERFORMED

1. *Laparoscopic adjustable gastric band*: Gastric banding is a purely restrictive procedure, meaning there is no malabsorption of micronutrients or macronutrients. Since the LAGB is restrictive, patients may report more hunger after the band procedure than after RYGB or SG.[23] Special attention should be made to foods that are satiating and well tolerated. The goals for protein intake should be based on a patient's individual needs during a rapid weight loss phase. Adequate fluid intake is essential, and patients taking in higher protein amounts should also increase fluid accordingly. Since the total amount of calories consumed is restricted, careful consideration to a healthy, well-balanced diet is essential. Tough or dry meats or poultry, if not well chewed, may "get stuck" in the restricted area and should be ground, diced, moist, and chewed thoroughly. Many patients also find that breads and other doughy products might get stuck, and are therefore not well tolerated. Because liquids and very soft foods pass through the restricted area easily, patients should be cautioned against consuming high-calorie soft foods, which include high-calorie beverages, cream-based soups, ice cream, etc.
   a. Starting about 6 weeks postband placement, patients will be scheduled for fills, also called adjustments. These fills will continue every few months over the course of a year or more, until the "sweet spot" is reached, which means that patients can consume small meals and planned snacks that create early satiety.[24] See Table 3.6 for post-LAGB diet stages and postadjustment diet.

2. *Roux-en-Y gastric bypass and sleeve gastrectomy*: Vegetarians can use soy milk or yogurt products, and patients who are lactose intolerant should be advised to use whey protein isolate powders and soy or lactaid milk products. Data on the nutritional needs of the patient undergoing the sleeve gastrectomy are limited. Most surgical centers that are performing the GS use the same diet stages and recommendations as the RYGB. There have been reports of postoperative micronutrient deficiencies following the SG; therefore, it is recommended that the same standard vitamin and mineral supplementation and biochemical surveillance recommended for the RYGB be recommended for patients post-SG.

Incidence rates of gastric esophageal reflux have been reported to be as high as 67% and higher at 1 month post-SG.[21] This typically decreases or resolves by 2 years postop. As with any WLS procedure, patients need to be taught how to prepare food so that it is a tolerable texture and to eat mindfully, stopping between bites to breathe and check in on their level of fullness. Avoid drinking large amounts of fluids with meals and until pouch/sleeve empties; a general guideline is to wait 30 min postmeal before resuming fluid intake. It is not necessary to avoid liquids 30 min before a meal.

3.4.7 POSTOPERATIVE MICRONUTRIENT STATUS

Data suggest that micronutrient deficiencies increase over time after WLS; however, the number of patients monitored over time decreases. It is very important that patients have their nutritional labs monitored. If patients are not being followed by their surgical center, the primary care provider should be educated regarding the appropriate post-WLS nutritional labs that need to be monitored. See Table 3.2 for biochemical surveillance. Micronutrients are discussed in detail elsewhere in this book.

3.4.8 SHORT-TERM POSTOP CHALLENGES (UP TO 18 MONTHS POST-WLS)

1. *Weight loss goals and expectations*: The most rapid weight loss typically occurs in the first 6 months postsurgery, with many patients continuing to lose weight up to 18 months. Many patients may be tempted to weigh daily, and some frequently throughout the day, especially in the early post-WLS; it is imperative that they be reminded of the emphasis on health and improvement in comorbidities rather than obsessing about the numbers on the scale. Emphasizing the changes in body measurements or clothing size is more indicative of fat loss than the number on the scale. The goal is to lose weight in as healthy a manner as possible, not as fast as possible; the rate and amount of weight loss will vary greatly among patients, and they should be encouraged not to compare weight losses. Health care providers should also be very careful about giving patient goals regarding the numbers on the scale.
2. *Healthy nutrition*: Most patients would say that they know what to eat, as many have been on numerous diets throughout their life. However, they also tend to learn about nutrition from popular diet books, food label claims, etc.

When quizzed about healthy eating, many patients admittedly respond with confusion as to what is healthy and what is not. A healthy diet should be designed to match an individual's life; it should be one that can be sustained over time and be based on factors that include cultural considerations, likes, dislikes, economical restraints, lifestyle, ethics etc. Nutritional needs are met by a healthy diet that incorporates lean protein sources, plant or animal, whole grain carbohydrates, fruits and vegetables, and low-fat healthy fats. Nutrition requirements can be met on a plant-based diet, and patients who choose to be vegetarian should be educated regarding a healthy vegetarian diet, be it lacto, lacto-ovo, or vegan.

There are many challenges to maintaining a healthy diet in today's environment; patients should be counseled to avoid introducing high-fat, high-salt, and highly sweetened processed foods. Guidelines for building a healthy diet include the following:
- Planning a breakfast within 2 h of waking.
- Plan and prepare for three meals and incorporate a planned snack if meals are longer than 5 h apart, paying close attention to physical hunger and satiety.
- Incorporate a protein source at each meal and snack.[12,22]
  - Protein has a high–diet-induced thermogenic effect.
  - Protein enhances satiety.
  - Protein utilization is a function at individual meals and should be distributed throughout the day.
  - Protein at meals and snacks enhances glycemic control.
- Incorporate a high-fiber food (fruit or vegetable) at each meal and snack.
- When incorporating grains, choose whole grains.
- Maintain hydration, avoiding high-calorie, highly sweetened beverages.
3. *Eating behaviors*: Initially, patients report diminished hunger and early satiety. However, as their weight stabilizes, hunger and satiety will increase since the body will no longer be relying on fat stores for daily energy needs. Patients are often highly motivated while achieving weight loss results, reducing or eliminating medications, fitting in smaller clothing sizes, etc. Motivation is a strong driver of making challenging behavior changes. This is an opportune time to educate patients and encourage healthy behaviors for long-term maintenance of a healthy weight. Referral to a dietitian for medical nutrition therapy, to assist patients in normalizing eating patterns, planning and preparing meals, learning to purchase healthy convenient foods, continuing or resuming a schedule of daily postsurgical vitamin and mineral supplementation, and incorporating a routine exercise schedule, may contribute to long-term success. Weight loss surgery influences the biological triggers to obesity; however, it does not change the environment.
4. Strategies for incorporating a healthy lifestyle include the following:
- Focusing on mindful eating
- Planning, preparing, and structuring meals and snacks throughout the day
- Avoiding large amounts of liquids at meals
- Paying attention to physical hunger and satiety and responding accordingly

- Recognizing nonhunger triggers to eating and incorporating alternative responses
- Cognitive restructuring—challenging distorted, negative thoughts related to eating and eating behaviors, especially all-or-nothing thinking related to eating and food choices

3.4.9 NUTRITIONAL CONSIDERATIONS IN WEIGHT MAINTENANCE

It is important for patients to understand the stages of weight loss and not to get discouraged as the rate of weight loss slows down and eventually stabilizes. Less than 5% of patients lose 100% of their excess body weight, and 10-year postop data show weight regain of approximately 20–25%.[26,27] Weight loss expectations should be addressed prior to a patient having weight loss surgery.[26,27] Unrealistic weight loss expectations may lead to unhealthful eating or overrestrictive dieting postsurgery. The RYGB and SG are metabolic procedures that have neural and hormonal influences that lead to decreased hunger and increased satiety. Teaching patients to trust their hunger, eat mindfully, and terminate a meal when comfortably full is a key element of successful weight maintenance. Long-term post-WLS support and education can be used to reinforce healthy eating habits, as well as lifestyle and behavior changes that promote weight maintenance.

3.4.10 GENERAL GUIDELINES DURING WEIGHT STABILIZATION[25]

1. Educating and involving the primary care provider in the long-term care, support, and monitoring of postop WLS patients, including:
   a. Mechanisms of weight loss for each procedure
   b. Weight loss expectations and variables that effect weight loss
   c. Biochemical surveillance of nutritional status (Table 3.4)
2. Periodic nutrition visits with the registered dietitian to reinforce healthy eating and behaviors; obesity is a chronic problem and therefore, all treatment therapies need to be lifelong.
3. If significant weight regain, especially in a short period of time, refer back to surgeon for assessment of surgical failure or complications of surgery.
4. Psychosocial variables, as well as sedentary lifestyle, poor attendance at postsurgery support groups, disordered eating patterns, and poor nutritional food choices, may contribute to suboptimal weight loss or weight regain.[28]
   a. Although there are environmental factors that influence weight loss and regain, it is important to assist patients to understand that obesity is a complex condition with multiple etiologies, and just as causes of obesity vary among individuals, so will treatment outcomes. Patients and providers need to think of obesity as a chronic problem, and that maintaining a healthier weight for some, even after WLS, may mean a lifetime of intermittent behavioral, medical, psychological, or nutritional therapy.

3.5 SPECIAL NUTRITION CONSIDERATIONS POST-WLS

3.5.1 DUMPING SYNDROME

Dumping syndrome is more common with the RYGB due to the lack of the pyloric sphincter and may occur after consumption of high sugar or highly processed carbohydrates, which create a hypertonic solution in the jejunum. This hypertonic solution leads to sudden distension of the jejunum, resulting in symptoms of *early dumping syndrome*, usually occurring 10–30 min after eating. Symptoms may include nausea, dizziness, weakness, rapid pulse, cold sweats, fatigue, frothing, cramps, and diarrhea.[33]

RYGB and SG patients may experience what is sometimes described as *late dumping syndrome*, which occurs 1–3 h after a meal, as a result of an exaggerated insulin release. This is caused by the rapid absorption of glucose triggering an exaggerated insulin release that results in rebound hypoglycemia (reactive hypoglycemia). Reactive hypoglycemia is discussed in the next section.

Patients should be counseled to avoid highly sweetened or processed carbohydrates. Slow, mindful eating, consuming a bite or two before consuming starches, and avoiding excessive fluid intake at meals and snacks may also help to prevent dumping syndrome. Foods containing natural sugars, such as dairy and fruit, do not commonly cause dumping.

There are varying reports of the occurrence of dumping syndrome in post-RYGB patients, ranging from 10 to 75% of patients.[29,30] It has traditionally been thought that it is uncommon for sleeve gastrectomy patients to experience dumping syndrome due to the preservation of the pyloric sphincter. However, more recent studies have demonstrated that when an oral glucose tolerance test was given to a set of patients with no history of diabetes and who were status post-SG, 33% of the patients experienced symptoms of dumping syndrome, but the same symptoms can also be a result of reactive hypoglycemia.[31,32]

3.5.2 REACTIVE HYPOGLYCEMIA

Reactive hypoglycemia, also known as late dumping syndrome, is a reaction that occurs after eating when blood glucose levels drop to below 70 mg/dl, causing symptoms of hypoglycemia (low blood glucose), which can be characterized by symptoms that include feeling shaky, sweaty, weak, and extreme fatigue. Reactive hypoglycemia is not a complication observed after adjustable gastric banding surgery, as the pylorus remains intact and the time it takes the food to reach the small intestine is not decreased.[33]

1. Possible etiologies of reactive hypoglycemia[34,35]:
   - Dumping syndrome
   - Beta cell hyperfunction
   - Underlying familial hyperinsulinism syndrome unmasked by weight loss
   - Increased beta cell mass that developed during obesity and did not regress postoperatively
   - Excessive secretion of GLP 1

TABLE 3.8

Pharmacological Treatments for Reactive Hypoglycemia

Drug	Administration	Mechanism of Action	Side Effects
• Acarbose	• Oral	• Delays the breakdown of starch into sugar	• Bloating • Flatulence • Diarrhea
• Somatostatin analogs	• Injection	• Delay gastric emptying • Slow transit through the bowel • Inhibit the release of gastrointestinal hormones, insulin secretion, and postprandial vasodilation	• Gall stone formation • Pain at injection site • Steatorrhea

Source: Data from Tack, J. et al., *Nat Rev Gastroenterol Hepatol*, 6, 583–590, 2009.

- Increased delivery of nutrients to the intestines seen after the RYGB and SG

2. Intervention for hypoglycemia: diet. Studies show that low-carbohydrate diets can prevent and improve symptoms of reactive hypoglycemia.[36] Treatment for patients with post-WLS hypoglycemia parallels treatment for patients with non-WLS hypoglycemia. Generally, consuming small, frequent meals and avoiding refined carbohydrates can help reduce the occurrence of reactive hypoglycemia. All patients who do not respond to diet treatment for reactive hypoglycemia should be referred to an endocrinologist for further evaluation.

3. Pharmacological treatment: In addition to diet treatment, drugs may also be used to treat reactive hypoglycemia. Pharmacological treatment is usually considered when the patient has made diet changes but continues to experience reactive hypoglycemia. The drugs often cause unpleasant side effects, so it is beneficial to weigh the pros and cons of this type of treatment. Table 3.8 lists the current drugs used for the management of hypoglycemia, their mechanism of action, and possible side effects.

4. Surgical treatments for hypoglycemia: Revision surgery to reverse the RYGB may be considered as a last resort if the patient has exhausted all other forms of treatment and continues to experience hypoglycemic symptoms that are compromising the patient's quality of life.[34] In severe cases of hyperplasia of the beta cells or nesidioblastosis, a partial or total pancreatic resection may be warranted.[29,34,35]

3.5.2.1 Reactive Hypoglycemia Monitoring and Evaluation

The patient should evaluate the frequency and occurrence of symptoms. Monitoring and evaluation for reactive hypoglycemia include any or all of the following:

- Tracking of food intake and symptoms—analyzing intake to determine patterns between food consumed and low blood glucose or symptoms of reactive hypoglycemia
- Self-monitoring blood glucose—tracking blood glucose levels before and after meals via a glucometer
- Continuous glucose monitoring—tracking device that measures blood glucose throughout the day and alerts patient of lows or drastic decreases in blood glucose

3.6 CONCLUSION

All WLS procedures have nutritional consequences. Since the risk of any surgery will never be completely eliminated, the role of the presurgical multidisciplinary team is to assess and prepare patients medically, nutritionally, and psychologically to reduce risks of surgery and improve surgical outcomes. The nutrition evaluation will guide the provider's presurgical treatment recommendations and provide valuable information regarding the nutritional and behavioral short- and long-term treatment needs of the individual patient. Registered dietitians are uniquely trained in both nutritional science and behavioral therapies and are an important member of the pre- and postmultidisciplinary team. Primary care providers also need to be aware of the nutritional implications of WLS, monitor the nutritional laboratory parameters influenced by each procedure, as well as nutrition-related comorbidities and environmental and behavioral factors that influence weight loss and maintenance.

REFERENCES

1. Aills L, Blankenship J, Buffington C, Furtado M, Parrott J. 2008. Bariatric nutrition: suggestions for the surgical weight loss patient. *SOARD* 4:S73–S108.
2. Mechanick JI, Kushner RF, Sugerman HJ, Gonzalez-Campoy JM, Collazo-Clavell ML, Guven S, Spitz AF, Apovian CM, Livingston EH, Brolin R, Sarwer DB, Anderson WA, Dixon J. 2008. American Association of Clinical Endocrinologists (AACE), The Obesity Society (TOS) and American Society of Metabolic and Bariatric Surgery (ASMBS). Clinical practice guidelines for the perioperative nutritional, metabolic and nonsurgical support of the bariatric surgery patient. *Endocr Pract* 14(Suppl 1).
3. Mechanick JI, Youdim A, Jones DB, Garvey WT, Hurley DL, McMahon MM, Heinberg LJ, Kushner R, Adams TD, Shikora S, Dixon JB, Brethauer S. 2013. Clinical practice guidelines for the perioperative nutritional, metabolic and nonsurgical support of the bariatric surgery patient—2013 update: cosponsored by the American Association of Clinical Endocrinologists, The Obesity Society and American Society of Metabolic and Bariatric Surgery. *SOARD* 9:159–191.
4. Endevelt R, Ben-Assuli O, Klain E, Zelber-Sagi S. 2013. The role of the dietician follow-up in the success of bariatric surgery. *SOARD*, published online January 24, 2013.
5. Cummings S. 2009. Surgery: Part B: Practical applications. In *Managing Obesity: A Clinical Guide*, chap. 9. ed. Nonas C, Foster G. Chicago, IL: American Dietetic Association.

6. Moize V, Andreu A, Flores L, Torres F, Ibarzabal A, Delgado S, Lacy A, Rodriguez L, Vidal J. 2013. Long-term dietary intake and nutritional deficiencies following sleeve gastrectomy or Roux-en-Y gastric bypass in a Mediterranean population. *JAND* 113:400–410.

7. Flancbaum L, Belsley S, Drake V, Colarusso T, Tayler E. 2006. Preoperative nutritional status of patients undergoing Roux-en-Y gastric bypass for morbid obesity. *J Gastrointest Surg* 10:1033–1037.

8. Damms-Machado A, Friedrich A, Kramer KM, Stingel K, Meile T, Küper MA, Königsrainer A, Bischoff SC. 2012. Pre- and postoperative nutritional deficiencies in obese patients undergoing laparoscopic sleeve gastrectomy. *Obes Surg* 22(6):881–889.

9. Benotti PN, Still CD, Wood C, Akmal Y, King H, Arousy H, Dancea H, Gerhard G, Patrick A, Strodel W. 2009. Preoperative weight loss before bariatric surgery. *Arch Surg* 144(12):1150–1155.

10. Still CD, Benotti P, Wood C, et al. 2007. Outcomes of preoperative weight loss in high risk patients undergoing gastric bypass surgery. *Arch Surg* 142(10):994–998.

11. Soeters PB, van de Poll MCG, van Gemert WG, Dejong CHC. 2004. Amino acid adequacy in pathophysiological states. *J Nutr* 134(6 Suppl):1575S–1582S.

12. Devkota S, Layman DK. 2010. Protein metabolic roles in treatment of obesity. *Curr Opin Clin Nutr Metab Care* 13:403–407.

13. Martin W, et al. 2006. Effects of dietary protein intake on indexes of hydration. *JADA* 106:587–589.

14. Lentine K, Wrone EM. 2004. New insights into protein intake and progression of renal disease. *Curr Opin Nephrol Hypertens* 13:333–336.

15. Litchford MD. 2006. *Practical applications in laboratory assessment of nutritional status.* Greensboro, NC: CASE Software. www.casesoft.com.

16. Castellanos V, Litchford M, Campbell W. 2006. Modular protein supplements and their application to long-term care. *Nutr Clin Pract* 21:485–504.

17. Cummings S, Furtado M. 2012. Nutritional care of the bariatric surgery patient. In *Psychosocial assessment and treatment of bariatric surgery patients*, ed. Mitchell JE, deZwaan M, 159–183. New York: Routledge Taylor and Francis Group.

18. Schaafsma G. 2000. The protein digestibility-corrected amino acid score. *J Nutr* 130(7):1865S–1867S.

19. Faria SL, Faria OP, Cardeal M, de Govea H, Buffinton C, Furtado M. 2013. Recommended levels of carbohydrate after bariatric surgery. *Bariatric Times* 10(3):16–21.

20. FAO/WHO Expert Consultation. The role of carbohydrates in maintenance of health. In *Carbohydrates in human nutrition.* http://www.fao.org/docrep/w8079e/w8079e00.htm (accessed April 30, 2013).

21. Weiner RA, Weiner S, Pomhoff I, Jacobi C, Makarewicz W, Weigand G. 2007. Laparoscopic sleeve gastrectomy—influence of sleeve size and resected gastric volume. *Obes Surg* 17:1297–1305.

22. Layman DK. 2009. Dietary guidelines should reflect new understandings about adult protein needs. *Nutr Metab* 6:12. http://www.nutritionandmetabolism.com/content/6/1/12 (accessed April 30, 2013).

23. Mariani LM, Fusco A, Turriziani M, Veneziani A, Marini MA, de Lorenzo A, Bertoli A. 2005. Transient increase of plasma ghrelin after laparoscopic adjustable gastric banding in morbid obesity. *Horm Metab Res* 37(4):242–245.

24. Valle E, Luu M, Autajay K, Francescatti AB, Fogg LF, Myers JA. 2012. Frequency of adjustments and weight loss after laparoscopic adjustable gastric banding. *Obes Surg* 22(12):1880–1883.

25. Pontiroli AE, Fossati A, Vedani P, Fiorilli M, Folli F, Paganelli M, Marchi M, Maffei C. 2007. Post-surgery adherence to scheduled visits and compliance, more than personality disorders predict outcome of bariatric restrictive surgery in morbidly obese patients. *Obes Surg* 17(11):1492–1497.
26. Himpens J, Cadiere GB, Bazi M, Vouche M, Cadiere B, Dapri G. 2011. Long-term outcomes of laparoscopic adjustable gastric banding. *Arch Surg* 146(7):802–807.
27. Sjostrom L, Lindroos AK, Peltonen M, Torgerson J, Bouchard C, Carlsson B, Dahlgren S, Larsson B, Narbro K, Sjostrom CD, Sullivan M, Wedel H. 2004. Swedish Obese Subjects Study Scientific Group. Lifestyle, diabetes, and cardiovascular risk factors 10 years after bariatric surgery. *N Engl J Med* 351:2683–2693.
28. Sarwar D, Wadden T, Moore R, Baker A, Gibbons L, Raper S, Williams N. 2008. Preoperative eating behavior, postoperative dietary adherence and weight loss following gastric bypass surgery. *Surg Obes Relat Dis* 4(5):640–646.
29. Z'graggen K, Guweidhi A, Steffen R, Potoczna N, Biral R, Walther F, Komminoth P, Horber F. 2008. Severe recurrent hypoglycemia after gastric bypass surgery. *Obes Surg* 18:981–988.
30. Laurenius A, Olbers T, Naslund I, Karlsson J. 2013. Dumping syndrome following gastric bypass: validation of dumping symptom rating scale. *Obes Surg* 23(6):740–55.
31. Papamargaritis D, Koukoulis G, Sioka E, Zachari E, Bargiota A, Zacharoulis D, Tzovaras G. 2012. Dumping symptoms and incidence of hypoglycemia after provocation test at 6 and 12 months after laparoscopic sleeve gastrectomy. *Obes Surg* 10:1600–1606.
32. Tzovaras G, Papamargaritis D, Sioka E, Zachari E, Baloyiannis I, Zacharoulis D, Koukoulis G. 2012. Symptoms suggestive of dumping syndrome after provocation in patients after laparoscopic sleeve gastrectomy. *Obes Surg* 22:23–28.
33. Tack J, Arts J, Caenepeel P, De Wulf D, Bisschops R. 2009. Pathophysiology, diagnosis and management of postoperative dumping syndrome. *Nat Rev Gastroenterol Hepatol* 6:583–590.
34. Patti ME, McMahon G, Mun EC, Bitton A, Holst JJ, Goldsmith J, Hanto DW, Callery M, Arky R, Nose V, Bonner-Weir S, Goldfine AB. 2005. Severe hypoglycemia post-gastric bypass requiring partial pancreatectomy: evidence for inappropriate insulin secretion and pancreatic islet hyperplasia. *Diabetologia* 48:2236–2240.
35. de Heide LJM, Glaudemans AWJM, Oomen PHN, Apers JA, Totte ERE, van Beek AP. 2012. Functional imaging in hyperinsulinemic hypoglycemia after gastric bypass surgery for morbid obesity. *J Clin Endocrinol Metab* 97(6):E963–E967.
36. Kellogg TA, Bantle JP, Leslie DB, Redmond JB, Slusarek B, Swan T, Buchwald H, Ikramuddin S. 2008. Postgastric bypass hyperinsulinemic hypoglycemia syndrome: characterization and response to modified diet. *Surg Obes Relat Dis* 4(4):492–499.

4 Anemia and Bariatric Surgery

Mark A. Marinella

CONTENTS

4.1 INTRODUCTION

Obesity is an ongoing problem within the United States and other Westernized countries and contributes to a variety of medical conditions, including diabetes mellitus, cardiovascular disease, sleep apnea syndrome, osteoarthritis, liver disease, and various cancers.[1-5] The discussion of the anatomic and technical aspects of bariatric procedures is not the goal of this chapter, but two widely performed procedures include the Roux-en-Y and the biliopancreatic diversion/duodenal switch (BPD). Restrictive and, to some degree, malabsorptive complications occur with the Roux-en-Y procedure, whereas malabsorptive complications dominate the nutritional deficiencies encountered in patients having BPD.[6] Anemia is common after bariatric surgery, approaching 40% in some series, and may be asymptomatic and incidental or severe and life altering.[7,8] The causes are many, but common general symptoms and signs include fatigue, lassitude, sleepiness, dyspnea, chest discomfort, systolic flow murmurs, and cutaneous/mucosal pallor. Some symptoms and signs may be peculiar to certain nutrient-related anemias and will be discussed in the appropriate sections of this chapter. A commonly used definition of anemia in general clinical practice is a hemoglobin of <13 g for males and <12 g for females, although individual laboratories may deviate slightly from these values.[1]

4.2   ANATOMIC AND PHYSIOLOGIC MECHANISMS FOR POST-BARIATRIC SURGERY ANEMIA

Patients undergoing purely restrictive procedures such as gastric banding may develop anemia from deficiencies of iron and folate resulting from meat intolerance and decreased grain and vegetable consumption, respectively.[1,6] This results from the physical inability to consume and tolerate an adequate diet. Indeed, it is the early satiety and discomfort that leads to weight loss from decreased caloric intake from the gastric banding procedure.[6] Restrictive-malabsorptive (Roux-en-Y) and malabsorptive (BPD) surgeries induce anemia in a more complicated fashion relating to malabsorption and maldigestion, although restriction of food intake can contribute to anemia in the Roux-en-Y patient.[1,3,9,10]

4.3   STOMACH

By surgically "bypassing" a significant portion of the gastric mucosa, the stage is set for anemia related to iron and B_{12} deficiency since the stomach is pivotal in the absorption of these nutrients.[1] A major contributor to postoperative iron deficiency anemia (IDA) is decreased availability of hydrochloric acid, which is necessary for optimal iron absorption.[1,6,11,12] An acidic milieu is needed for conversion of dietary ferric (Fe^{+3}) to ferrous (Fe^{+2}).[6] In addition, many patients take proton pump inhibitors for acid-related conditions, and this dramatically decreases acid production. As such, consumption of ascorbic acid with an iron supplement may help enhance absorption.[13] Bypassing the stomach may also lead to copper deficiency since this is a site of copper absorption in addition to the proximal small bowel.[1] Adequate copper stores are necessary for optimal iron absorption and, in the form of haphaestin, conversion of iron to the Fe^{+3} state for transferrin transport.[14,15] As such, copper deficiency from decreased intake or absorption can lead to a functional iron deficiency state from suboptimal transferrin function. Since adequate gastric mucosa is required for optimal vitamin B_{12} status, patients undergoing Roux-en-Y may develop deficiency from decreased gastric acid and pepsin availability resulting from impaired cleavage of B_{12} from food.[16,17] Intrinsic factor (IF) is secreted by gastric parietal cells in the distal stomach and deficiency may ensue due to impaired binding of B_{12} by IF, which is necessary for absorption in the terminal ileum.[1,6,16,17]

Another anatomic reason for anemia involving the stomach is IDA resulting from bleeding from a marginal ulcer at the gastrojejunal anastamosis, which can affect

3–23% of patients undergoing Roux-en-Y.[2] Marginal ulceration may result from *Helicobacter* infection, anastamotic ischemia from staple or suture tension, nonsteroidal drugs, or local acid-induced erosions.[2,18–21] Bacterial overgrowth may uncommonly occur in the gastric-duodenal pouch following Roux-en-Y caused by stagnation of contents and subsequent bacterial proliferation.[6,22] Overgrowth of nonresident flora may lead to alteration of normal enteric flora culminating in diarrhea, steatorrhea, and anemia from bacterial usurpation of vitamin B_{12}. This syndrome, however, is more common in patients undergoing BPD since the intestinal limb is longer than the gastric-duodenal limb with Roux-en-Y, but should be on the differential diagnosis of anemia in the Roux-en-Y patient in the appropriate clinical scenario.[1,6,22]

4.4 SMALL BOWEL

The small bowel is the primary site of absorption of several nutrients. Table 4.1 displays the various anatomic segments of the small bowel that are responsible for absorption of the most relevant nutrients involved in bariatric-related anemia. As noted, early satiety and dyspepsia can lead to decreased intake of iron-rich foods, especially red meat, which can contribute to IDA.[6] The duodenum is the primary site of iron absorption, and bypass of this segment contributes to IDA. Bypass of the duodenum and jejunum can also result in anemia related to deficiency of copper, vitamin C, and the vitamin B-complex (anemia due to specific vitamin deficiencies will be discussed later in this chapter). The jejunum is also responsible for absorption of most of the dietary protein load, and severe protein depletion, as can occur following BPD, may result in an anemia.[2,3,23] Furthermore, excessive vomiting in the setting of a postoperative anastomotic stricture can contribute to malnutrition. Protein deficiency in rats results in anemia due to blunted erythropoietin and thyroxine synthesis leading to impaired erythropoiesis.[24,25] The anemia of protein-malnutrition is typically normochromic and normocytic with an inappropriately low reticulocyte count.[23] Bone marrow biopsy in severely malnourished patients has demonstrated hypocellularity.

TABLE 4.1
Anatomic Areas of Vitamin and Trace Element Absorption in the Small Bowel

Nutrient	Area
Iron	Duodenum
Copper	Duodenum, jejunum
Vitamin C	Duodenum, jejunum
Thiamine	Duodenum, jejunum
Riboflavin	Duodenum, jejunum
Niacin	Duodenum, jejunum
Pyridoxine	Duodenum, jejunum
Folate	Duodenum, jejunum, ileum
Vitamin B_{12}	Ileum

Another potential mechanism of anemia is a blind-pouch syndrome that most often occurs following BPD, due to the long excluded segment of small bowel in the biliopancreatic limb. Bowel contents may become overgrown with pathogenic bacteria that alter the normal enteric flora population, resulting in diarrhea, abdominal pain, steatorrhea, and anemia.[22] Bacterial overgrowth competes with luminal vitamin B_{12}, which leads to deficiency and megaloblastic anemia.

4.5 CAUSES OF ANEMIA IN THE IMMEDIATE POSTOPERATIVE SETTING

Etiologies of post-bariatric surgery anemia differ in the early and later postoperative periods. Although there is no accepted definition of early versus late anemia, for the sake of this chapter, early-onset anemia will refer to that which occurs during the immediate postoperative hospitalization and the ensuing days after discharge.[1] Surgical blood loss is the most significant cause of acute anemia and is more common following prolonged BPD procedures than laparoscopic Roux-en-Y. Bleeding complications leading to anemia occur in about 4% of gastric bypass patients and may result from vascular injury, breakdown of an anastomotic suture or staple line, or acidic erosions within the gastric remnant.[2] Postoperative vomiting may result in a Mallory–Weiss tear and hematemesis. Uncommonly, venous thromboembolism prophylaxis or treatment may result in retroperitoneal hematoma and anemia.

Uncommon causes of postoperative anemia that need to be considered in the appropriate clinical scenario are displayed in Table 4.2. Hemolytic anemia due to an acute transfusion reaction is rare, but should be considered if sudden back pain, hypotension, anemia, and hemoglobinuria develop during or immediately following a red cell transfusion. Other uncommon causes of hemolysis in the immediate postoperative setting include disseminated intravascular coagulation (DIC) complicating infection or sepsis, drugs, hypophosphatemia, and thrombotic thrombocytopenic

TABLE 4.2
Causes of Acute Anemia Following Bariatric Surgery

Blood loss from surgery
Intra-abdominal/retroperitoneal hematoms
Surgical injury, anticoagulant therapy
Esophagitis, gastritis
Ulceration of anastamosis
Marrow suppression from sepsis/infection
Hemolysis
Drugs, transfusion therapy, hypophosphatemia/refeeding syndrome
Disseminated intravascular coagulation (DIC)
Thrombotic thrombocytopenic purpura (TTP)
Acute folate deficiency
B_{12} deficiency from nitrous oxide anesthesia

purpura (TTP).[1,2,26] Sepsis can lead to anemia and other cytopenias due to bone marrow suppression and a hypoproliferative state. Postoperative vomiting, nasogastric suction, and poor oral intake can occasionally induce acute folate depletion and sudden anemia. A peculiar etiology of acute postoperative anemia is B_{12} deficiency resulting from inhaled nitrous oxide anesthesia.[27] Nitrous oxide is an oxidizing agent that interferes with methionine synthetase and subsequent inactivation of methylcobalamin, a cofactor of methionine synthase. The end result is impaired conversion of homocysteine to methionine—a key reaction in the metabolism of B_{12}. Severe megaloblastic anemia can occur suddenly following nitrous oxide administration in patients with marginal reserves.[27–29]

4.6 LATE-ONSET ANEMIA FOLLOWING BARIATRIC SURGERY

The most common causes of anemia occurring months to years following bariatric surgery are due to deficiencies of one or more nutrients.[1] Deficiencies of water-soluble vitamins may develop within weeks of surgery if intake is poor, or months to years later in the case of vitamin B_{12} deficiency since body stores are often adequate for long time periods. Anemia in the late postoperative setting is common following Roux-en-Y and BPD, occurring in up to 40% of patients in some published series.[7,8,30] Some patients may require blood transfusions if anemia is severe. Most cases of symptomatic anemia occur within 8 weeks to 2 years of surgery and most commonly result from deficiencies of iron, vitamin B_{12}, and folate.[1–5] As noted earlier, iron deficiency can result from not only malabsorption, but also from decreased intake of meat products, anastomotic ulceration, and gastritis. Menstruating women are at an especially high risk of IDA due to ongoing iron losses in menstrual fluid; decreased absorption of dietary iron can rapidly lead to symptomatic iron deficiency. Less common causes include copper deficiency and various B-complex deficiencies.[31,32] The primary mechanism of late-onset anemia is decreased contact of food with the excluded small bowel absorptive area within the afferent limb of the Roux-en-Y or BPD.[1,2,6,9,10] Table 4.3 lists etiologies of late-onset anemia.

4.7 SPECIFIC CAUSES OF ANEMIA FOLLOWING BARIATRIC SURGERY

4.7.1 IRON DEFICIENCY

Iron deficiency is common following both Roux-en-Y and BPD for reasons described earlier. Iron is required not only for adequate erythropoiesis and erythrocyte hemoglobinization, but also for optimal cellular function, and is a component of myoglobin and cytochromes.[33] As such, iron deficiency can lead to nonanemia symptoms, such as oral pain, pagophagia (ice eating), pica, leg cramps, and myalgia.[1,34] Disrupted cellular energetics due to altered cytochrome synthesis may induce some of the nonspecific symptoms of iron deficiency, such as weakness and fatigue.[33] Prolonged iron deficiency eventually leads to overt anemia with its attendant symptoms (i.e., dyspnea, fatigue, angina, dizziness, syncope) and signs (i.e., cheilitis, smooth tongue, pallor, systolic flow murmur, tachycardia). Typical laboratory findings associated

TABLE 4.3

Nutrient Deficiencies Associated with Late-Onset Anemia Following Bariatric Surgery

Deficiency	Clinical Features
Iron	Fatigue, pica, dyspnea, koilonychia, pallor, microcytic anemia, low serum ferritin, elevated RDW
Copper	Ataxia, reflex changes, microcytic anemia, neutropenia
B_{12}	Ataxia, decreased sensation, impaired proprioception, macrocytic anemia, hypersegmented neutrophils
Folate	Glossitis, macrocytic anemia
Riboflavin	Glossitis
Niacin	Diarrhea, dermatitis, dementia
Thiamine	Confusion, tachycardia (high-output failure), parasthesia, lactic acidosis (severe)
Pyridoxine	Microcytic anemia
Vitamin C	Gingival bleeding, perifollicular keratosis, corkscrew hairs, ecchymosis
Protein	Weight loss, sarcopenia, low albumin

with IDA include decreased hematocrit, low mean corpuscular volume (MCV < 80), elevated red cell distribution width (RDW), decreased intracellular hemoglobin concentration (MCHC), low serum ferritin, and elevated total iron binding capacity.[1,35] The serum ferritin is the most simple and accurate way to diagnose or exclude iron deficiency. The classic picture of IDA is a hypochromic and microcytic anemia with an elevated RDW; the peripheral smear should be assessed as well to exclude findings suggestive of folate or B_{12} deficiency, such as macrocytosis and hypersegmented neutrophils.

Heme iron from red meat is more bioavailable than plant-based nonheme iron. As such, poor intake or intolerance to red meat can contribute to iron deficiency, especially in a menstruating woman or in the absence of adequate iron supplementation. Amaral et al. noted hypoferremia and overt anemia in 51% of females and 20% of males following gastric bypass surgery.[30] Females with menorrhagia may require gynecologic evaluation to limit menstrual blood losses, as this complicates the ability to replenish marrow iron stores. Treatment of gastric ulcerations with an acid suppressing agent such as a proton pump inhibitor may be necessary to limit occult blood loss. Bariatric patients should routinely receive oral iron supplements unless there is an underlying iron overload state such as hemachromotosis. Brolin et al. reported that 320 mg of oral ferrous sulfate twice daily prevented iron deficiency in menstruating females who had prior gastric bypass.[36] Other iron salts such as ferrous gluconate or fumarate can be tried depending on the patient's individual tolerance. Taking vitamin C or orange juice with an iron tablet enhances absorption significantly by providing an acidic milieu, which is often lacking in this population.[13] Patients with profound IDA or severe symptoms can be treated with a variety of intravenous iron preparations such as iron sucrose, which, although safe, carry a small risk of allergic anaphylactoid reactions.[1,6] Due to the risk of virally transmitted infection and immunologic and allergic complications, transfusion of red blood cells should be utilized as a last resort for patients with profound or symptomatic IDA, especially in the setting of cerebrovascular or cardiac ischemia.

4.7.2 FOLATE DEFICIENCY

Folic acid (pteroylmonoglutamic acid) is the primary compound of a large family of compounds collectively referred to as folates.[1,2,6] Intracellular folates are vital for DNA synthesis and cellular proliferation, especially hematopoietic and epithelial cells. Folate deficiency leads to impaired red cell nuclear development and results in a megaloblastic anemia.[37] Impaired proliferation of oral and gastrointestinal epithelium may result in glossitis and mucositis.[6,37] The biochemistry of folates is beyond the scope of this chapter, but these compounds are water soluble and primarily found in green vegetables, mushrooms, and liver. Cooking readily destroys dietary folates and demands increase during pregnancy, hemolysis, and a variety of inflammatory diseases. Folate-deficient pregnant women who have undergone gastric bypass surgery have a higher risk of neural tube defects in their offspring.[38,39] The body stores of folate are limited, and overt megaloblastic anemia can occur within days to weeks if severe depletion is not corrected.[37] In the bariatric population, prolonged postoperative vomiting from any cause can lead to rapid folate deficiency, especially if stores were marginal before surgery. Folate deficiency has been reported in up to almost 40% of patients undergoing Roux-en-Y surgery, and is primarily due to prolonged vomiting and poor intake of folate-rich foods and supplements.[40,41] Malabsorption of folate is less common following Roux-en-Y since the nonbypassed small bowel is usually adequate to absorb dietary folate; deficiency is more common following BPD due to limited absorption.[1]

Folate deficiency is usually suspected when macrocytosis with or without anemia is present. The MCV is typically elevated (>100) unless a concurrent IDA is present, in which case the MCV may be normal. The red cell folate level is low and serum homocysteine is elevated since folate is involved in homocysteine metabolism.[33,37] Differentiating between folate and B_{12} deficiency can be difficult since both entities can result in macrocytic anemia with elevated homocysteine.[37] In such cases, serum methylmalonic acid should be measured since this will be normal with folate deficiency and elevated with B_{12} deficiency.[1,6,37]

Treatment of overt and severe folate deficiency should include high-dose oral folic acid (2–5 mg daily for several weeks) or intravenous folic acid (1–2 mg daily for several days) followed by daily oral supplementation.[42,43] Otherwise, oral doses of of 400–1000 µg daily are recommended to prevent deficiency. Pregnant women who have undergone bariatric surgery should receive extra folic acid in addition to multivitamin supplements to prevent neural tube defects.

4.7.3 VITAMIN B_{12} DEFICIENCY

Vitamin B_{12} (cobalamin) is a complicated compound vital for normal hematologic and neurologic function. This vitamin is composed of a porphyrin ring surrounding a cobalt atom and is a key component of nuclear DNA production.[37] Vitamin B_{12} deficiency typically develops after 2–4 years of poor intake or absorption since liver stores are usually adequate in the typical Western diet. Vitamin B_{12} physiology is complex, but basically begins when dietary B_{12} is liberated by gastric acid and subsequently bound by salivary and gastric R-binders in the stomach lumen.[37,43] Once within the duodenal lumen, exposure to pancreatic enzymes cleaves B_{12} from R-binders, allowing B_{12} to attach to intrinsic factor (IF) that is produced by gastric parietal cells. The B_{12}-IF complex is subsequently absorbed in the terminal ileum.[37,43] The mechanisms of B_{12} deficiency following Roux-en-Y and BPD are complex but include decreased exposure of the food bolus to gastric mucosa, impairing acid-induced release of B_{12} from R-binders and exposure to parietal cell IF, which is necessary for distal absorption of B_{12}.[6,44] Blind-pouch syndrome can also contribute to B_{12} deficiency due to usurpation of B_{12} by overgrowth of nonresident enteric bacteria.[45] Dietary deficiency due to poor intake of B_{12} may occur especially in vegetarians or if meat intolerance is present. Yale and colleagues monitored B_{12} levels in gastric bypass patients, noting subnormal values and impaired absorption.[46] In fact, Smith et al. monitored absorption of radiolabeled food-bound B_{12} and noted markedly decreased absorption in bariatric patients compared to control patients; oral crystalline B_{12}, however, was well absorbed by both groups.[12] Some authors have reported B_{12} deficiency in up to 70% of gastric bypass patients 2 years after surgery.[47–50]

Clinical manifestations of overt B_{12} deficiency include fatigue, dyspnea, oral pain, pallor, and in severe cases, neurologic symptoms such as parasthesias, gait instability, and confusion.[1,6,43] Indeed, it is vital to always consider B_{12} deficiency in any patient with macrocytic anemia and not attribute this to folate deficiency alone since failure to replenish B_{12} can lead to permanent neurologic injury such as neuropathy, dementia, or spinal cord dysfunction.[43] Deficiency typically manifests as macrocytic anemia (MCV < 100); however, the MCV may be normal if concomitant iron deficiency is present.[1] Hypersegmented neutrophils (>5 lobes) are frequently noted on the peripheral blood smear and are a valuable clue to B_{12} deficiency; macroovalocytes are characteristically present as well. In severe cases, leukopenia and thrombocytopenia may occur as well as ineffective erythropoiesis, which can present with low haptoglobin and elevated serum lactate dehydrogenase (LDH).[6,43] Serum homocysteine and methylmalonic acid are typically elevated and may be measured if the diagnosis is not clear.

Rapid treatment of B_{12} deficiency is especially important in severe cases to prevent neurologic sequelae. Patients with severe anemia may have cardiovascular instability and also require rapid parenteral replenishment. The clinician needs to be cognizant for acute hypokalemia during initial B_{12} administration to patients with severe deficiency, as brisk hematopoiesis can deplete potassium stores, leading to ventricular arrhythmias.[43] Deficiency of iron and folate can occur from brisk hematopoiesis in patients with marginal stores of these elements.[51] Subcutaneous administration of 1000 μg of cyanocobalamin for several days followed by monthly injection of the same dose is usually adequate to treat and prevent later deficiency.[1,6] Mild cases can be treated with oral crystalline B_{12} in doses of 350–1000 μg daily. Supplementation of monthly parenteral B_{12} or oral crystalline B_{12} 350–1000 μg daily is usually adequate to prevent deficiency in those with normal postoperative stores.[52,53] An intranasal preparation is also available.[1]

4.7.4   COPPER DEFICIENCY

Copper deficiency is an important, but often overlooked, cause of anemia in patients who have undergone obesity surgery.[54,55] Copper is a component of a variety of enzyme systems, including cytochrome C oxidase, tyrosinase, and superoxide dismutase.[14] Absorbed in the stomach and proximal small bowel, copper is carried by cerruloplasmin, an alpha-2-globulin.[15] In addition to malabsorption, ingestion of zinc supplements can lead to impaired small bowel copper absorption and deficiency.[56] Adequate copper stores aid in iron absorption; indeed, deficiency of both iron and copper may be present.[6,14,15] Copper converts iron into the Fe^{+3} state for subsequent transport by transferrin.[14] Deficiency therefore results in altered iron transport and an iron deficiency state. Decreased production of the copper-containing enzyme superoxide dismutase impedes superoxide removal with subsequent damage to the red cell membrane.[15] In addition, impaired erythroblast proliferation may occur from deficiency of intracellular copper-containing enzyme systems. Neutrophil production is also impaired by copper deficiency and may lead to significant neutropenia.[57,58]

Symptoms of copper deficiency may be subtle but include fatigue and general anemic symptoms. Severe copper deficiency has been described to cause a myeloneuropathic syndrome and should be considered if neurologic symptoms are present.[32] Diagnosis is established by a low serum copper or cerruloplasmin level. Low serum ferritin may be noted. Typical hematologic findings include microcytic anemia and neutropenia—a valuable clue.[54,55] Bone marrow biopsy reveals vacuolization of myeloid and erythroid precursors; dyserythropoiesis is often present.[57]

Treatment of copper deficiency is with oral copper salts such as copper sulfate (2–4 mg daily) or intravenous copper chloride if severe cytopenia or neurologic symptoms are present. A clue to copper deficiency is the failure of a microcytic anemia to respond to iron therapy. In such cases, copper deficiency must be suspected and appropriately treated to reverse the anemia.[59]

4.7.5   THIAMINE DEFICIENCY

Acute deficiency of thiamine produces the Wernicke encephalopathy syndrome, which has been described in many patients undergoing bariatric surgery, especially those with prolonged vomiting and scant oral intake.[60–62] Thiamine (vitamin B_1) is a member of the B-complex group and is a component of many intracellular enzyme systems that regulate oxidative decaroxylation of ketoacids and transketolase in the hexose and pentophosphate shunt reactions.[63] Although uncommon, severe thiamine deficiency has been reported to cause a macrocytic anemia with dyserythropoiesis of marrow precursor cells.[64] Acute high-output cardiac failure due to thiamine deficiency (beriberi) may cause dilutional anemia.[1,62] All patients who have undergone Roux-en-Y or BPD should receive thiamine supplementation as part of a B-complex or multivitamin to prevent deficiency. Treatment of overt deficiency is with 50–100 mg of parenteral thiamine for several days, followed by oral administration in similar doses to prevent further deficiency.[1,2]

4.7.6   RIBOFLAVIN DEFICIENCY

Riboflavin, a B-complex vitamin, functions as a component of flavin adenine dinucleotide (FAD) and flavin mononucleotide (FMN)—coenzymes involved in oxidation-reduction reactions and electron transport.[63] Riboflavin deficiency results in decreased erythrocytic glutathione reductase acitivity, since this enzyme requires FAD.[63] Although hemolysis has not been reported, studies have demonstrated that subjects administered a riboflavin-void diet and the riboflavin antagonist galactoflavin developed pure red cell aplasia manifesting as anemia and reticulocytopenia.[65] Bone marrow findings in these subjects showed erythroid hypoplasia with pronormoblastic vacuolization. Foy and Kondi reported a case of riboflavin deficiency-induced red cell aplasia that resolved with riboflavin.[66] Riboflavin deficiency most often occurs in the context of other B-complex or iron deficiency, and as such, checking levels is usually not warranted. However, if a bone marrow biopsy is performed and reveals hypoplasia and vaculozation of erythroid element, riboflavin deficiency should be considered (as well as copper deficiency; see above section). Treatment of suspected or confirmed deficiency is with oral B-complex supplements or as monotherapy.[1]

4.7.7   NIACIN DEFICIENCY

Niacin, another member of the B-complex, is a vital component of a variety of intracellular coenzymes, most notably nicotinamide adenine dinucleotide (NAD), which is essential for macronutrient metabolism.[63] Absorbed in the small bowel, niacin deficiency, if severe, can lead to the classic syndrome of pellagra: dermatitis, diarrhea, and dementia.[67] Macrocytic anemia has been described and responds to oral niacin supplements.[63,67] Since laboratory assays are expensive and may be misleading, niacin deficiency should be considered in the bariatric surgery patient who develops anemia in conjunction with rash or diarrhea. Empiric administration of B-complex should prevent overt deficiency, but if niacin deficiency or pellagra is confirmed, larger amounts of niacin can be administered orally with improvement in anemia.[67]

4.7.8   PYRIDOXINE DEFICIENCY

Pyridoxine, vitamin B_6, functions as a coenzyme in heme synthesis and is converted within the red cell to pyridoxal-5-phosphate, which assists in the formation of aminolevulinic acid, a porphyrin precursor involved in hemoglobin synthesis.[23] Deficiency typically occurs with low intake and malabsorption syndromes and usually coexists with other B-complex deficiencies. Symptoms are usually nonspecific (e.g., fatigue), and the hemogram classically reveals a hypochromic and microcytic anemia due to impaired heme synthesis.[23,68] Indeed, pyridoxine deficiency can resemble iron and copper deficiencies, both of which can cause microcytic anemia. A clue to pyridoxine deficiency is the presence of ringed sideroblasts on bone marrow examination. Treatment with oral vitamin B_6 100 mg daily is adequate for treatment, but prevention with daily B-complex supplementation should be the rule in bariatric patients.[1] An intravenous form is available if deficiency is severe or oral administration is not plausible. Finally, pyridoxine deficiency should also be considered in any patient with microcytic anemia who fails to respond to iron therapy.

4.7.9 Ascorbic Acid Deficiency

Ascorbic acid, vitamin C, is a water-soluble vitamin with a well-described deficiency known as scurvy. Clements and colleagues discovered low levels of this vitamin in approximately 35% of bariatric patients at years 1 and 2 postoperatively.[69] Ascorbic acid serves as an electron donor for several enzyme systems, including those involved with collagen synthesis, carnitine and tyrosine metabolism, and the metabolism of other amino acids.[63] This vitamin is required for proper activity of folic acid reductase in the reduced (active) form, which is necessary for formation of tetrahydrofolic acid, the metabolically active form of folic acid.[23] Ascorbic acid likely prevents oxidation and inactivation of tetrahydrofolic acid, which can result in megaloblastic anemia from functional folate deficiency.[23,70] Ascorbic acid can only reverse the megaloblastosis if adequate folic acid levels are present. Intramedullary hemolysis may complicate severe deficiency. Another pathophysiologic mechanism for anemia due to ascorbic acid deficiency is iron deficiency from bleeding (often occult gastrointestinal) due to capillary fragility from impaired collagen formation and poor absorption of dietary iron.[71] Dietary iron deficiency often complicates dietary ascorbic acid deficiency, especially in children. Poor absorption of ascorbic acid and iron is common in patients undergoing Roux-en-Y and BPD, so it is vital for clinicians caring for these patients to consider the importance ascorbic acid plays in preventing anemia.[6,69] Further, vitamin C facilitates gastrointestinal absorption of dietary and supplemental oral iron preparations.[13]

The clinician must maintain a high index of suspicion to diagnose ascorbic acid deficiency. Risk factors in the bariatric population include poor absorption, vomiting, and decreased oral intake of fruits and vegetables.[1,6] Although overt scurvy is uncommon in the United States, clinical manifestations include fatigue, glossitis, gingival bleeding, perifollicular hemorrhage, "corkscrew" hairs, hyperkeratosis, pallor, and large subcutaneous ecchymoses, and heme-positive stool if occult intestinal bleeding is present.[71] Deficiency states can be prevented with a vitamin C supplement or a B-complex-containing supplement. Treatment with 100–200 mg daily typically corrects the hematologic derangements. As noted above, ascorbic acid taken with oral iron increases absorption.

4.7.10 Protein Deficiency

Most patients who undergo Roux-en-Y and BPD are followed in multidisciplinary clinics, and as such, protein-calorie malnutrition is relatively uncommon. However, in noncompliant patients or in those with protracted vomiting from any cause, protein loss and subsequent overt deficiency may develop. Protein-energy malnutrition produces a hypometabolic state that may result in a hypoproliferative anemia, which in experimental animals is characterized by blunted erythropoietin and thyroxine synthesis.[24,25] Indeed, hypoproliferative anemia is common in advanced renal failure and hypothyroidism, respectively. In addition to physical findings of poor nutrition, such as pallor and sarcopenia, the bone marrow examination reveals hypocellularity.[23,72] Consequently, a normochromic and normocytic anemia with reticulocytopenia is noted on the hemogram. Treatment entails correction of the macronutrient deficit with adequate feeding. However, the clinician needs to monitor for refeeding syndrome during nutritional repletion since hypophosphatemia can result in hemolytic anemia.[73]

4.8 SUMMARY

With the increasing popularity of bariatric surgery for treating morbid obesity, clinicians of all specialties who encounter this population of patients need to be cognizant of the hematologic consequences complicating these procedures. Bypass and malabsorptive procedures are most apt to induce micronutrient and protein deficiencies that may manifest as anemia in conjunction with a specific syndromic picture (e.g., pellagra, scurvy) or with nonspecific symptoms such as asthenia and weakness. To prevent anemia, daily administration of a well-balanced multiple vitamin with trace elements and a B-complex is required. Menstruating females should also take a daily oral iron supplement (320 mg or more) to prevent overt iron deficiency. Patients with documented specific deficiencies can be prescribed individual vitamins or trace elements, and those with severe iron deficiency can be treated with parenteral iron compounds. Adequate protein is also vital to prevent complications related to malnutrition.

REFERENCES

1. Marinella MA. Anemia following Roux-en-Y surgery for morbid obesity: a review. *South Med J* 2008;101:559–564.
2. Brethauer SA, Chand B, Schauer PR. Risks and benefits of bariatric surgery: current evidence. *Cleve Clin J Med* 2006;73:993–1007.
3. Hedley AA, Ogden CL, Johnson CL, et al. Prevalence of overweight and obesity among US children, adolescents, and adults, 1999–2002. *JAMA* 2004;291:2847–2850.
4. Podnos YE, Jimenez JC, Wilson SE, et al. Complications after laparoscopic gastric bypass: a review of 3464 cases. *Arch Surg* 2003;138:957–961.
5. Blume CA, Boni CC, Casagrande DS, et al. Nutritional profile of patients before and after Roux-en-Y gastric bypass: 3-year follow up. *Obes Surg* 2012;11:1767–1685.
6. Shankar P, Boylan M, Sriram K. Micronutrient deficiencies after bariatric surgery. *Nutrition* 2010;26:1031–1037.
7. Ruz M, Carrasco F, Rojas P, et al. Iron absorption and iron status are reduced after Roux-en-Y gastric bypass. *Am J Clin Nutr* 2009;90:527–532.
8. Cable CT, Colbert CY, Showalter T, et al. Prevalence of anemia after Roux-en-Y gastric bypass surgery: what is the right number? *Surg Obes Relat Dis* 2011;7:134–139.
9. Brolin RE, LaMarca LB, Kenler HA, et al. Malabsorptive gastric bypass in patients with superobesity. *J Gastrointest Surg* 2002;6:195–205.
10. Nelson WK, Fatima J, Houghton SG, et al. The malabsorptive very, very long limb Roux-en-Y gastric bypass for super obesity: results in 257 patients. *Surgery* 2006;140:517–523.
11. Parkes E. Nutritional management of patients after bariatric surgery. *Am J Med Sci* 2006;331:207–213.

12. Smith CD, Herkes SB, Behrns KE, et al. Gastic acid secretion and vitamin B_{12} absorption after vertical Roux-en-Y gastric bypass for morbid obesity. *Ann Surg* 1993;218:91–96.

13. Rhode BM, Shustic C, Christou NV, et al. Iron absorption and therapy after gastric bypass. *Obes Surg* 1999;9:17–21.

14. Vulpe CD, Kuo YM, Murphy TL, et al. Hephaestin, a ceruloplasmin homologue implicated in intestinal iron transport, is defective in the sla mouse. *Nat Genet* 1999;21:195–199.

15. Nagano T, Toyada T, Tanabe H, et al. Clinical features of hematological disorders caused by copper deficiency during long-term enteral nutrition. *Intern Med* 2005;44:554–559.

16. Tucker ON, Szomstein S, Rosenthal RJ. Nutritional consequences of weight-loss surgery. *Med Clin North Am* 2007;91:499–514.

17. Simon SR, Zemel R, Betancourt S, et al. Hematologic complications of gastric bypass for morbid obesity. *South Med J* 1989;82:1108–1110.

18. Lubin M, McCoy M, Waldrep DJ. Perforating marginal ulcers after laparoscopic gastric bypass. *Surg Endosc* 2006;20:51–54.

19. Frezza EE, Herbert H, Ford R, et al. Endoscopic suture removal at gastrojejunal anastomosis after Roux-en-Y gastric bypass to prevent marginal ulceration. *Surg Obes Relat Dis* 2007;3:619–622.

20. Rasmussen JJ, Fuller W, Ali MR. Marginal ulceration after laparoscopic gastric bypass: an analysis of predisposing factors in 260 patients. *Surg Endosc* 2007;21:1090–1094.

21. Sapala JA, Wood MH, Sapala MA, et al. Marginal ulcer after gastric bypass: a prosective 3-year study. *Obes Surg* 1998;8:505–516.

22. Oxentenko AS, Litin SC. Clinical pearls in gastroenterology. *Mayo Clin Proc* 2009;84:906–911.

23. Beutler E. Anemia due to other nutritional deficiencies. In Beutler E, Coller BS, Lichtman MA, et al., eds., *Williams hematology*, 471–475. 6th ed. New York: McGraw-Hill, 2002.

24. Caro J, Silver R, Erslev AJ, et al. Erythropoietin production in fasted rats. Effects of thyroid hormones and glucose supplementation. *J Lab Clin Med* 1981;98:860–868.

25. Delmonte L, Aschkenasy A, Eyquem A. Studies on the hemolytic nature of protein-deficiency anemia in the rat. *Blood* 1964;24:49–68.

26. Naqvi TA, Baumann MA, Chang JC. Postoperative thrombotic thrombocytopenic purpura. *Int J Clin Pract* 2004;58:169–172.

27. Hoffbrand AV, Moss PAH, Petit JE. Megaloblastic anaemias and other macrocytic anemias. In *Essential haematology*, 44–57. 5th ed. Malden, MA: Blackwell Publishing, 2006.

28. Krajewski W, Kucharska M, Pilacik B, et al. Impaired vitamin B_{12} metabolic status in health-care workers occupationally exposed to nitrous oxide. *Br J Anaesth* 2007;99:812–818.

29. Marie RM, Le Biez E, Busson P, et al. Nitrous oxide anesthesia-associated myelopathy. *Arch Neurol* 2000;57:380–382.

30. Amaral JF, Thompson WR, Caldwell MD, et al. Prospective hematologic evaluation of gastric exclusion surgery for morbid obesity. *Ann Surg* 1985;201:186–193.

31. Prodan CI, Bottomley SS, Vincent AS, et al. Copper deficiency after gastric surgery: a reason for caution. *Am J Med Sci* 2009;337:256–258.

32. Juhasz-Pocsine K, Rudnicki SA, Archer RL, Harik SI. Neurologic complications of gastric bypass surgery for morbid obesity. *Neurology* 2007;68:1843–1850.

33. DeBiasse-Fortin MA. Mineral and trace elements. In Matarese LE, Gottschlich MM, eds., *Contemporary nutrition support practice: a clinical guide*, 164–172. 2nd ed. Philadelphia: Saunders, 2003.

34. Marinella MA. "Tomatophagia" and iron-deficiency anemia. *N Engl J Med* 1999;341:60–61.

35. Toskes PP. Hematologic abnormalities following gastric resection. *Major Probl Clin Surg* 1976;20:119–128.

36. Brolin RE, Gorman JH, Gorman RC, et al. Prophylactic iron supplementation after Roux-en-Y gastric bypass: a prospective, double-blind, randomized study. *Arch Surg* 1998;133:740–744.

37. Munker R. Anemias: general considerations and microcytic, and megaloblastic anemias. In Munker R, Hiller E, Glass J, et al., eds., *Modern hematology: biology and clinical management*, 83–99. 2nd ed. Totowa NJ: Humana Press, 2007.

38. Martin L, Chavez GF, Adams MJ Jr, et al. Gastric bypass surgery as maternal risk factor for neural tube defects. *Lancet* 1988;1:640–641.

39. Knudsen LB, Kallen B. Gastric bypass, pregnancy, and neural tube defects. *Lancet* 1986;2:227.

40. Halverson JD. Micronutrient deficiencies after gastric bypass for morbid obesity. *Am Surg* 1986;52:594–598.

41. Kushner R. Managing the obese patient after bariatric surgery: a case report of severe malnutrition and review of the literature. *JPEN* 2000;24:126–132.

42. Elliot K. Nutritional considerations after bariatric surgery. *Crit Care Nurs Q* 2003;26:133–138.

43. Hoffbrand AV, Moss PAH, Pettit JE. Haemolytic anaemias. In *Essential haematology*, 58–71. 5th ed. Malden, MA: Blackwell Publishing, 2006.

44. Marcuard SP, Sinar DR, Swanson, MS, et al. Absence of luminal intrinsic factor after gastric bypass surgery for morbid obesity. *Dig Dis Sci* 1989;34:1238–1242.

45. Evers BM. Small intestine. In Townsend CM, Beauchamp RD, Evers BM, eds., *Sabiston textbook of surgery: the biological basis of modern surgical practice*, 1323–1380. 17th ed. Philadelphia: Elsevier Saunders, 2004.

46. Yale CE, Gohdes PN, Schilling RF. Cobalamin absorption and hematologic status after two types of gastric surgery for obesity. *Am J Hematol* 1993;42:63–66.

47. Rhode BM, Arseneau P, Cooper BA, et al. Vitamin B_{12} deficiency after gastric surgery for obesity. *Am J Clin Nutr* 1996;63:103–109.

48. Schilling RF, Gohdes PN, Hardie GH. Vitamin B_{12} deficiency after gastric bypass surgery for obesity. *Ann Intern Med* 1984;101:501–502.

49. Halverson JD, Zuckerman GR, Koehler RE, et al. Gastric bypass for morbid obesity: a medical-surgical assessment. *Ann Surg* 1981;194:152–160.

50. Crowley LV, Seay J, Mullin G. Late effects of gastric bypass for obesity. *Am J Gastroenterol* 1984;79:850–860.

51. Hvas AM, Nexo E. Diagnosis and treatment of vitamin B_{12} deficiency—an update. *Haematologica* 2006;91:1506–1512.

52. Rhode BM, Tamin H, Gilfix BM, et al. Treatment of B_{12} deficiency after gastric surgery for severe obesity. *Obes Surg* 1995;5:154–158.

53. Butler CC, Vidal-Aball J, Cannings-John R, et al. Oral vitamin B_{12} for vitamin B_{12} deficiency: a systematic review of randomized controlled trials. *Fam Pract* 2006;23:279–285.

54. Balsa JA, Botella-Carretero JI, Gomez-Martin JM, et al. Copper and zinc serum levels after derivative bariatric surgery: differences between Roux-en-Y gastric bypass and biliopancreatic diversion. *Obes Surg* 2011;6:744–750.

55. Gletsu-Miller N, Broderius M, Rediani JK, et al. Incidence and prevalence of copper deficiency following Roux-en-Y gastric bypass surgery. *Int J Obes (Lond)* 2011;36:328–335.

56. Hoffman HN II, Phyliky RL, Fleming CR. Zinc-induced copper deficiency. *Gastroenterology* 1988;94:508–512.

57. Gregg XT, Reddy V, Prchal JT. Copper deficiency masquerading as myelodysplastic syndrome. *Blood* 2002;100:1493–1495.

58. Kumar N, Ahlskog JE, Gross JB Jr. Acquired hypocupremia after gastric surgery. *Clin Gastroenterol Hepatol* 2004;2:1074–1079.

59. Chen CC, Takeshima F, Miyazaki T, et al. Clinicopathological analysis of hematologic disorders in tube fed patients with copper deficiency. *Intern Med* 2007;46:839–844.
60. Bozbora A, Coskun H, Ozarmagan S, et al. A rare complication of adjustable gastric banding: Wernicke's encephalopathy. *Obes Surg* 2000;10:274–275.
61. Aasheim ET. Wernicke encephalopathy after bariatric surgery—a systematic review. *Ann Surg* 2008;248:714–720.
62. Marinella MA. Wernicke's encephalopathy. In *Recognizing clinical patterns: clues to a timely diagnosis*, 102. Philadelphia: Hanley and Belfus, 2002.
63. Boosalis MG. Vitamins. In Matarese LE, Gottschlich MM, eds., *Contemporary nutrition support practice: a clinical guide*, 145–163. Philadelphia: Saunders, 2003.
64. Bazarbachi A, Muakkit S, Ayas M, et al. Thiamin-responsive myelodysplasia. *Br J Haematol* 1998;102:1098–1100.
65. Lane M, Alfrey CP Jr. The anemia of human riboflavin deficiency. *Blood* 1965;25:432–442.
66. Foy H, Kondi A. A case of true red cell aplastic anemia successfully treated with riboflavin. *J Pathol Bacteriol* 1953;65:559–564.
67. Spivak JL, Jackson DL. Pellagra: an analysis of 18 patients and a review of the literature. *Johns Hopkins Med J* 1977;140:295–309.
68. Clayton PT. B_6-responsive disorders: a model of vitamin dependency. *J Inherit Metab Dis* 2006;29:317–326.
69. Clements RH, Katasani VG, Palepu R, et al. Incidence of vitamin deficiency after laparoscopic Roux-en-Y gastric bypass in a university hospital setting. *Am Surg* 2006;72:1196–1204.
70. Cox EV, Meynell MJ, Northam BE, et al. The anemia of scurvy. *Am J Med* 1967;42:220–227.
71. Hansen EPK, Metzsche C, Henningsen E, Toft P. Severe scurvy after gastric bypass surgery and a poor postoperative diet. *J Clin Med Res* 2012;4:135–137.
72. Borelli P, Blatt S, Pereira J, et al. Reduction of erythroid progenitors in protein-energy malnutrition. *Br J Nutr* 2007;97:307–314.
73. Marinella MA. The refeeding syndrome and hypophosphatemia. *Nutr Rev* 2003;61:320–323.

5 Metabolic Bone Disease Following Bariatric Surgery

Stephanie F. Deivert and Christopher D. Still

CONTENTS

A 47-year-old premenopausal woman, Anna, who underwent Roux-en-Y gastric bypass (RYGB) surgery for morbid obesity 5 years ago presents to her obesity medicine specialist after being lost to follow-up since 2 months after surgery with complaints of gradually worsening symptoms of fatigue, weakness, back pain, and muscle and joint pain. Before surgery she weighed 386 pounds and now weighs 224 pounds with a body mass index (BMI) of 34. She has no history of fractures, thyroid disease, and does not smoke or drink alcohol. She reports that she is happy with her weight loss and that it has been stable over the past 3 years. She takes a bariatric multivitamin that contains calcium and vitamin D two tablets twice daily, and gives herself vitamin B_{12} injections every 6 months as prescribed by her primary care doctor. She reports discomfort in her muscles and is visibly weak in her movements and rising from her chair. The physical and neurologic examinations are otherwise unremarkable. Her diet history equates to approximately 45–50 g of protein intake daily. She reports that she does not tolerate dairy products since the surgery. She reports that 4 years ago she was diagnosed with an ulcer and was started on a proton pump inhibitor (PPI), but did not think she needed to call her surgeon. She has recently been diagnosed with fibromyalgia.

Biochemical markers were significant for hypocalcemia, undetectable 25-hydroxyvitamin D, elevated alkaline phosphatase, mild hypophosphatemia, hypoalbuminemia, intact parathyroid hormone (PTH) level two times the upper range of normal, and very low urine calcium.

Dual-energy x-ray absorptiometry (DXA) data lumbar spine: T score, –2.3; Z score, –2.2
DXA data of left total hip: T score, –2.1; Z score: –2.5

This case is a typical presentation of metabolic bone disease in a bariatric patient, many of whom have been lost to follow-up for several years postoperatively. They typically report vague symptoms of fatigue, myalgias, and arthralgias that are often misdiagnosed for many months or even years as fibromyalgia, rheumatoid arthritis, polymyalgia rheumatica, Paget's disease, or even depression. Many patients have developed osteopenia or osteoporosis with hypocalcemia, very low or undetectable 25-hydroxyvitamin D levels, secondary hyperparathyroidism, increased 1,25-dihydroxyvitamin D levels, and increased serum alkaline phosphatase.[1] Muscle weakness or complaints of loss of muscle mass, dull poorly localized bone pain, gait impairments such as a waddling gait, and difficulty arising from a chair or going down a flight of stairs all serve as clues to the possible presence of metabolic bone disease. Obtaining a dietary and supplementation history is crucial in bariatric patients, and clinicians should have a high index of suspicion for the presence of metabolic bone disease in those who have suboptimal doses or forms of supplementation, especially when combined with poor dietary intake.[2,3]

This case emphasizes the importance for bariatric patients to have regular postoperative follow-up with a provider who is familiar with proper monitoring of nutrients and biochemical markers following surgery. Monitoring these parameters on an ongoing basis, as well as proper education, will allow for early detection of nutritional deficiencies and ultimately help to prevent the development of metabolic bone disease in the bariatric population.

5.1 ESSENTIAL NUTRIENTS FOR BONE HEALTH

Many nutrients play an essential role in bone health. This chapter will focus on those that are pertinent for the obese or bariatric surgery patient.

5.1.1 VITAMIN D

Vitamin D is a fat-soluble vitamin that has been appreciated for its role in calcium homeostasis and bone health since its identification.[4] Vitamin D consists of two bioequivalent forms that must undergo two successive hydroxylations in the liver and kidney to become biologically active. Vitamin D_2, also known as ergocalciferol, is obtained from dietary sources such as yeast and plants. Vitamin D_2 has been shown to be about 30% as effective as vitamin D_3 at maintaining vitamin D status.[5] Vitamin D_3, also known as cholecalciferol, is found in oily fish, cod liver oil, or fortified foods. The other main source of vitamin D_3 is production in the skin through exposure to ultraviolet B (UVB) radiation in sunlight. The provitamin 7-dehydrocholesterol (7-DHC, or provitamin D_3) is converted from cholesterol in our bodies. Provitamin D_3 is found in the epidermis, where it absorbs UVB radiation, transforming it into previtamin D_3, and then undergoes a rapid isomerization to form vitamin D_3. Once vitamin D_2 or D_3 enters the circulation, it is bound to the vitamin D binding protein and transported to the liver, where it is hydroxylated on carbon 25 to produce 25-hydroxyvitamin D_3 [25(OH)D], or calcidiol. Calcidiol is not tightly regulated and is the major circulating form of vitamin D; an increase in cutaneous production or ingestion will result in an increase in serum levels. Therefore, this is the most widely accepted measurement that should be used to determine if a patient is deficient. However, calcidiol is biologically inert and is transported to the kidney to be further hydroxylated, yielding 1,25-dihydroxyvitamin D_3 [1,25(OH)$_2$D], or calcitriol, which is the metabolically active form of vitamin D.[4-7]

Because dietary vitamin D is fat soluble, once ingested it is incorporated into the chylomicron fraction and absorbed through the lymphatic system. It is estimated that approximately 80% of the ingested vitamin D is absorbed by this mechanism.[4,7] Vitamin D is principally absorbed in the small intestine, preferentially in the jejunum and ileum, in a process that is highly dependent of bile salts.[8] Malabsorption of vitamin D after bariatric surgery occurs by bypassing or altering these segments of intestine or decreasing fat absorption.

5.1.1.1 Role of Vitamin D in Maintaining Calcium Levels

Vitamin D's major function is to maintain serum calcium levels within very tight physiological values by several complex mechanisms. It acts in the small intestine to enhance calcium entry through active transport mechanisms when calcium intake is low. Calcitriol works in various ways: it induces calcium channels and also activates several calcium binding proteins to facilitate transport. In addition to calcium absorption, calcitriol also enhances absorption of dietary phosphorus. In vitamin D deficiency, 10–15% or less of dietary calcium and 60% of dietary phosphorus is absorbed by the gastrointestinal tract. When dietary calcium intake is lacking, calcitriol interacts with osteoblasts in a way that results in osteoclast maturation. The osteoclasts release hydrochloric acid and proteolytic enzymes to dissolve bone mineral and matrix, which allows for the release of calcium into extracellular space.[6]

5.1.1.2 Role of Vitamin D in Bone Health

Vitamin D does not have a direct active role in the bone mineralization process; its main responsibility is to maintain serum calcium and phosphorus levels in the normal range to allow proper bone mineralization to occur. However, it does have a direct effect on bone cell homeostasis in a variety of ways. $1,25(OH)_2D$ is involved with multiple interactions that affect osteoblast activity, including increasing expression of bone-specific alkaline phosphatase, osteocalcin, osteonectin, osteprotogerin, and a variety of cytokines. It is also known for altering proliferation and apoptosis of skeletal cells.[6]

5.1.1.3 Food Sources of Vitamin D

Vitamin D is rare in foods, except for oily fish such as salmon and mackerel, which provide about 400 IU per 3.5 oz, or fish liver oils such as cod liver oil. However, fortified foods provide most of the vitamin D in the American diet. For example, almost all of the U.S. milk supply is voluntarily fortified with 100 IU/8 oz or 1/6 of the Recommended Dietary Allowance (RDA) per serving. Other fortified foods include yogurt, and some cereals, bread products, and orange juice.[9–11] However, a sampling study from the U.S. Department of Agriculture (USDA) showed inconsistencies from nondetectable to almost twice the reported amount of vitamin D in fortified products.[12] Despite obvious concerns with inconsistencies in fortification practices, bariatric patients also may not tolerate the foods most often fortified and naturally high in vitamin D postoperatively. Malabsorptive procedures can cause lactose intolerance, which sometimes leads to patient avoidance or the use of products that may not be fortified. Other fortified foods—cereals, breads, and orange juice—are not recommended or tolerated in quantities that would provide adequate amounts of daily dietary vitamin D. Oily fish also may not be tolerated after malabsorptive procedures, and if tolerated, is generally not consumed on a daily basis to reach recommended amounts of vitamin D.

5.1.1.4 Factors Influencing Vitamin D

Other than dietary intake, vitamin D is also synthesized in the skin. However, a variety of factors can influence the cutaneous production of vitamin D_3. Melanin competes with 7-DHC for UVB photons in the skin and reduces the amount of vitamin D_3 that is produced, and therefore people with darker pigmentation are more likely to become vitamin D deficient if dietary intake is inadequate. Also, aging diminishes the concentration of 7-DHC in the skin available for conversion to vitamin D_3, thus increasing risk of vitamin D deficiency in older individuals.[13] Other factors that have been shown to play a role are latitude, time of day, seasonal variations, in additions to amount of exposed skin, as well as sunscreen usage.[6] Most pertinently in the bariatric surgery population, vitamin D insufficiency has also been associated with obesity (BMI ≥ 30) in both men and women. Although data are not conclusive, it is likely due to decreased bioavailability of D_3 from both cutaneous and food sources because it is deposited in body fat.[14–16] In addition to obesity likely being a direct causal factor for vitamin D deficiency, it may be compounded by less sun exposure of those affected by obesity. Those undergoing bariatric surgery may already have vitamin D deficiency before malabsorptive and dietary consequences of the surgery even come in to play.

5.1.1.5 Vitamin D Requirements

Dietary vitamin D can be essential at maintaining nutritional status, especially in the presence of decreased solar exposure and efficiency of synthesis. A wide optimal range for 25(OH)D is reported (25–80 ng/ml), and differences of opinion exist as to the definition of vitamin D insufficiency (sometimes reported as <30 ng/ml) and deficiency (<20 ng/ml).[17] Other sources suggest that deficiency should be considered below a serum 25(OH)D value of 30–32 ng/ml (75–80 nM).[18] However, in 2010, the Institute of Medicine (IOM) committee concluded that a serum concentration of 20 ng/ml (50 nmol/L) was sufficient for most individuals. The current RDA for oral intake of vitamin D is 600 IU from 1 year of age up to age 70, and increases to 800 IU after the age of 71. These 2010 guidelines are increases from the previous standards. These updated guidelines are based on minimal sun exposure.[9]

In 2008 the American Association of Clinical Endocrinologists (AACE), The Obesity Society (TOS), and American Society for Metabolic and Bariatric Surgery (ASMBS) developed medical guidelines for perioperative nutritional support of the bariatric surgery patient, which were recently updated in 2013. These guidelines include evidence-based recommendations for supplementation postoperatively. Grade C evidence exists that supplementation of ergocalciferol (D_2) or cholecalciferol (D_3) at a level of 400–800 IU/day is indicated in bariatric surgical patients who have undergone RYGB, biliopancreatic diversion (BPD), or biliopancreatic diversion with duodenal switch (BPD/DS) to prevent or minimize secondary hyperparathyroidism without inducing hypercalcemia.[19,20] However, some studies and clinicians have suggested that 800–6000 IU/day or more of vitamin D is needed to maintain serum 25(OH)D levels in the optimal range.[5,21,22] Studies have also found that biochemical bone markers show a negative remodeling balance, characterized by an increase in bone resorption following purely restrictive procedures, despite no evidence of secondary hyperparathyroidism.[23,24] This may be due in part to reduced intake, but may indicate a necessity to supplement vitamin D following purely restrictive surgeries as well.

5.1.2 CALCIUM

5.1.2.1 Calcium Distribution

Total body calcium content in the body of an adult is approximately 1000 g, most of which (99%) is in the form of hydroxyapatite crystal $[Ca_{10}(PO4)_6 (OH)_2]$ in bone. The crystal allows for the weight-bearing properties of the bone and also acts as a reservoir of calcium and phosphorus (PO_4) to maintain appropriate intra- and extracellular levels. The remaining calcium in the body is in extracellular fluid, including blood and soft tissue. Total serum calcium ranges from 8.8 to 10.4 mg/dl and consists of about 50% free ions, 40% protein-bound, and 10% as part of citrate and PO_4 ions. The major calcium binding proteins include albumin and globulin in the serum, and calmodulin and other calcium binding proteins in the cell. The main ionic complexes found in the serum are calcium phosphate, calcium carbonate, and calcium oxalate.[7,25]

5.1.2.2 Calcium Absorption

Dietary intake is necessary to provide enough calcium to maintain health body stores. With adequate calcium intake the duodenum and jejunum are responsible for about 90% of calcium absorption. During periods of increased calcium requirement or low calcium intake, calcium active transport in the duodenum and ileum is stimulated. Also in this phase, the jejunum and also the colon will participate in absorption, but to a lesser extent than the duodenum and ileum. Fractional absorption rates will be increased from 25–45% to about 55–70%. Calcium intake of at least 400 mg/day is required to maintain neutral or positive calcium balance in adults. When diets fall below 200 mg/day, calcium balance is negative. Calcium absorption begins to plateau around 1000 mg/day. The relationship between calcium absorption and calcium intake can be explained by two absorptive mechanisms: a cell-mediated active transport and a passive, diffusional absorption when intake exceeds needs. Calcium active transport is stimulated by $1,25(OH)_2D_3$ when calcium intake is lower. When calcium intake is very high, primarily passive absorption is stimulated due to low serum levels of $1,25(OH)_2D_3$. Permeability of each intestinal segment allows for diffusional calcium flow along the paracellular pathway. Permeability is similar throughout the duodenum, jejunum, and ileum, while it is intermediate throughout the colon, and is lowest in the cecum. The wide variation of calcium absorption in healthy adults for levels of adequate consumption is mainly thought to be due to variation in the active component of the absorptive process.[7,25]

5.1.2.3 Calcium Homeostasis

Calcium homeostasis is tightly controlled, and as such, a normal serum calcium level does not at all mean intake or absorption is adequate. Parathyroid hormone (PTH) and $1,25(OH)_2D_3$, or calcitriol, are the most important hormones in calcium homeostasis. The major regulator is PTH, which is part of a negative feedback loop to maintain serum calcium levels. PTH secretion is regulated by parathyroid cell plasma membrane Ca-sensing receptor (CaSR). PTH secretion is stimulated by hypocalcemia and works in three primary ways to increase serum calcium levels. Indirectly, it increases calcium absorption in the small intestine by stimulating renal synthesis of calcitriol in the renal proximal tubule, about 24 h after PTH secretion. This active form of vitamin D works in the small intestine to promote calcium absorption. PTH also works in the kidney within minutes to directly decrease urinary calcium losses by stimulating renal tubule reabsorption of the filtered calcium. PTH also inhibits phosphate reabsorption in the renal tubules. PTH has a rapid effect, within minutes to hours, stimulating bone resorption via increased osteoclastic and osteocytic-mediated mechanisms. Hypercalcemia suppresses CaSR signaling and therefore suppresses PTH secretion that causes reductions in renal tubule Ca reabsorption, and increases urine calcium excretion allowing for calcium to return to normal levels.[7,25] PTH and vitamin D are also interrelated in that the parathyroid chief cell has a vitamin D receptor that responds to calcitriol by decreasing the expression of the PTH gene and decreasing the synthesis and secretion of PTH.[6]

5.1.2.4 Factors That Influence Calcium Absorption

5.1.2.4.1 Ratio of Calcium to Phosphorus

The relationship between calcium and phosphate metabolism is very complex, in some cases unclear, and remains a subject of some controversy. Like calcium, most of the body's PO_4 content is found in bone, with a ratio of calcium to phosphorous of 2.2:1.0, by weight. Phosphorus balance, like calcium, is maintained through intestinal absorption, renal excretion, and bone accretion, and includes both organic and inorganic forms of phosphate. Absorption is also through passive and active transport mechanisms stimulated by 1, $25(OH)_2D_3$ primarily in the proximal duodenum, jejunum, and to a lesser extent, distal ileum. Differences between calcium and phosphorus balance include phosphorus absorption is not limited, and is absorbed almost twice as efficiently as dietary calcium, with absorption rates ranging from 60 to 80% of dietary PO_4 intake, with a normal intake of 775–1860 mg. Also, dietary phosphorus is found in abundance in meat, poultry, and fish, which provide about 15–20 times more phosphorus than calcium, by weight. Essentially, some amounts of phosphorus are found in most foods, whereas only a few types of foods provide adequate dietary calcium. Polyphosphate additives are also used as stabilizers in all popular cola beverages and as chemical additives. As a result, phosphorus deficiency is rarely seen as a nutritional problem, unlike calcium. Although phosphorus requirements have not officially been determined for humans, a one-to-one ratio of calcium to phosphorus, by weight, in the diet is recommended, while typical American diets are estimated to be about 1:2.[7] The RDA for adults ranges by age from 580 to 1250 mg.[8] A delicate balance between calcium and phosphorus is necessary for maintaining proper bone density and prevention of osteoporosis. Sufficient phosphorus intake is important to ensure the proper balance of essential minerals in order to promote bone remineralization.[7] Some studies have shown high phosphorus intakes to cause hypocalcemia, nutritional secondary hyperparathyroidism, and progressive bone loss in several animal models.[26,27] However, others suggest, given a typical Western diet having a Ca/P ratio well below 1, that as long as dietary calcium intake is adequate, excess phosphorous does not reduce calcium absorption.[28]

Consideration must be made for the role of phosphorus in bone health after bariatric surgery. As mentioned, phosphorus absorption occurs primarily in the small intestine, which is a concern following malabsorptive procedures. However, post-operatively all bariatric surgery patients are encouraged to consume diets rich in phosphorus through addition of lean meats, poultry, and fish. As a result, phosphorus deficiency is unlikely if dietary goals are being tolerated and met. Similarly, portion sizes of these foods are generally not large enough to cause much concern for excess dietary phosphorus. In some instances, post-bariatric surgery patients are not able to tolerate these types of food and may have a hard time reaching adequate goals. Low phosphorus levels can occur in the setting of malabsorption, malnutrition, vitamin D deficiency, and metabolic bone disease.[29] Oral supplementation may be necessary in these instances.

5.1.2.4.2   *The Anion's Influence on the Rate of Calcium Absorption*

The solubility of the specific calcium influences the rate and level of calcium absorption. Calcium oxalate is relatively insoluble and is poorly absorbed by the human gut, with only about 10% being absorbed. Only about 5% of calcium oxalate from spinach has been shown to be absorbed, although it is not clear why this is even less absorbed than pure calcium oxalate.[7]

Calcium salts have an absorption range of 25–40% when taken with meals. The absorbability of milk calcium also falls at the upper end of this range. Calcium carbonate, which generally is the most commonly consumed form of calcium for supplementation, has about a 30% rate of absorption. The reason why this form is used in supplementation is because the pills are smaller and made at less cost due to a relatively lower molecular weight of the anion when compared to other calcium salts, even though the absorbability is lower. Calcium carbonate absorption is highly dependent on an acidic environment, and therefore recommended to be given with meals to get to the 30% absorption rate. Highly soluble calcium salts such as those with citrate, malate, or glycine as the counterion have also been used in supplementation. Calcium citrate is more rapidly absorbed than calcium carbonate, but more importantly, it has been shown not to be dependent on the acidic environment for absorption.[7]

5.1.2.4.3   *Achlorhydria and Calcium Absorption*

Calcium must be ionized and in solution to be absorbed. In a normal individual, secreted gastric acid lowers the pH of the stomach, which allows for improved absorption of calcium because calcium salts are more soluble in acid than at a neutral pH. If calcium compounds are not solubilized in the stomach and enter the small intestine's alkaline environment, they are less available for absorption and not likely to be broken down further. In low acid environments, supplements in the form of calcium carbonate have been shown to have absorption rates as low as 4%. Absorption increases if supplements are taken with food, in both soluble and less soluble forms of calcium, in healthy individuals. In addition to stimulating gastric acid production, some have theorized that food may slow the entry of calcium into the intestines, allowing for more complete absorption.[7] When calcium carbonate was given with skim milk, achlorhydric patients absorbed as much calcium as control subjects with normal stomach acidity.[30] Although the labeled calcium was in the form of calcium carbonate, an exchange between the supplemental calcium and milk calcium could have occurred; therefore, one can conclude that achlorhydria can play a minimal role in calcium absorption only if solubilized calcium is available.[7]

5.1.2.5   Calcium Requirements

As mentioned previously, calcium intake of 400 mg/day is considered adequate; however, the RDA for adult men of <71 years and premenopausal adult women is 1000 mg/day, increasing to 1200 mg for postmenopausal women and men over the age of 71 years. Recommendations are different for those younger than 18 years.[31] Calcium requirements do increase with age to compensate for decreased intestinal absorption. Higher rates of absorption occur during childhood, adolescence, and the young adult years, as well as during pregnancy or lactation for healthy people. When diets are low in calcium, absorptive efficiency increases, although efficiency rates decline with age or when calcium intake is high. Typically only about 20–60% of dietary calcium is absorbed in a healthy individual, depending on factors such as age, calcium intake, skeletal requirements, vitamin D status, and bioavailability in foods.[7]

According to the AACE/TOS/ASMBS guidelines, grade B evidence exists that supports a maintenance dose of 1200–1500 mg calcium/day for bariatric surgery, and preferentially in the form of calcium citrate, primarily due to the effect of achlorhydria and the improved rate of absorption with the anion of citrate. Also, long-term use of proton pump inhibitors in patients for treatment of or protection against anastomotic ulcers can result in more pronounced achlorhydria.[19,20] Optimal daily intake of calcium based on the specific bariatric surgical procedure is currently not well defined; however, in most studies this dosing can be applied to most bariatric procedures with the exception of the BPD with or without duodenal switch, which requires up to 2000 mg. Also, some have suggested increasing maintenance calcium to 2000 mg for bariatric surgeries during the rapid weight loss phase.[3,32] Generally, calcium citrate is well tolerated by patients as far as the gastrointestinal side effects reported with calcium supplementation. However, compliance can be an issue due to expense, as well as the practicality of the forms of citrate that pose an issue and large size of the pill. Tablets are often extremely large and only have 240 mg calcium/tablet, which often needs to be broken or crushed. Powder or chewable forms are available at an increased cost. If calcium citrate cannot be taken, calcium carbonate should be encouraged with meals and, ideally, low-fat dairy products to provide sufficient solubilized calcium. Supplementation should be recommended even in purely restrictive operations due to decreased dietary intake of calcium. Overall absorption can be an issue in some patients; therefore, regular monitoring is recommended. Urine calcium can assist in assessing the adequacy of calcium intake in that abnormally low urine calcium in the presence of normal renal function suggests inadequate intake or absorption.[3,32]

5.1.3   Protein

5.1.3.1   Considerations in Bone Health

Studies have shown that increasing dietary protein, especially that with a high sulfur–amino acid content such as animal protein, can induce excessive losses of urine calcium and cause a negative calcium balance. This effect is called the calciuric effect of protein. This is particularly a concern when animal protein intake is high and calcium intake is low, as with many American diets. The effects have been shown to be minimized with the higher phosphorus and adequate calcium content of food sources.[7] Nonetheless, epidemiological studies have shown a positive relationship between incidence of hip fracture and level of animal protein intake; those consuming animal-based foods excrete more calcium than subjects ingesting plant-based foods at comparable calcium intakes.[33,34] The exact mechanism by which protein induces urinary calcium losses is unknown, although it was presumed due, in part, to the catabolism of sulfur-containing amino acids. When plasma sulfur levels are high, a compound is formed with calcium, perhaps buffering from bone. This compound passes into the renal tubule and is poorly reabsorbed, which results in the excretion into urine. This constant buffering from the bone results in longer-term skeletal loss and decreases in bone mineral density.[35]

This issue is a consideration for bariatric surgery patients and the risk of metabolic bone disease, as patients are generally encouraged to consume a high-protein diet in the early postoperative period to prevent malnutrition. However, recent studies have shown urinary calcium losses associated with high protein intake may result from increased intestinal calcium absorption because no changes were noted with bone turnover in the short term. This finding suggests that bone structure may not be impacted by high protein intake at all.[36,37]

On the contrary, other epidemiological studies have shown increased rates of bone loss as well as reduced bone density in individuals who maintain a low-protein diet. Although exact mechanisms are not known, it has been theorized that it could play a role in bone resorption, bone formation, or both. These studies have demonstrated that a low-protein diet can actually reduce intestinal calcium absorption, which results in a rise in PTH.[38] The effects of various intakes of protein (0.7, 0.8, 0.9, and 1.0 g/kg of body weight) have been studied, demonstrating decreased calcium absorption and increased PTH levels by day 4 in the 0.7 and 0.8 g/kg diets, but not with 0.9 and 1.0 g/kg.[39]

5.1.3.2 Protein Recommendations

A review of protein and bone health actually concluded that diets containing 1.0 to 1.5 g protein/kg should be recommended as ideal for bone health despite current recommendations for protein being only 0.8 g/kg.[40] Recommendations for bariatric surgery patients postoperatively are 60–120 g protein/day, which may or may not fall at or above the 1.0 g protein/kg of ideal body weight or adjusted body weight. Considerations should be made for the use of adjusted body weight in order to approximate metabolically active tissue when calculating protein needs due to the link between protein intake, calciuria, and fracture risk. Protein intakes can be inadequate for all types of bariatric surgery due to intolerances or decreased intake. Moreover, BPD patients may be at increased risk of protein malnutrition through increased malabsorption.[41] AACE/TOS/ASMBS guidelines encourage intake of 80–120 g/day for patients with either BPD or BPD/DS, and 60 g/day or more for those with RYGB. They also encourage protein intakes to be quantified periodically.[19,20]

5.1.4 Magnesium

5.1.4.1 Magnesium Distribution

Total body concentration of magnesium (Mg) is approximately 25 g, of which about 65% is found in bone, 33% is intracellular, and 1% is in extracellular compartments. Only 20–30% of bone Mg is freely exchangeable; the remaining is associated with the apatite crystal and is nonexchangeable, even in a magnesium-deficient diet. Most of the Mg associated with the hydroxyapatite crystal is found on the bone surface and is not integrated into the structure. Normal plasma Mg ranges are from 1.7 to 2.2 mg/dl, about half in the ionic state, about one-third is protein-bound, and the remainder occurs in the form of complexes. Ionic Mg is the portion that is most closely correlated to Mg-dependent actions.[7,25] Magnesium appears to play an important role in calcium and bone metabolism, which may affect bone remodeling and strength, and it has also been associated with increased bone mineral density.[32,42,43]

5.1.4.2 Magnesium Homeostasis

Unlike the hormonal system that was described with calcium, magnesium levels are regulated largely by the quantitative influx and efflux of Mg across the intestine, bone, and kidney. The kidney primarily regulates serum levels and is able to adjust to attain a high-efficiency tubular reabsorption rate. Ionic magnesium in the blood is a factor in regulating PTH secretion, but to a lesser extent than calcium.[7,25]

5.1.4.3 Magnesium Absorption

Magnesium is plentiful in plant and animal foods, and therefore intake is generally adequate. With typical dietary intake of 168–720 mg/day of magnesium, absorption averages around 35–40%, with rates varying from 20 to 70%. However, when dietary magnesium is in the form of a complex with phosphorus, it is less absorbed. Intestinal magnesium absorption is directly proportional to dietary intake. Magnesium is absorbed by specific transport systems in both the small intestine and colon, by both cellular and paracellular pathways. Magnesium absorption is not dependent on vitamin D, and there is no correlation between serum vitamin D levels and Mg absorption.[7,25]

5.1.4.4 Magnesium Deficiency

Magnesium deficiency is rare and primarily only occurs in prolonged diarrhea or intestinal diseases, with malabsorption that accompanies chronic alcoholism, in those who are taking loop diuretics or proton pump inhibitors, or in those with surgical removal of the small intestine. In conditions associated with steatorrhea, the magnesium is lost due to reduced absorption and chelation with unabsorbed fatty acids in the bowel lumen. Thus, patients who have undergone a malabsorptive bariatric surgery are at risk for magnesium deficiency, especially those with substantial diarrhea.[7,25] A well-designed 2-year controlled trial has shown postmenopausal women may benefit from magnesium supplementation for bone health.[43] However, studies are lacking in the area of magnesium supplementation after bariatric surgery.[32] Nonetheless, it is important to be aware of this when assessing laboratory data for bone disease because magnesium deficiency can cause plasma calcium levels to drop even when the diet is adequate in calcium and vitamin D.[7] However, in magnesium deficiency, unlike calcium or vitamin D deficiency, impaired PTH secretion will occur. Decreased PTH secretion results in further calcium and vitamin D abnormalities, which in turn decrease jejunal absorption of magnesium.[40] It appears magnesium is needed for proper formation and secretion of PTH.[7] In this instance of plasma calcium reduction it is important to replace magnesium and not just calcium and vitamin D.

5.1.4.5 Magnesium Requirements

The current RDA for magnesium is between 310 and 420 mg/day, increasing with age and also higher in males. Green vegetables, some legumes, nuts, seeds, and whole unrefined grains are good sources of magnesium. According to the AACE/TOS/ASMBS guidelines, there is currently insufficient data to recommend empiric supplementation of magnesium after bariatric surgery beyond what is included in a mineral-containing multivitamin. These preparations usually provide the RDA of magnesium.[19,20]

5.1.5 B VITAMINS

5.1.5.1 Considerations in Bone Health

B vitamins and perhaps homocysteine levels may be a contributing factor to metabolic bone disease following bariatric surgery. Both vitamin B_{12} and folate deficiencies have been documented following all types of bariatric surgeries, although they are less likely in purely restrictive surgeries. Malabsorption due to bypass or altering of the gut, and inadequacy of intrinsic factor secretion are thought to be the main mechanisms for deficiencies. Those with pernicious anemia have been shown to have lower bone mineral density, not related to achlorhydria.[44] Vitamin B_{12} deficiency has been noted as a potential important modifiable risk factor for osteoporosis.[45] Other data have shown at the cellular level that high homocysteine levels, perhaps caused by B vitamin deficiencies, may have adverse affects on the extracellular bone matrix by stimulating bone resorption and disturbing collagen.[46,47] However, most recently a meta-analysis of 27 studies regarding B vitamins, homocysteine levels, and bone mineral density showed no associations.[48] Until future studies shed more light on this topic, B vitamins should be considered a potential contributing factor in metabolic bone disease following bariatric surgery.

5.1.5.2 Monitoring and Supplementation

Monitoring, in addition to vitamin B_{12} supplementation, and a multivitamin containing folate are recommended for all patients after bariatric surgery.[49] Some patients with mild malabsorption have been shown to maintain serum B_{12} levels above 150 pmol/L with 350 µg/day, whereas others may require lifelong subcutaneous injections.[50,51] In addition to regular monitoring, the AACE/TOS/ASMBS guidelines recommend supplementation with crystalline vitamin B_{12} at a dosage of 500 µg/weekly intranasally, or oral 1000 µg daily or more can be used to maintain adequate serum vitamin B_{12}. If sufficiency cannot be maintained using oral or intranasal routes, then 1000 µg every month, or 1000–3000 µg every 6–12 months intramuscularly or

TABLE 5.1

Bone Health Nutrient Recommendations for Bariatric Patients

Nutrient	RDA	Supplementation for Bariatric Surgery Patients	Variations and Considerations
Vitamin D	600–800 IU/day	400–800 IU/day for all bariatric surgery patients	800–6000 IU/day has been shown to be needed to maintain adequate levels, particularly in malabsorptive procedures
Calcium	1000–1200 mg/day	1200–1500 mg/day; citrate form is recommended, especially for RYGB, BPD w/wo DS	Up to 2000 mg/day has been shown to be needed in BPD w/wo DS and in some cases RYGB
Phosphorus	580–1250 mg/day	Generally very abundant in food sources and absorption is efficient; empiric supplementation is generally not necessary	Supplementation may be needed for correction of mild to moderate hypophosphatemia (1.5–2.5 mg/dl); excessive intakes may also be a concern
Magnesium	310–420 mg/day	Standard MVI containing 310–420 of Mg daily	Correction of hypomagnesemia may be indicated
Vitamin B$_{12}$	2.4–2.8 µg/day	500 µg/weekly, intranasally, or 1000 µg/day orally	1000 µg/month IM or sub-Q or 1000–3000 µg every 6–12 months IM or sub-Q
Folate	400–600 µg/day	A multivitamin preparation that has 400–800/day	Additional folate may be needed in a setting of elevated homocysteine levels
Protein	0.8 g/kg/day; AIBW should be used	Dietary intakes of 60–120g/day; 80–120 g/day for BPD w/wo DS and 60+ g/day for RYGB	It is recommended to aim for a range of 1.0–1.5 g/kg AIBW

subcutaneously is indicated. Folic acid supplementation of 400–800 µg/day is provided daily through the use of the routine multivitamin at 1–2 tablets/day.[19,20]

A summary of diet and supplementation recommendations for bariatric patients for bone health can be found in Table 5.1.

5.2 OBESITY, WEIGHT LOSS, AND BONE HEALTH

Many people often associate obesity with being "overnourished." Obesity itself should never be used as a surrogate marker for nutritional status.[3] Morbidly obese individuals often have preexisting nutritional deficiencies even prior to bariatric surgery. Similarly, many people think that morbid obesity is protective against metabolic bone disease, when in fact, being obese has been found to be an independent risk factor for vitamin D deficiency, as discussed. Calcium deficiency and elevated parathyroid hormone have also been found to be common in obese individuals presenting for bariatric surgery, placing them at further risk for bone disease. These studies have shown deficiency rates for vitamin D in excess of 60%, and prevalence of elevated PTH in this population ranges from 25 to 48%.[52] Weight loss itself also induces bone loss that correlates with the amount and rate at which it occurs. A voluntary loss of 10% of body weight can result in a 1–2% decrease of bone density at all sites, although this can vary among populations.[53] Another study found that weight loss of 0.7 kg/week caused an activation of the calcium-PTH axis more so than a loss of 0.3 kg/week.[54]

All of this puts the patient at risk even prior to bariatric surgery. After surgery, restricted intake, possible intolerances, rapid weight loss, and possible malabsorption put many bariatric surgery patients at high risk for metabolic bone disease. Many studies have examined metabolic bone disease after bariatric surgery and have shown that it develops in greater than 70% of patients undergoing a malabsorptive procedure, whereas others have shown detection of increased markers for bone resorption as soon as 8 weeks after any type of bariatric surgery. One study showed that 48% of patients who underwent gastric banding had significant bone loss of greater than 3% 1 year after surgery.[25,55,56]

5.3 FOLLOW-UP

One risk factor in the development of complications following bariatric surgery is lack of follow-up with a clinician knowledgeable about the intricacies of the surgery. Rigorous evaluation for long-term follow-up is necessary in order to prevent potentially serious consequences, including metabolic bone disease. This should be a multidisciplinary approach that involves surgeons, obesity medicine specialists, dietitians, and endocrinologists, as well as psychological follow-up for compliance issues. Lifelong monitoring of biochemical markers and bone densitometry, as well as assessing dietary and supplement status, is crucial after bariatric operations for early detection and perhaps prevention of metabolic bone disease.

5.3.1 MONITORING

There have been several recommendations published in the literature for perioperative screening, risk stratification, and management of metabolic bone disease (MBD) in bariatric patients. In 2010, the Endocrine Society published its own version of clinical practice guidelines for the post-bariatric surgery patients. These combined with the AACE/TOS/ASMBS guidelines now provide evidence-based practice guidelines that include recommendations for testing and management of skeletal and mineral disorders. Although these sets of guidelines serve as an excellent general tool, essential information specifically addressing bone disease in this population is still lacking. Proposed future research topics and areas in need of evidence-based practice guidelines include, but are not limited to, postsurgical/post-weight loss bone assessment, the use of cholecalciferol (D3) over D_2 or D analogs specific to the bariatric population, the efficacy of UVB light in bariatric patients resistant to oral repletion, and both the risks and questionable efficacy of oral bisphosphonates in this population.[3]

5.3.1.1 Laboratory Data

Biochemical indices for diagnostic testing for metabolic bone disease recommended by the AACE/TOS/ASMBS guidelines include serum Ca, phosphorus, magnesium, 25(OH)D (and 1,25(OH)D if renal function is compromised), bone-specific alkaline phosphatase or osteocalcin, PTH, and a bone marker of resorption such as urine N-telopeptide (NTX), 24 h Ca excretion, vitamin A and K_1 levels, and albumin and prealbumin. Regular monitoring suggestions include only PTH, 25(OH)D every 3–6 months for the first year and annually thereafter for patients undergoing RYGB. For those who have undergone BPD with or without switch, the following are recommended: PTH and 24 h urine calcium monitoring every 6–12 months, urine N-telopeptide annually, and osteocalcin as needed.[19] In contrast, the Endocrine Society recommends following vitamin D, calcium, phosphorus, PTH, and alkaline phosphatase levels every 6 months in patients who have undergone malabsorptive procedures.[21] Also, some studies have found that serum telopeptides seem to be a reliable marker of bone metabolism after restrictive procedures due to decreased weight bearing after surgery.[21,23,24]

A summary of laboratory and clinical markers for bariatric patients regarding bone health can be found in Tables 5.2 and 5.3.

5.3.1.2 Dual-Energy X-Ray Absorptiometry

Dual-energy x-ray absorptiometry (DXA) is the gold standard for measuring bone density; the results are reported in T and Z score. The Z score should be used for premenopausal women and men younger than 50 years of age. This score is the patient's bone mineral density expressed in standard deviations (SD) from the mean in an age- and sex-matched reference population. A Z score greater than –2.0 is generally considered within expected range, and that lower than –2.0 is below the expected range for that age and sex. Whereas the T score is also calculated as a SD from the mean, the comparison group is that of young healthy adults. The World Health Organization (WHO) classifies T scores above –1 SD as normal, between –1 and –2.5 SD as osteopenia, and below –2.5 SD as osteoporosis.[57–59] The Endocrine Society recommends baseline DXA preoperatively and annually thereafter until stable in patients who have undergone a malabsorptive bariatric surgery, although no

---

TABLE 5.2

Metabolic Bone Workup (AACE/TOS/ASMBS Guidelines)

Serum calcium, phosphorus, magnesium

25(OH)D, and 1,25(OH)D if renal function is compromised

Bone-specific alkaline phosphatase or osteocalcin

Intact PTH

Resorption bone marker (urine N-telopeptide)

24 h calcium excretion

Vitamin A and K_1 levels

Albumin and prealbumin

DXA (at 3 sites) at baseline and 2-year follow-up per ISCD and NOF recommendations

---

TABLE 5.3

Regular Monitoring for Metabolic Bone Disease for Bariatric Patients

Guidelines	RYGB	BPD w/wo DS
AACE/TOS/ASMBS	Every 3–6 months for the first year and annually thereafter: 25(OH)D Serum B$_{12}$ Optional: RBC folate, MMA, HCy Intact PTH DXA monitoring may be indicated at baseline and at about 2 years	Every 3 months for first year, every 3–6 months thereafter: Serum B$_{12}$ (MMA, HCy optional) 25(OH)D Albumin/prealbumin RBC folate Every 6–12 months: Intact PTH 24 h urine Ca Annually: Urine N-telopeptide As needed: Osteocalcin DXA monitoring may be indicated at baseline and at about 2 years
Endocrine Society	25(OH)D, serum calcium, phosphorus, PTH, and alkaline phosphatase every 6 months	25(OH)D, serum calcium, phosphorus, PTH, and alkaline phosphatase every 6 months

Serum telopeptides have been shown to be a reliable marker for bone metabolism in restrictive procedures; however, not enough evidence supports regular monitoring at this time.

data show that such monitoring will actually improve outcomes.[21] The AACE/TOS/ASBMS guidelines stated there is insufficient evidence to warrant routine preoperative assessment.[19,20] A baseline measurement will, however, provide valuable information to the patient and provider, in addition to offering a comparison postsurgery, especially in a higher-risk population. If the presurgery DXA is abnormal, it will allow the clinician to pursue further investigation and treatment as appropriate, prior to the compounding effects of the surgery. With regard to postsurgery surveillance, a convincing amount of data exist that significant changes may be detected through DXA after 12 months. These changes in the first year following surgery could influence clinical decisions.[3] The AACE/TOS/ASMBS guidelines do, however, suggest DXA at 2 years postoperatively for all types of bariatric surgeries.[19,20]

A limitation in the bariatric population is the weight capacity of the machines, with most being approximately 275–350 pounds, and some newer machines going up to 450 pounds. Forearm measurements and a peripheral bone density test of the heel, wrist, or hand are suggested by the National Osteoporosis Foundation to give a more complete picture than just using a forearm measurement in patients who exceed weight capacities.[59] Another limitation in the bariatric surgery population is that there is the potential for biases in the setting of weight loss because changes in soft tissue may cause spurious results.[3]

5.4 TREATMENT

Abnormal DXA may be indicative of both primary and secondary disease. In the bariatric surgery patient one should first suspect secondary bone disease due to nutritional deficiencies. Those deficiencies should be the primary focus of treatment interventions; focusing on the underlying cause of the secondary disease can result in significant improvements in bone marrow density (BMD). The etiology of confirmed vitamin D deficiency, hypocalcemia, hypomagnesemia, hypophosphatemia, elevated alkaline phosphatase, secondary hyperparathyroidism, and even protein or vitamin B_{12} deficiency should be clearly defined, and appropriate treatment interventions should be initiated.

5.4.1 CORRECTION OF BIOCHEMICAL MARKERS

A primary area of treatment will no doubt be correction of vitamin D deficiency. For treatment of deficiency, the Endocrine Society recommends a dose two to three times higher (6000–10,000 IU/day) for obese patients, patients with malabsorptive syndromes, and patients on medications affecting vitamin D metabolism. A maintenance therapy of at least 3000–6000 IU/day is recommended.[2] Correction of vitamin D deficiency in bariatric surgery patients generally requires more than this, particularly in the malabsorptive procedures. Repletion has been recommended for as high as 50,000 to 150,000 IU of D_2 or D_3 daily for 1 to 2 weeks, and more recalcitrant cases may require concurrent oral administration of calcitriol according to the AACE/TOS/ASMBS guidelines.[19,20] A maintenance dose of up to 50,000 IU one to three times per week has been suggested in the literature.[3,17] Cholecalciferol has demonstrated superiority in the literature at maintaining 25(OH)D levels and has been recommended particularly if dosing is less than once weekly. It is recommended that both D_2 and D_3 be taken with a meal containing fat to ensure maximum absorption. In patients who are unable to achieve normal levels of 25(OH)D with oral supplementation, UVB phototherapy has been shown to be an effective alternative.[17] However, these studies have primarily been done in a population of low to normal BMI, and the effects have not been well studied in the obese or bariatric population.

5.4.2 BISPHOSPHONATE USE

In the case of clinical and biochemical resolution of secondary bone disease coupled with persistently abnormal DXA, other treatment considerations should be considered for osteoporosis. Resolution of secondary bone disease indices include a normal parathyroid hormone level, 25(OH)D level of 30–60 ng/ml, normal serum calcium level, normal phosphorus level, and 24 h urine calcium excretion between 70 and 250 mg/24 h. Therapy considerations should be based on National Osteoporosis Foundation–World Health Organization 2008 guidelines.[19,20] However, safety and efficacy data are lacking for antiresorptive or anabolic medications in bariatric surgery patients. The decision to prescribe these types of medications must take into consideration the patient's risk-benefit profile. Some concerns are a higher risk of

TABLE 5.4

Corrective Supplementation and Treatment

Treatment	Dosage	Frequency	Maintenance Dosing	Potential Biochemical Markers Influenced	Considerations
Vitamin D	50,000–150,000 IU of D_2 or D_3 D_3 may be superior	Daily to weekly for 2–12 weeks	50,000 IU 1–3 times per week to month may be needed	↓ PTH ↑ serum vitamin D ↑ phosphorus ↑ calcium and improve related markers	Concurrent oral calcitriol may be needed in some cases; dosages dependent on laboratory data and resistance to correction
Phosphorus	1000 mg orally	Daily, until repletion	Usually not necessary	↑ phosphorus	Usually due to vitamin D deficiency
Magnesium	20–50 mEq orally for mild, asymptomatic disease	Daily, until repletion	Usually not necessary	↑ calcium improve impaired PTH secretion	Usually due to chronic PPI use or excessive vomiting and/or diarrhea
Bisphosphonates	Intravenous is preferential Zoledronic acid 5 mg or Ibandronate 3 mg	Yearly or every 3 months	Yearly or every 3 months	n/a	Only should be considered in patients with osteoporosis once underlying biochemical markers are normal

anastomotic ulceration, tolerance in the postsurgical gut, and absorption of drug following surgery. Intravenous preparations are available for those patients who are not absorbing or tolerating oral antiresorptive medications.[20] AACE/TOS/ASMBS guidelines recommend using intravenous therapy, unless concerns for anastomotic ulceration or absorption do not exist. Dosages for oral bisphosphonates include alendronate, 70 mg/week; risedronate, 35 mg/week or 150 mg/month; and ibandronate, 150 mg/month. Recommended intravenous dosages of bisphosphonates are zoledronic acid, 5 mg once a year; or ibandronate, 3 mg every 3 months.[20]

A summary for corrective supplementation and treatments for bariatric patients regarding bone health can be found in Table 5.4.

5.5 CASE STUDY CONCLUSION: THE PLAN FOR ANNA

Initial treatment of Anna, our patient presented at the beginning of this chapter, should begin with vitamin D repletion. A suggested regimen would be to give cholecalciferol 50,000 IU along with 1500 mg calcium daily for 2 weeks, followed by a maintenance dose of 50,000 IU weekly and continuing the daily calcium. Biochemical markers should be repeated in 6–12 weeks, and dosing could be adjusted based on the response to initial treatment. Further lab studies could include serum B_{12}, as well as serum magnesium, to rule out hypomagnesemia-induced hypocalcemia. Nutritional counseling should be revisited to improve dietary protein intake, and also foods high in calcium and vitamin D. Biochemical markers should be checked every 3 months until normalized. Once biochemical markers are normalized, the patient should be maintained on a daily supplementation schedule. At this time, the use of bisphosphonate could be considered. Laboratory data should be rechecked every 6 months to ensure adequacy, and DXA should be repeated in 1–2 years to monitor the effectiveness of the interventions taken.

5.6 SUMMARY

Metabolic bone disease following bariatric surgery is a multifactorial process. A number of metabolic factors conspire to predispose this population to problems with bone health. Preexisting conditions are exacerbated by reduced intake, decreased or altered absorption, and potentially poor compliance with vitamin and mineral supplementation. At the same time, the use of common medications for the prevention or treatment of conditions such as anastomotic ulcer may further alter absorption of key nutrients for bone health. The weight loss (and in many cases rapid) in and of itself further compounds the problem. The signs and symptoms associated with metabolic bone disease often are under- or misdiagnosed. Treatments involved should focus on underlying nutritional causes of the disease first, and then treatments with bisphosphonates can be considered. Future research is needed to further understand the issues involved with bone disease after bariatric surgery. Until more data are available, diligent screening and prevention in the form of proper maintenance supplementation are critical in the care of bariatric patients in hopes of preventing or alleviating the effects of bariatric surgery on bone health.

REFERENCES

1. DePrisco C, Levine SN. 2005. Metabolic bone disease after gastric bypass surgery for obesity. *Am J Med Sci* 329(2):57–61.
2. Holick MF, Binkley NC, Bischoff-Ferrari HA, et al. 2011. Evaluation, treatment and prevention of vitamin D deficiency: an Endocrine Society clinical practice guideline. *J Clin Endocrinol Metab* 96(7):1911–1930. Available at http://www.endo-society.org/guidelines/final/upload/final-standalone-vitamin-d-guideline.pdf (accessed April 1, 2013).
3. Williams SE. 2011. Metabolic bone disease in the bariatric surgery patient. *J Obes*, article 634614. doi: 10.1155/2011/634614 (accessed April 1, 2013).

4. Holick MF. 1995. Environmental factors that influence the cutaneous production of vitamin D. *Am J Clin Nutr* 61(3 Suppl):638S–645S.

5. Holick MF. 2007. Vitamin D deficiency. *N Engl J Med* 357:266–281.

6. Holick MF, Garabedian M. 2006. Vitamin D: photobiology, metabolism, mechanism of action, and clinical applications. In *Primer on the metabolic bone diseases and disorders of mineral metabolism*, ed. MJ Favus, 106–114. 6th ed. Washington, DC: American Society for Bone and Mineral Research.

7. Brody T. 1999. *Nutritional biochemistry*. 2nd ed. San Diego: Academic Press.

8. U.S. Department of Agriculture. 1997. National Agricultural Library. Dietary Reference Intakes for calcium, phosphorus, magnesium, vitamin D and flouride. Calcium. Available at http://fnic.nal.usda.gov/dietary-guidance/dri-reports/calcium-phosphorus-magnesium-vitamin-d-and-fluoride (accessed March 20, 2013).

9. Institute of Medicine, Food and Nutrition Board. *Dietary Reference Intakes for calcium and vitamin D*. Washington, DC: National Academy Press, 2010.

10. Gebhardt SE, Thomas RG, Exler J, Lemar LE, Holden JM. 2009. Estimation of the vitamin D content of foods for the assessment of dietary intake. Presented at International Conference on Diet and Activity Methods, Washington, DC, June 5–7.

11. National Institutes of Health. 2011. Office of Dietary Supplements. Vitamin D fact sheet. Available at od.od.nig.gov/factsheets/VitaminD-HealthProfessional (accessed April 1, 2013).

12. Patterson KY, Philips KM, Horst RL, et al. 2010. Vitamin D content and variability in fluid milks form a US Department of Agriculture nationwide sampling to update values in the National Nutrient Database for Standard Reference. *J Dairy Sci* 93(11):5082–5090. doi: 10.3168/jds.2010–3359 (accessed April 1, 2013).

13. Holick MF. 2003. Calciotropic hormones and the skin: a millennium prospective. *J Cell Biochem* 88:296–307.

14. Earthman CP, Beckman LM, Masodkar K, Sibley SD. 2012. The link between obesity and low circulating 25-hydroxyvitamin D concentrations: considerations and implications. *Int J Obes (Lond)* 36:387–396. doi: 10.1038/ijo.2011.119 (accessed March 20, 2013).

15. Wortsman J, Matsuoka LY, Chen TC, Lu Z, Holick MF. 2000. Decreased bioavailability of vitamin D in obesity. *Am J Clin Nutr* 72:690–693.s

16. Ginde AA, Liu MC, Camargo CA. 2009. Demographic differences and trends of vitamin D insufficiency in the US population, 1988–2004. *Arch Intern Med* 169:626–632. doi: 10.1001/archinternmed.2008.604.

17. Kennel KA, Drake MT, Hurley DL. 2010. Vitamin D deficiency in adults: when to test and how to treat. *Mayo Clin Proc* 85(8):752–758. doi: 10.4065/mcp.2010.0138 (accessed April 1, 2013).

18. Dawson-Hughes B, Heaney RP, Holick MF, Lips P, Meunier PJ, Vieth R. 2005. Estimates of optimal vitamin D status. *Osteopros Int* 16:713–716.

19. Mechanick JI, Kushner RF, Sugerman HJ, et al. 2008. American Association of Clinical Endocrinologists, The Obesity Society, and American Society for Metabolic and Bariatric Surgery Medical guidelines for clinical practice for the perioperative nutritional, metabolic, and nonsurgical support of the bariatric patient. *Endocr Pract* 14(Suppl 1):1–83.

20. Mechanick JI, Youdim A, Jones DB, et al. 2013. Clinical practice guidelines for the perioperative nutritional, metabolic, and nonsurgical support of the bariatric surgery patient—2013 update: cosponsored by American Association of Clinical Endocrinologists, The Obesity Society, and American Society for Metabolic and Bariatric Surgery. *Obesity* 21(Suppl 1):1–27.

21. Heber D, Greenway FL, Kaplan LM, Livingston E, Salvador J, Still CD. 2010. Endocrine and nutritional management of the post bariatric surgery patient: an Endocrine Society clinical practice guideline. *J Clin Endocrinol Metab* 95(11):4823–4843. Available at http://endo-society.org/guidelines/final/upload/final-standalone-post-bariatric-surgery-guideline-color.pdf (accessed April 1, 2013).
22. Goldner WS, Stoner JA, Lyden E, et al. 2009. Finding the optimal dose of vitamin D following Roux-en-Y gastric bypass: a prospective, randomized pilot clinical trial. *Obes Surg* 19(2):173–179. doi: 10.1007/s11695-008-9680-y (accessed April 1, 2013).
23. Pugnale N, Giusti V, Suter M, et al. 2003. Bone metabolism and risk of secondary hyperparathyroidism 12 months after gastric banding in obese pre-menopausal women. *Int J Obes* 27(1):110–116.
24. Giusti V, Gasteyger C, Suter M, Heraief E, Gaillard RC, Burckhardt P. 2005. Gastric banding induces negative bone remodelling in the absence of secondary hyperparathyroidism: potential role of serum C telopeptides for follow-up. *Int J Obes* 29(12):1429–1435.
25. Favus MJ, Bushinsky DA, Lemann Jr J. 2006. Regulation of calcium, magnesium, and phosphate metabolism. In *Primer on the metabolic bone diseases and disorders of mineral metabolism*, ed. MJ Favus, 76–83. 6th ed. Washington, DC: American Society for Bone and Mineral Research.
26. Calvo MS, Park YK. 1996. Changing phosphorus content of the U.S. diet: potential for adverse effects on bone. *J Nutr* 126:1168S–1180S.
27. Calvo MS. 1994. The effects of high phosphorus intake on calcium homeostatis. In *Advances in nutritional research*, ed. H Draper, 183–207. New York: Plenum Press.
28. Gueguen L, Pointillart A. 2000. The bioavailability of dietary calcium. *JACN* 19(2):119S–136S.
29. Agus ZS. 2013. Causes of hypophosphatemia. In *UpToDate*, ed. S Goldfarb and JP Forman. Waltham, MA: UpToDate. http://www.uptodate.com/contents/causes-of-hypophosphatemia (accessed March 20, 2013).
30. Recker RR. 1985. Calcium absorption and achlorhydria. *N Engl J Med* 313:70–73. As referenced in Brody T. 1999. *Nutritional biochemistry*. 2nd ed. San Diego: Academic Press.
31. National Institutes of Health. 2013. Office of Dietary Supplements. Calcium fact sheet. Available at od.od.nig.gov/factsheets/Calcium-HealthProfessional/#h2 (accessed April 1, 2013).
32. Williams SE, Cooper K, Richmond B, Schauer P. 2008. Perioperative management of bariatric surgery patients: focus on metabolic bone disease. *Cleve Clin J Med* 75(5):333–334, 336, 338 passim.
33. Abelow BJ, Holford TR, Insogna KL. 1992. Cross-cultural association between dietary protein and hip fracture: a hypothesis. *Calcif Tissue Int* 50:14–18.
34. Hu J-F, Zhao X-H, Parpia B, Campbell T. 1993. Dietary intakes and urinary excretion of calcium and acids: a cross-sectional study of women in China. *Am J Clin Nutr* 58:398–406.
35. Barzel US, Massey LK. 1998. Excess dietary protein can adversely affect bone. *J Nutr* 128:1051–1053.
36. Kerstetter JE, O'Briend KO, Caseria DM, Wall DE, Insogna KL. 2005. The impact of dietary protein on calcium absorption and kinetic measures of bone turnover in women. *J Clin Endocrinol Metab* 90(1):26–31.
37. Bihuniak JD, Simpson CA, Sullivan RR, Caseria DM, Kerstetter JE, Insogna KL. 2013. Dietary protein-induced increases in urinary calcium are accompanied by similar increases in urinary nitrogen and urinary urea: a controlled clinical trial. *J Acad Nutr Diet* 113(3):447–451.
38. Kerstetter JE, O'Brien KO, Insogna KL. 2003. Low protein intake: the impact on calcium and bone homeostasis in humans. *J Nutr* 133(3):855S–861S.

39. Kerstetter J, Svastisalee C, Caseria D, et al. 2000. A threshold for low protein diet induced elevations in parathyroid hormone. *Am J Clin Nutr* 72:168–173.

40. Ilich JZ, Kerstetter JE. 2000. Nutrition in bone health revisited: a story beyond calcium. *J Am Coll Nutr* 19:715–737.

41. Sugarman HJ. 2001. Bariatric surgery for severe obesity. *J Assoc Acad Minor Phys* 12(3):129–136.

42. Ryder KM, Shorr RI, Bush AJ, et al. 2005. Magnesium intake from food and supplements is associated with bone mineral density in healthy older white subjects. *J Am Geriatr Soc* 53(11):1875–1880.

43. Stendig-Lindberg G, Tepper R, Leicher I. 1993. Trabecular bone density in a two year controlled trial of peroral magnesium in osteoporosis. *Magnes Res* 6(2):153–163.

44. Eastell R, Vieira NE, Yergey AL, et al. 1992. Pernicious anaemia as a risk factor for osteoporosis. *Clin Sci (Lond)* 82(6):681–685.

45. Tucker KL, Hannan MT, Qiao N, et al. 2005. Low plasma vitamin B_{12} is associated with lower BMD: the Framingham Osteoporosis Study. *J Bone Miner Res* 20(1):152–158.

46. Herrmann M, PeterSchmidt J, Umanskaya N, et al. 2007. The role of hyperhomocysteinemia as well as folate, vitamin B(6) and B(12) deficiencies in osteoporosis: a systematic review. *Clin Chem Lab Med* 45(12):1621–1632.

47. Ozdem S, Samanci S, Tasatargil A, et al. 2007. Experimental hyperhomocysteinemia disturbs bone metabolism in rats. *Scand J Clin Lab Invest* 67(7):748–756.

48. van Wijngaarden JP, Doets EL, Szczecińska A, et al. 2013. Vitamin B_{12}, folate, homocysteine, and bone health in adults and elderly people: a systematic review with meta-analyses. *J Nutr Metab* 2013:486186. doi: 10.1155/2013/486186 (accessed March 20, 2013).

49. Shankar P, Boylan M, Sriram K. 2010. Micronutrient deficiencies after bariatric surgery. *Nutrition* 26(11–12):1031–1037. doi: 10.1016/j.nut.2009.12.003 (accessed March 20, 2013).

50. Rhode BM, Tamin H, Gilfix BM, Sampalis JS, Nohr C, MacLean LD. 1995. Treatment of vitamin B_{12} deficiency after gastric surgery for severe obesity. *Obes Surg* 5:154–158.

51. Fujioka K. 2005. Follow-up of nutritional and metabolic problems after bariatric surgery. *Diabetes Care* 28(2):481–484. doi: 10.2337/diacare.28.2.481 (accessed March 13, 2013).

52. Carlin AM, Rao DS, Rao DS. 2006. Prevalence of vitamin D depletion among morbidly obese patients seeking gastric bypass surgery. *Surg Obes Relat Dis* 2(2):98–103.

53. Shapses SA, Riedt CS. 2006. Bone, body weight, and weight reduction: what are the concerns. *J Nutr* 136(6):1453–1456.

54. Shapses SA, Cifuentes M, Sherrell R, et al. 2002. Rate of weight loss influences calcium absorption. *J Bone Miner Res* 17:S471.

55. Collazo-Clavell ML, Jimenez A, Hodgson SF, Sarr MG. 2004. Osteomalacia after Roux-en-Y gastric bypass. *Endocr Pract* 10(3):287–288

56. Parikh SJ, Edelman M, Uwaifo GI, et al. 2004. Gastric bypass surgery for morbid obesity leads to an increase in bone turnover and a decrease in bone mass. *J Clin Endocrinol Metab* 89:1196–1199.

57. Kanis JA, Melton L, Christiansen C, Johnston CC, Khaltaev N. 1994. The diagnosis of osteoporosis. *J Bone Miner Res* 9:1137–1141.

58. WHO Study Group. 1994. *Assessment of fracture risk and its application to screening for postmenopausal osteoporosis.* WHO Technical Report Series, no. 843. Geneva: World Health Organization.

59. National Osteoporosis Foundation. 2008. Clinician's guide to prevention and treatment of osteoporosis. Available at http://www.fitbones.org/Documents/NOF_Clinicians_Guide.pdf (accessed March 24, 2013).

6 Neurological Disorders

Neeraj Kumar

CONTENTS

6.1 INTRODUCTION

Optimal functioning of the central and peripheral nervous system is dependent on a constant supply of appropriate nutrients. Particularly important for optimal functioning of the nervous system are the B-group vitamins (thiamine, vitamin B_{12}, niacin, pyridoxine, folate), vitamin E, copper, and vitamin D. The epidemic of obesity and limited efficacy of available medical treatments has resulted in increasing utilization of bariatric surgical procedures for treatment of medically complicated obesity. This has been accompanied by an increased incidence and awareness of neurologic complications resulting from bariatric surgery. These are often related to nutrient deficiencies. The preventable and potentially treatable nature of these disorders makes this an important subject. Prognosis depends on prompt recognition and institution of appropriate therapy.

A number of reviews address the issue of neurologic complications of bariatric surgery.[1–6] The interested reader is directed to these for detailed bibliographies. The bibliography that accompanies this chapter is biased toward review articles and case series rather than individual case reports.

Not infrequently, laboratory evidence of a nutrient deficiency is not accompanied by clinical manifestations associated with that particular nutrient deficiency. For many nutrients, the clinical manifestations associated with the deficiency state that have been discussed in this chapter have not been reported in context of bariatric surgery itself. Further, many deficiencies and related clinical manifestations described here are from the gastrectomy literature rather than literature that deals with gastric bypass for obesity.

6.2 NEUROLOGIC COMPLICATIONS FOLLOWING BARIATRIC SURGERY: FREQUENCY, NATURE, AND TIMING

Complications related to the central or peripheral nervous system may be seen in approximately 5–16% of patients after surgery for peptic ulcer disease or obesity.[1–5,7–16] Neurologic complications following bariatric surgery can involve any level of the neuraxis. Frequently, more than one part of the nervous system is involved. Commonly recognized neurologic complications related to bariatric surgery include encephalopathy, optic neuropathy, myelopathy or myeloneuropathy, radiculoplexus neuropathy, polyneuropathy, and mononeuropathy (resulting in carpal tunnel syndrome or meralgia paresthetica or foot drop). Rarely reported complications include a clinical presentation that mimics Guillain–Barré syndrome, rhabdomyolysis, and myotonia.[1,13,17,18] Some patients have more than one site of involvement (e.g., encephalopathy and peripheral neuropathy). Encephalopathy and polyradiculopathy are commonly early complications; myelopathy and polyneuropathy are generally delayed complications.[4]

6.3 NEUROLOGIC COMPLICATIONS FOLLOWING BARIATRIC SURGERY: RISK FACTORS AND MECHANISMS

Risk factors for neurologic complications after bariatric surgery include rate and amount of weight loss, prolonged gastrointestinal symptoms (nausea, vomiting, diarrhea, dumping syndrome), postsurgical complications, subclinical preoperative deficiency, inadequate nutritional follow-up and failure to take recommended supplements, food avoidance, postoperative loss of appetite, reduced serum albumin and transferrin, and type of procedure (greater with malabsorptive procedures like biliopancreatic diversion with duodenal switch).[1,3–5,11,12,19,20]

Despite their obesity, patients may have nutritional deficiencies prior to bariatric surgery.[21] Commonly implicated nutrient deficiencies in patients with neurologic disease include B-group vitamins (thiamine, vitamin B_{12}), vitamin D, copper, and iron. Multiple nutrient deficiencies may coexist. Often a specific nutrient deficiency is not identified.[1] The precise clinical significance of neurologic manifestations related to deficiencies of pyridoxine, folate, niacin, and riboflavin in patients who have undergone bariatric surgery is unclear.

The most common mechanism of neurologic complications following bariatric surgery is directly related to the nutrient deficiency.[22–24] Some have also suggested a possible immune-mediated or inflammatory basis.[12] Weight loss may predispose to compression mononeuropathies like common peroneal nerve involvement at the fibular head.[25] This likely is due to loss of fat, which otherwise protects the common peroneal nerve against compression at the fibular head. The presence of a widespread polyneuropathy is an additional risk factor for development of a superimposed peroneal neuropathy.[25] In some cases meralgia paresthetica may result from extrinsic pressure from an abdominal retractor.[26]

Table 6.1 summarizes the neurologic manifestations seen after bariatric surgery and the implicated nutrient deficiency.

TABLE 6.1

Neurologic Complications Associated with Bariatric Surgery and Implicated Nutrient Deficiency

Neurologic Complication	Implicated Nutrient Deficiency
Encephalopathy	Thiamine, B_{12} (rarely folate, niacin)
Myelopathy	B_{12}, copper (rarely folate, vitamin E)
Optic neuropathy	B_{12}, thiamine, copper (rarely folate)
Polyradiculopathy	Thiamine
Neuropathy	B_{12}, thiamine, copper (rarely pyridoxine, folate, niacin, vitamin E)
Myopathy (rare)	Vitamin D, vitamin E

6.4 NUTRIENT DEFICIENCY AND RELATED NEUROLOGIC MANIFESTATIONS

6.4.1 THIAMINE (B_1) (TABLE 6.2)

6.4.1.1 Thiamine Deficiency and Bariatric Surgery

Thiamine deficiency is frequently seen following bariatric surgery.[11,14,19,23,27–37] In one study the incidence of thiamine deficiency 2 years following bariatric surgery was estimated to be approximately 18%.[23] Preoperative thiamine deficiency in patients undergoing bariatric surgery has also been recognized.[38,39]

Due to a short half-life and absence of significant storage amounts, a continuous dietary supply of thiamine is necessary. It has been suggested that given the daily requirement of thiamine of approximately 1–2 mg per day, and body stores of approximately 30–50 mg, it takes approximately 4–6 weeks for body stores to be depleted.[40] Most cases of thiamine deficiency-related neurologic manifestations are seen 4–12 weeks after bariatric surgery.[14] Cases have been reported as early as 2 weeks or as late as 18 months after gastric bypass.[30,31]

Thiamine deficiency can be seen in conditions associated with decreased intake, decreased absorption, defective transport, increased losses, and enhanced requirements.[41] Thiamine deficiency following bariatric surgery may be due to intractable vomiting, rapid weight loss, inadequate vitamin repletion, glucose administration without thiamine, parenteral feeding, and bacterial overgrowth.[19] Thiamine requirement is related to the total caloric intake and proportion of calories provided as carbohydrates. A high-caloric and high-carbohydrate diet increases the demand for thiamine. The thiamine requirement is also dependent on the body's metabolic rate, with the requirement being the greatest during periods of high metabolic demand. In patients with a marginal nutritional status, the increased metabolic demand associated with various diseases can precipitate symptoms of thiamine deficiency.

6.4.1.2 Physiologic Role of Thiamine

Thiamine functions as a coenzyme in the metabolism of carbohydrates, lipids, and amino acids.[41] It has a role in energy production by adenosine triphosphate synthesis, in myelin sheath maintenance, and in neurotransmitter production. Following cellular uptake, thiamine is phosphorylated into thiamine diphosphate, the metabolically active form that is involved in several enzyme systems. Thiamine diphosphate is a cofactor for the pyruvate dehydrogenase complex, α-ketoglutarate dehydrogenase, and transketolase. Pyruvate dehydrogenase and α-ketoglutarate dehydrogenase are involved in the tricarboxylic acid cycle in oxidative decarboxylation of α-ketoacids such as pyruvate and α-ketoglutarate to acetyl coenzyme A and succinate, respectively. α-Ketoglutarate dehydrogenase is the rate-limiting enzyme in the tricarboxylic acid cycle, which is involved in the synthesis of high-energy phosphates. Transketolase transfers activated aldehydes in the hexose monophosphate shunt (pentose-phosphate pathway) in the generation of nicotinamide adenine dinucleotide phosphate for reductive biosynthesis. Thiamine diphosphate may be further phosphorylated to thiamin triphosphate, which may activate high-conductance chloride channels and have a role in regulating cholinergic and serotonergic neurotransmission. Thiamine deficiency results in reduced synthesis of high-energy phosphates and lactate accumulation. Thiamine-deficient membranes are unable to maintain osmotic gradients. Intracellular and extracellular swelling results and astrocyte-related functions are impaired. Proposed mechanisms that lead to neurotoxicity also include glutamate-mediated excitotoxicity, DNA fragmentation and apoptotic cell death, decreased synaptic transmission, mitochondrial dysfunction, and intracellular oxidative stress with free radical and cytokine production.

6.4.1.3 Clinical Manifestations of Thiamine Deficiency

Thiamine deficiency affects the central nervous system, peripheral nervous system, and cardiovascular system.[41–43] These may be involved in various combinations. Cardiac involvement may manifest as high-output or low-output cardiac failure. The two major forms of beriberi are dry beriberi and wet beriberi. Dry beriberi is characterized by a sensorimotor, distal, axonal peripheral neuropathy often associated with calf cramps, muscle tenderness, and burning feet. Autonomic neuropathy may be present. A rapid progression of the neuropathy mimicking Guillain–Barré syndrome has also been described.[44–46] Wet beriberi is peripheral neuropathy associated with a high-output congestive heart failure. The terms *wet* and *dry beriberi* have been used to describe the presence or absence of edema in neuropathic beriberi. Peripheral neuropathy attributable to thiamine deficiency following bariatric surgery has been referred to as bariatric beriberi.[47]

The best characterized central nervous system neurological disorders related to thiamine deficiency are Wernicke encephalopathy and Korsakoff syndrome (also referred to as Korsakoff psychosis).[41,43] Because of the close relationship between Wernicke encephalopathy and Korsakoff psychosis, the term *Wernicke-Korsakoff syndrome* is commonly used. Wernicke encephalopathy often results from severe, short-term thiamine deficiency, while peripheral neuropathy is more often a consequence of prolonged mild to moderate thiamine deficiency.[41] Wernicke encephalopathy related to alcoholism is more common in men. Wernicke encephalopathy related to bariatric surgery is more commonly reported in women. It is unclear if this relates to a female predisposition for Wernicke encephalopathy or is a reflection of the higher rates of bariatric surgery in women. The symptoms of subclinical thiamine deficiency are often vague and nonspecific and include fatigue, lethargy, irritability, restlessness, and headaches.[41]

The clinical features of Wernicke encephalopathy include a subacute onset of the classic triad of ocular abnormalities, gait ataxia, and mental status changes.[34,41-43,48-51] The onset may be gradual, and the classic triad is frequently absent.[48,49] Ocular abnormalities include nystagmus (horizontal more common than vertical), ophthalmoparesis (commonly involving the lateral recti), and conjugate gaze palsies (usually horizontal). Complete ophthalmoplegia is rare. Other reported findings include sluggish pupillary reactivity, anisocoria, light-near dissociation, optic neuropathy, central scotomas, sudden bilateral blindness, retinal hemorrhages or papilledema, macular edema, and a Miller Fisher syndrome-like presentation. The gait and trunk ataxia is a consequence of cerebellar and vestibular dysfunction. In some patients the ataxia may be accompanied by dysarthria. A coexisting chronic peripheral neuropathy may be an additional contributing factor for the gait difficulty. Mental status changes include inability to concentrate, apathy, impaired awareness of the immediate situation, spatial disorientation, and confusion, delirium, and frank psychosis.[32,33,48] If untreated, this can progress to stupor, coma, and death. Rarely, coma may be the sole manifestation of Wernicke encephalopathy. Involvement of the hypothalamic and brainstem autonomic pathways may be associated with hypothermia or hyperthermia, hypotension, or bradycardia. Other unusual manifestations include seizures, asterixis, chorea, myoclonus, hypertonia, quadriparesis, dysphagia, or hearing loss.[14,29,41,43]

About 80% of patients with Wernicke encephalopathy who survive develop Korsakoff syndrome.[48,52-54] Korsakoff syndrome is an amnestic-confabulatory syndrome characterized by severe anterograde and retrograde amnesia that follows Wernicke encephalopathy; Korsakoff syndrome emerges as ocular manifestations and encephalopathy subside. Korsakoff syndrome is probably more likely to occur when Wernicke encephalopathy is a consequence of alcohol abuse.[55] In Korsakoff syndrome, memory is disproportionately impaired relative to other aspects of cognitive function. Alertness, attention, social behavior, and other aspects of cognitive functioning are generally preserved.

6.4.1.4   Diagnosis

Wernicke encephalopathy is largely a clinical diagnosis.[14,51] Urinary thiamine excretion and serum thiamine levels may be decreased in Wernicke encephalopathy, but they don't accurately reflect tissue concentrations and are therefore not reliable indicators of thiamine status. A normal serum thiamine level does not exclude Wernicke encephalopathy. Whole blood thiamine levels are more sensitive than plasma thiamine. The preferred tests are the erythrocyte transketolase activation assay or measurement of thiamine diphosphate in red blood cells.[56] Since these laboratory abnormalities normalize quickly, a blood sample should be drawn before initiation of treatment. Pyruvate accumulates during thiamine deficiency, and elevated serum lactate provides additional confirmation. An anion-gap metabolic acidosis accompanied by a primary respiratory alkalosis may be present.[57] Thiamine deficiency may manifest as unexplained metabolic acidosis.[58]

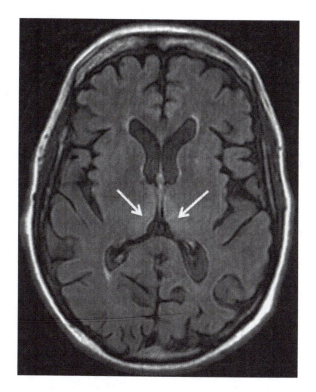

FIGURE 6.1 Brain MRI in thiamine deficiency. Brain MRI showing increased FLAIR signal in the medial thalami consistent with the clinical impression of Wernicke encephalopathy.

Cerebrospinal fluid analysis may show raised protein concentration in later stages.[41] Electroencephalogram may show nonspecific slowing.[41] Computed tomography is of limited utility. Low-density abnormalities may be seen in the paraventricular regions of the thalamus.[59] Magnetic resonance imaging (MRI) is the imaging modality of choice.[29,41–43,50,51,59–61] Not infrequently, no radiographic abnormalities are present.[14] Typical MRI findings include increased T2 or proton density or FLAIR signal in the paraventricular regions (Figure 6.1). Involved areas include the thalamus, hypothalamus, mammillary body, periaqueductal midbrain, tectal plate, red nucleus, pons, fourth ventricle floor, medulla, midline cerebellum, dentate, and rarely, the splenium of the corpus callosum or basal ganglia structures. Increased signal may involve the hypoglossal, medial vestibular, facial, and dentate nuclei.[62] Involvement of cortical regions on MRI has also been reported and may indicate irreversible lesions and poor prognosis. Contrast enhancement may be present in the early stages. Hemorrhagic lesions are rare. The signal abnormalities resolve with treatment, but shrunken mammillary bodies may persist as sequelae. Additional findings in the chronic stages include dilated aqueduct and third ventricles with atrophy of the midbrain tegmentum, paramedian thalamic nuclei, mammillary bodies, and frontal lobes. Frontal atrophy may also be seen. Diffusion-weighted imaging MRI abnormalities may be seen in the early stages. Both cytotoxic and vasogenic edema may be concurrently present. Proton magnetic resonance spectroscopy may show evidence of lactate accumulation.

6.4.1.5 Management

Patients with a history of bariatric surgery who present with signs of gastrointestinal distress should receive thiamine preventively.[19] Intravenous glucose infusion in patients with thiamine deficiency may consume the available thiamine and precipitate an acute Wernicke encephalopathy. At-risk patients should therefore receive parenteral thiamine prior to administration of glucose or parenteral nutrition.[63]

Patients suspected of having beriberi or Wernicke encephalopathy should promptly receive parenteral thiamine. It has been suggested that patients with signs of Wernicke encephalopathy should receive higher doses than the commonly used regimen of 100 mg intravenously given every 8 h (Table 6.2).[40,41,64,65] Magnesium deficiency may make a patient resistant to thiamine replacement.[66]

In wet beriberi a rapid improvement is seen with clearing of symptoms within days. Improvement in motor and sensory symptoms takes weeks or months. Response in Wernicke encephalopathy is variable. Ocular signs improve in a few hours. A fine horizontal nystagmus may persist. Improvement in gait ataxia is prompt, and memory is often delayed.[27] Mental status changes improve over days or weeks. As the global confusional state recedes, some patients are left with Korsakoff syndrome.[19] Prompt treatment of Wernicke encephalopathy prevents the development of Korsakoff syndrome. Korsakoff syndrome does not respond to thiamine therapy. Recovery of consciousness may be seen even in patients in deep coma. Even with thiamine treatment, the mortality may be high and is possibly related to coexisting medical conditions.

TABLE 6.2
Thiamine (Vitamin B$_1$) Deficiency and Bariatric Surgery

Pathophysiology	Intractable vomiting, rapid weight loss, inadequate vitamin supplementation, glucose administration without thiamine
Clinical manifestations	Wernicke encephalopathy (ocular abnormalities, gait ataxia, mental status changes: classic triad rarely seen)
	Korsakoff syndrome (amnestic–confabulatory syndrome)
	Peripheral neuropathy, dry beriberi, wet beriberi (peripheral neuropathy with congestive heart failure)
	Polyradiculopathy (may mimic Guillain–Barré syndrome)
Diagnosis	Largely clinical diagnosis; erythrocyte transketolase activation assay or red blood cell thiamine diphosphate; MRI may show abnormal signal in paraventricular regions
Management	Wernicke encephalopathy: 500 mg of thiamine given intravenously three times a day for 2–3 days, followed by 250 mg/day intravenously or intramuscularly for 3–5 days, followed by long-term oral maintenance with 50–100 mg orally
Additional comments	Manifestations seen within weeks of bariatric surgery; body thiamine stores can be depleted in 4–6 weeks

Sudden death can occur and may be related to hemorrhagic brainstem lesions.[67,68] Those with Korsakoff syndrome who do improve do so after a delay of a month or so. Occasionally patients may not achieve maximal improvement for more than a year.

6.4.2 Vitamin B_{12} (B_{12}, Cobalamin) (Table 6.3)

6.4.2.1 B_{12} Deficiency and Bariatric Surgery

Gastric bypass leaves the stomach essentially intact. Despite that, B_{12} deficiency is commonly seen following gastric surgery (gastrectomy and bariatric surgery).[4,22,69–72] Laboratory evidence of B_{12} deficiency is often unaccompanied by clinical manifestations.[73] Following gastric bypass surgery, reduced B_{12} levels at 1 year may be seen in up to two-thirds of patients.[22,70] A study noted B_{12} deficiency in approximately 40% of gastric bypass patients at 7 years.[70] In another study, 30% of patients developed B_{12} deficiency within a year despite receiving a daily multivitamin containing the recommended daily allowance of B_{12}.[71]

The estimated daily losses of B_{12} (mainly in the urine and feces) are minute (1–3 μg) compared with body stores (2–5 mg). The body does not have the ability to degrade B_{12}. Hence, even in the presence of severe malabsorption, 2–5 years may pass before B_{12} deficiency develops.[74] Deficient B_{12} levels and neurologic complications related to B_{12} deficiency are generally not seen until months to years after bariatric surgery.

B_{12} deficiency following gastric surgery may result from inadequate intake, impaired hydrolysis of vitamin B_{12} from dietary protein due to reduction in gastric acid and pepsin, intrinsic factor loss, abnormal intrinsic factor and vitamin B_{12}

TABLE 6.3
Vitamin B_{12} Deficiency and Bariatric Surgery

Pathophysiology	Impaired hydrolysis of vitamin B_{12} from dietary protein due to reduction in gastric acid and pepsin, intrinsic factor loss, decreased contact time in the ileum
	Other causes of B_{12} deficiency like pernicious anemia may coexist
Clinical manifestations	Myelopathy with involvement of dorsal column and corticospinal tract
	Peripheral neuropathy
	Myeloneuropathy (subacute combined degeneration)
	Optic neuropathy
	Neuropsychiatric manifestations
Diagnosis	Serum vitamin B_{12}, serum methylmalonic and plasma homocysteine, hematologic abnormalities (anemia, macrocytosis, hypersegmented neutrophils, megaloblastic marrow); MRI may show abnormal signal in the dorsal column or lateral corticospinal tract
Management	A common regimen is 1000 μg intramuscular injections for 5–7 days followed by monthly 500–1000 μg intramuscular injections
Additional comments	Manifestations seen years after bariatric surgery; body stores depleted in 2–5 years in the absence of supplementation

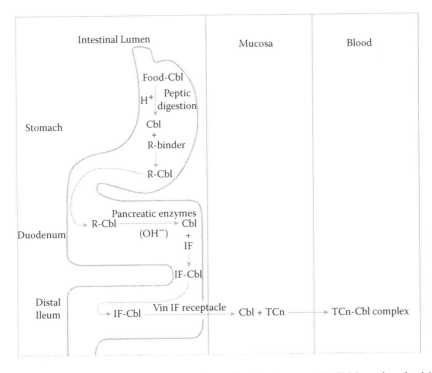

FIGURE 6.2 Physiology of cobalamin absorption. In the stomach, Cbl bound to food is dissociated from proteins in the presence of acid and pepsin. The released Cbl binds to R proteins secreted by salivary glands and gastric mucosa. In the small intestine, pancreatic proteases partially degrade the R proteins–Cbl complex at neutral pH and release Cbl, which then binds with intrinsic factor (IF). IF is a Cbl binding protein secreted by gastric parietal cells. The IF-Cbl complex binds to specific receptors in the ileal mucosa and is internalized. In addition to the IF-mediated absorption of ingested Cbl, there is a nonspecific absorption of Cbl that occurs by passive diffusion at all mucosal sites. This is a relatively inefficient process by which 1–2% of the ingested amount is absorbed. Cbl, cobalamin; H+, acidic; OH-, alkaline; IF, intrinsic factor. (Reproduced from Tefferi, A., and Pruthi, R. K., *Mayo Clin. Proc.*, 69, 1994, 181–186. With permission.)

interaction, decreased contact time in the ileum, duodenal bypass, or bacterial overgrowth.[5,22] Other causes of B_{12} deficiency may coexist. These include pernicious anemia, atrophic gastritis, *Helicobacter pylori* infection, antacid therapy, gastrointestinal diseases associated with malabsorption, pancreatic disease, and vegetarianism. Figure 6.2 illustrates the steps involved in absorption of B_{12}.

6.4.2.2   Physiologic Role of B_{12}

Figure 6.3 illustrates the key pathways that are dependent on B_{12}.[75] Methylcobalamin is a cofactor for a cytosolic enzyme, methionine synthase, in a methyl-transfer reaction that converts homocysteine to methionine. Methionine is adenosylated to S-adenosylmethionine, a methyl group donor required for neuronal methylation reactions involving proteins, nucleic acids, neurotransmitters, myelin, and phospholipids.

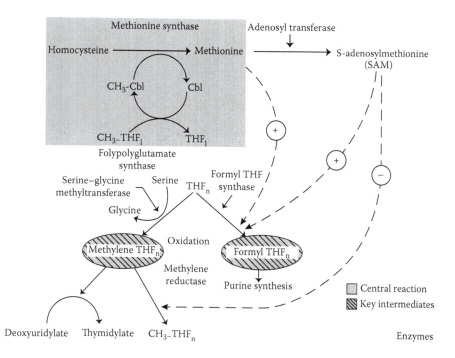

FIGURE 6.3 Biochemistry of cobalamin and folate deficiency. CH_3, methyl group; Cbl, cobalamin; THF_1 and THF_n, monoglutamated and polyglutamated forms of tetrahydrofolate. (Reproduced from Tefferi, A., and Pruthi, R. K., *Mayo Clin. Proc.,* 69, 1994, 181–186. With permission.)

Decreased S-adenosylmethionine production possibly leads to reduced myelin basic protein methylation and white matter vacuolization in B_{12} deficiency. Methionine also facilitates the formation of formyltetrahydrofolate, which is involved in purine synthesis. The biologically active folates are in the tetrahydrofolate form. Methyl tetrahydrofolate is the predominant folate and is required for the B_{12}-dependent remethylation of homocysteine to methionine. During the process of methionine formation methyl tetrahydrofolate donates the methyl group and is converted into tetrahydrofolate, a precursor for purine and pyrimidine synthesis. Methionine also facilitates the formation of formyltetrahydrofolate, which is involved in purine synthesis. Impaired deoxyribonucleic acid synthesis could interfere with oligodendrocyte growth and myelin production. Methylation of deoxyuridylate to thymidylate is mediated by methylene tetrahydrofolate. Impairment of this reaction results in accumulation of uracil, which replaces the decreased thymine in nucleoprotein synthesis and initiates the process that leads to megaloblastic anemia. Adenosylcobalamin is a cofactor for mitochondrial L-methylmalonyl coenzyme A mutase, which catalyzes the conversion of L-methylmalonyl coenzyme A to succinyl coenzyme A in an isomerization reaction. Accumulation of methylmalonate and propionate may provide abnormal substrates for fatty acid synthesis. Succinyl coenzyme A enters the citric acid cycle and participates in gluconeogenesis.

6.4.2.3   Clinical Manifestations of B$_{12}$ Deficiency

Neurological manifestations may be the earliest and often the only manifestation of B$_{12}$ deficiency.[42,76–79] The severity of the hematologic and neurologic manifestations may be inversely related in a particular patient. Relapses are generally associated with the same neurological phenotype. The commonly recognized neurological manifestations include a myelopathy with or without an associated neuropathy, optic neuropathy (impaired vision, optic atrophy, centrocecal scotomas), and paresthesias without abnormal signs.

The best characterized neurological manifestation of B$_{12}$ deficiency is a myelopathy that has commonly been referred to as subacute combined degeneration. The neurological features typically include a spastic paraparesis, extensor plantar response, and impaired perception of position and vibration. Accompanying peripheral nerve or rarely optic nerve involvement may be present. Asymmetry should prompt search for other causes.

Neuropsychiatric manifestations of B$_{12}$ deficiency include impaired memory, personality change, psychosis, emotional lability, and rarely delirium or coma.[43,76,77] A concomitant encephalopathy may obscure a coexisting myelopathy.

Unusual, and therefore poorly characterized, neurologic manifestations possibly related to B$_{12}$ deficiency include cerebellar ataxia, leukoencephalopathy, orthostatic tremors, myoclonus, ophthalmoplegia, catatonia, vocal cord paralysis, a syringomyelia-like distribution of motor and sensory deficits, and autonomic dysfunction.[42] Symptoms like fatigue, irritability, and lethargy are nonspecific but not uncommonly reported in the older literature.

Clinical, electrophysiological, and pathological involvement of the peripheral nervous system has been described with B$_{12}$ deficiency.[80] In most cases the clinical features of a B$_{12}$ deficiency polyneuropathy are similar to those of a cryptogenic sensorimotor polyneuropathy. Clues to possible B$_{12}$ deficiency in a patient with polyneuropathy included a relatively sudden onset of symptoms, findings suggestive of an associated myelopathy, onset of symptoms in the hands, concomitant involvement of upper and lower limbs, macrocytic red blood cells, and the presence of a risk factor for B$_{12}$ deficiency.

6.4.2.4   Diagnosis

Though a widely used screening test, serum B$_{12}$ measurement has technical and interpretive problems and lacks sensitivity and specificity for the diagnosis of B$_{12}$ deficiency.[74,78,79,81–85] A proportion of B$_{12}$-deficient patients may have B$_{12}$ levels that are on the lower side of the normal range. Some patients with low B$_{12}$ levels don't have clinically or metabolically significant B$_{12}$ deficiency. Levels of serum methylmalonic acid and plasma total homocystine are useful as ancillary diagnostic tests. The specificity of methylmalonic acid is superior to that of homocystine. Though homocystine is a very sensitive indicator of B$_{12}$ deficiency, its major limitation is its poor specificity.

A rise in the mean corpuscular volume may precede development of anemia. The presence of neutrophil hypersegmentation may be a sensitive marker for B$_{12}$ deficiency and may be seen in the absence of anemia or macrocytosis. Megaloblastic bone marrow changes may be seen.

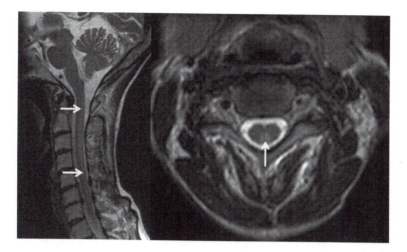

FIGURE 6.4 Cord MRI in copper or B_{12} deficiency myelopathy. Sagittal (left) and axial (right) T2-weighted MRI showing increased signal involving the dorsal column in the cervical cord. This patient had copper deficiency myelopathy. Similar findings are also seen in myelopathy due to vitamin B_{12} deficiency.

Electrophysiologic abnormalities include nerve conduction studies suggestive of a sensorimotor axonopathy, and abnormalities on somatosensory evoked potentials, visual evoked potentials, and motor evoked potentials.[80] Somatosensory evoked potential abnormalities may be commonly seen in patients with a B_{12} deficiency neuropathy and indicate a subclinical myelopathy.

MRI abnormalities in B_{12} deficiency include a signal change in the posterior and lateral columns and less commonly subcortical white matter[42] (Figure 6.4). Contrast enhancement involving the dorsal or lateral columns may be present.[86] The dorsal column may show a decreased signal on T1-weighted images.[86] Other reported findings include cord atrophy and anterior column involvement. Treatment may be accompanied by reversal of cord swelling, contrast enhancement, and signal change. Also reported is increased T2 signal involving the cerebellum. Rarely, striking diffuse white matter abnormalities (supratentorial and very rarely infratentorial) suggestive of a leukoencephalopathy may be seen. Brain T2 hyperintensities seen in B_{12} deficiency may show significant improvement with vitamin B_{12} replacement.

6.4.2.5 Management

The goals of treatment are to reverse the signs and symptoms of deficiency, replete body stores, and monitor response to therapy. A short course of daily or weekly therapy is often followed by monthly maintenance therapy (Table 6.3).[74] The role of oral therapy in patients with severe neurologic disease has not been well studied.[87]

In the absence of controlled studies, the most recommend routine is initiation of B_{12} supplementation following bariatric surgery. Oral crystalline B_{12} in a dose of at least 350 μg/day should suffice.[88–90]

Response to treatment may relate to extent of involvement and delay in starting treatment.[77] Remission correlates inversely with the time elapsed between symptom onset and therapy initiation. Response of the neurologic manifestations is variable, may be incomplete, often starts in the first week, and is complete in 6 months. The neuropathy may be slow to respond or may not respond at all.[80] This is not unexpected given the underlying axonal degeneration. Response of the hematologic derangements is prompt and complete. Reticulocyte count begins to rise within 3 days and peaks around 7 days. Red blood cell count begins to rise by 7 days and is followed by a decline in mean corpuscular volume with normalization by 8 weeks. Methylmalonic acid and plasma total homocystine levels normalize by 10–14 days.

6.4.3 COPPER (TABLE 6.4)

6.4.3.1 Copper Deficiency and Bariatric Surgery

The most common cause of acquired copper deficiency is a prior history of gastric surgery (for peptic ulcer disease or bariatric surgery).[4,91–105] In a review of reported cases of copper deficiency myelopathy, a prior history of gastric surgery has been present in nearly half the cases.[103]

A study of neurologic complications related to bariatric surgery identified delayed onset myelopathy due to copper or B_{12} deficiency as the most common and disabling complication.[4] The duration between gastric surgery and onset of neurologic symptoms may range from less than a year to 24 years.[96,97]

Gastric surgery results in copper deficiency because copper is absorbed from the proximal intestines and stomach. The acidic environment in the stomach facilitates solubilization of copper by dissociating it from copper-containing dietary macromolecules. Bacterial overgrowth has also been implicated as a cause of copper deficiency in a patient with a prior history of gastric surgery.[98] Other causes of copper deficiency

---

TABLE 6.4
Copper Deficiency and Bariatric Surgery

Pathophysiology	Copper is absorbed from the proximal intestines and stomach
	The acidic environment in the stomach facilitates solubilization of copper by dissociating it from copper-containing dietary macromolecules
	Other causes of copper deficiency like zinc ingestion or bacterial overgrowth may coexist
Clinical manifestations	Myelopathy with involvement of dorsal column and corticospinal tract
	Peripheral neuropathy
	Myeloneuropathy (subacute combined degeneration)
	Optic neuropathy
Diagnosis	Serum and urinary copper, serum ceruloplasmin, hematologic abnormalities; MRI shows increased signal involving the dorsal column
Management	8 mg of elemental copper every day orally for a week, 6 mg a day for the second week, 4 mg a day for the third week, and 2 mg a day thereafter
	2 mg of elemental copper given intravenously every day for 5 days
Additional comments	Manifestations seen years after bariatric surgery, copper and vitamin B_{12} deficiency may coexist

include excessive zinc ingestion, gastrointestinal diseases associated with malabsorption like celiac disease or inflammatory bowel disease, and prolonged parenteral nutrition.[42,106,107] The coexistence of multiple causes of copper deficiency increases the chances of development of a clinically significant deficiency state.[98] Other nutrient deficiencies like B_{12} or vitamin E can coexist with copper deficiency.[98,108]

6.4.3.2 Physiologic Role of Copper

Copper is a component of enzymes that have a critical role in the structure and function of the nervous system.[42] Copper permits electron transfer in key enzymatic pathways. These copper-associated enzymes include cytochrome c-oxidase for electron transport and oxidative phosphorylation, copper-zinc superoxide dismutase for antioxidant defense, tyrosinase for melanin synthesis, dopamine β-hydroxylase for catecholamine biosynthesis, lysyl oxidase for crosslinking of collagen and elastin, peptidylglycine α-amidating monooxygenase for neuropeptide and peptide hormone processing, monoamine oxidase for serotonin synthesis, and ceruloplasmin for brain iron homeostasis.

6.4.3.3 Clinical Manifestations of Copper Deficiency

Copper deficiency-associated myelopathy has been described in ruminants and other animal species and has been called swayback or enzootic ataxia. The hematological hallmarks of copper deficiency are anemia and neutropenia.[99,109] The anemia may be microcytic, macrocytic, or normocytic. Thrombocytopenia and resulting pancytopenia are relatively rare. Typical bone marrow findings include a left shift in granulocytic and erythroid maturation with cytoplasmic vacuolization in erythroid and myeloid precursors and the presence of ringed sideroblasts or hemosiderin-containing plasma cells. Erythroid hyperplasia with a decreased myeloid-to-erythroid ratio and dyserythropoiesis including megaloblastic changes may be seen. Patients may be given a diagnosis of sideroblastic anemia or myelodysplastic syndrome or aplastic anemia.

The most common neurologic manifestation is that of a myelopathy or myeloneuropathy that resembles the subacute combined degeneration seen with B_{12} deficiency.[94,96] It presents with a spastic gait and prominent sensory ataxia. The sensory ataxia is primarily due to dorsal column dysfunction. Clinical or electrophysiological evidence of an associated axonal peripheral neuropathy is common. A wrist drop or foot drop may be present.

Peripheral neuropathy without myelopathy, peripheral neuropathy followed by a myeloneuropathy, central nervous system demyelination, myopathy with myelopathy, optic neuropathy (including acute and bilateral blindness) with myelopathy, optic neuritis with peripheral neuropathy, a sensory ganglionopathy, myelo-optico-neuropathy with hyposmia and hypogeusia, and cognitive impairment have also been described in association with copper deficiency, but the precise significance of these reported associations is unclear and needs further study.[42] Also reported is progressive, asymmetric weakness or electrodiagnostic evidence of denervation suggestive of lower motor neuron disease.[95,106]

Copper and vitamin B_{12} deficiency may coexist. Continued neurological deterioration in patients with a history of B_{12}-related myelopathy who have a normal B_{12}

level while on replacement should be evaluated for copper deficiency. A prior history of vitamin B$_{12}$ deficiency may be present, particularly in patients with a prior history of gastric surgery. A history of anemia or leukopenia, or anemia or leukopenia at presentation is commonly present. Hematological manifestations may not accompany the neurological syndrome.[94,96]

6.4.3.4   Diagnosis

Laboratory indicators of copper deficiency include decrease in serum copper or ceruloplasmin, and in 24 h urinary copper excretion. These parameters are not sensitive to marginal copper status and are inadequate for assessing body copper stores. Urinary copper declines only when dietary copper is very low. Changes in serum copper usually parallel the ceruloplasmin concentration. Ceruloplasmin is an acute-phase reactant, and the rise in ceruloplasmin is probably responsible for the increase in serum copper seen in conditions like pregnancy, oral contraceptive use, liver disease, malignancy, hematologic disease, myocardial infarctions, smoking, diabetes, uremia, and various inflammatory and infectious diseases. Copper deficiency could be masked under these conditions. Serum zinc and 24 h urinary zinc excretion levels should be obtained, and an elevation in these should prompt an aggressive search for an exogenous source of zinc.

A low serum copper or ceruloplasmin can be seen in Wilson disease or in the Wilson disease heterozygote state. A significant elevation in urinary copper excretion should prompt consideration of Wilson disease or the Wilson disease heterozygote state as a cause for low serum copper levels. Serum ceruloplasmin is absent in aceruloplasminemia and is low in carriers with a mutation in the ceruloplasmin gene. Hence, the laboratory detection of a low serum copper does not imply copper deficiency.[110]

Evoked potential studies may provide electrophysiologic evidence of posterior column dysfunction.[94,96,111] Axonal loss predominates on nerve conduction studies. Myopathic potentials may be rarely seen. Other reported electrophysiological abnormalities noted in patients with copper deficiency and neurological manifestations include prolonged visual evoked potentials and impaired central conduction on transcranial magnetic stimulation.[111]

The commonest abnormality on the spine MRI is increased T2 signal involving the dorsal column (Figure 6.4).[94,96,112] Additionally, signal change involving the lateral column has also been reported.[113] This is similar to the spine MRI changes seen in patients with vitamin B$_{12}$ deficiency. The cervical cord is most commonly involved and contrast enhancement is not present. A recent report noted symmetric hyperintensities involving the pyramidal tract in the medulla, pons, and midbrain.[114] Nonspecific areas of increased signal involving the subcortical white matter have been reported but are of uncertain significance.[94,96,112] Also reported is a more confluent subcortical white matter signal change or periventricular lesions suggestive of demyelination.[94,98]

6.4.3.5   Management

There have been no studies that address the most appropriate dose, duration, route, and form of copper supplementation. At times prolonged oral therapy may not result in improvement; parenteral therapy may be required. Some have employed initial parenteral administration followed by oral administration. Copper supplements may not be adequately absorbed when administered through a jejunostomy tube necessitating parenteral therapy. Other situations in which parenteral therapy may be required include severely depleted patients or significant malabsorption. The presence of rapid deterioration or significant hematologic derangement may also prompt consideration of parenteral therapy. In most cases, however, oral administration of 2 mg of elemental copper a day seems to suffice. The same dose of elemental copper may be given intravenously; a commonly used regimen is 2 mg of elemental copper administered intravenously (over 2 h) daily for 5 days and periodically thereafter. Subcutaneous or intramuscular supplementation has also been employed. The standard dose of 2 mg a day may not be adequate in all patients. Doses up to 9 mg/day orally have been used (Table 6.4). Commonly used copper salts include copper gluconate, copper sulfate, and copper chloride.

Despite a suspected absorption defect, oral copper supplementation is generally the preferred route of supplementation (Table 6.4). Periodic assessment of serum copper is essential to determine adequacy of replacement and to decide on the most appropriate long-term administration strategy. Because of the need for long-term replacement, parenteral therapy is not preferred and is generally not required.

Response of the hematological parameters (including bone marrow findings) is prompt and often complete.[42,94,96] Hematological recovery may be accompanied by reticulocytosis. Recovery of neurological signs and symptoms is variable. Normalization of serum copper with improvement in neurological symptoms, electrophysiology, and imaging has been reported, but the more common outcome is cessation of progression. Improvement is often subjective and involves sensory symptoms. Periodic monitoring of copper status should be considered in high-risk patients after bariatric surgery.[105] Long-term supplementation is often required.

6.4.4   Vitamin B$_6$ (B$_6$, Pyridoxine)

6.4.4.1   B$_6$ Deficiency and Bariatric Surgery

Laboratory evidence of B$_6$ deficiency has been recognized before and after bariatric surgery.[23,115]

Additional causes of B$_6$ deficiency include gastrointestinal diseases associated with malabsorption, alcoholism, and use of B$_6$ antagonists like isonicotinic acid hydrazide, cycloserine, hydralazine, and penicillamine. Individuals at risk of developing B$_6$ deficiency include pregnant and lactating women and elderly individuals.

6.4.4.2   Physiologic Role of B$_6$

Pyridoxal and pyridoxamine are two other naturally occurring compounds that have biological activity comparable to pyridoxine. All three compounds are readily converted to pyridoxal phosphate. Pyridoxal phosphate serves as a coenzyme in many reactions involved in the metabolism of amino acids, lipids, nucleic acid, and one carbon units, and in the pathways of gluconeogenesis, and neurotransmitter and heme biosynthesis. The interconversion and metabolism of B$_6$ are dependent on riboflavin, niacin, and zinc. Niacin, carnitine, and folate require B$_6$ for their metabolism.

6.4.4.3 Clinical Significance of B_6 Deficiency

Adults are much more tolerant of pyridoxine deficiency than infants. Even with low levels symptoms are rare. Up to 50% of slow activators may develop a dose-related peripheral neuropathy due to B_6 deficiency when treated with isonicotinic acid hydrazide.[42] Chronic B_6 deficiency results in a microcytic hypochromic anemia. Chronic vitamin B_6-deficient patients may develop secondary hyperoxaluria and thus are at higher risk for nephrolithiasis. As with other B vitamin deficiencies, glossitis, stomatitis, cheilosis, and dermatitis may be seen.

6.4.4.4 Diagnosis

Vitamin B_6 status can be assessed by measuring its levels in the blood or urine. The most commonly used measure is plasma pyridoxal phosphate. Functional indicators of vitamin B_6 status are based on pyridoxal phosphate-dependent reactions.

6.4.4.5 Management

Vitamin B_6 may be supplemented in a dose of 50–100 mg/day to prevent development of the neuropathy. Higher doses of B_6 have been associated with a sensory neuronopathy.

6.4.5 Folate

6.4.5.1 Folate Deficiency and Bariatric Surgery

Folate deficiency following gastric bypass is a relatively rare occurrence.[72,116] Folate deficiency may be due to bacterial overgrowth associated with gastric bypass surgery.[117,118] Preoperative folate deficiency has also been recognized.[115,116] Folate deficiency rarely exists in the pure state. It may coexist with other nutrient deficiencies. Hence, attribution of neurological manifestations to folate deficiency requires exclusion of other potential causes. A review of neurologic complications following bariatric surgery failed to show a correlation between folate deficiency and neurologic complications.[4] Serum folate falls within 3 weeks after decrease in folate intake or absorption, red blood cell folate declines weeks later, and clinically significant depletion of folate stores may be seen within months. Clinical features of folate deficiency occur more rapidly with low stores or coexisting alcoholism.

6.4.5.2 Physiologic Role of Folate

Folate functions as a coenzyme or cosubstrate by modifying, accepting, or transferring one carbon moieties in single-carbon reactions involved in the metabolism of nucleic and amino acids. The biologically active folates are in the tetrahydrofolate form. Methyl tetrahydrofolate is the predominant folate and is required for the cobalamin-dependent remethylation of homocystine to methionine (Figure 6.3). Methylation of deoxyuridylate to thymidylate is mediated by methylene tetrahydrofolate. Impairment of this reaction results in accumulation of uracil, which replaces the decreased thymine in nucleoprotein synthesis and initiates the process that leads to megaloblastic anemia.

6.4.5.3 Clinical Manifestations of Folate Deficiency

Theoretically folate deficiency could cause the same deficits as those seen with B_{12} deficiency because of its importance in the production of methionine, S-adenosylmethionine, and tetrahydrofolate. For unclear reasons, neurologic manifestations like those seen in B_{12} deficiency are rare in folate deficiency. The myeloneuropathy or neuropathy or megaloblastic anemia seen in association with folate deficiency is indistinguishable from B_{12} deficiency.[42] The relationship between folate deficiency in pregnancy and neural tube defects is well established. Folate deficiency has been associated with affective disorders, but the precise significance of this is unclear.[119,120] In recent years there has been some evidence that suggests that chronic folate deficiency may increase risk of cardiovascular disease, cerebrovascular disease, peripheral vascular disease, and venous thrombosis, and may cause cognitive impairment.[121,122] The precise significance of these observations awaits further studies.

6.4.5.4 Diagnosis

Plasma homocysteine levels have been shown to be elevated in patients with clinically significant folate deficiency.[83] Serum folate fluctuates daily and does not correlate with tissue stores. Red blood cell folate is more reliable than plasma folate because its levels are less affected by short-term fluctuations in intake.[123] However, red blood cell folate assay is subject to greater variation depending on the method and laboratory.[124]

6.4.5.5 Management

With documented folate deficiency, an oral dose of 1 mg three times a day may be followed by a maintenance dose of 1 mg a day. Acutely ill patients may need parenteral administration in a dose of 1–5 mg. A reasonable maintenance dose is 400 µg/day. Coexisting B_{12} deficiency should therefore be ruled out before instituting folate therapy. Plasma homocysteine is likely the best biochemical tool for monitoring response to therapy; it decreases within a few days of instituting folate therapy but does not respond to inappropriate B_{12} deficiency therapy.[125] Since folate deficiency is generally seen in association with a broader dietary inadequacy, the associated comorbidities need to be addressed.

6.4.6 Vitamin E

6.4.6.1 Vitamin E Deficiency and Bariatric Surgery

Low vitamin E levels have been recognized before and very rarely following bariatric surgery.[115,126] When present, it is generally in the context of procedures associated with fat-soluble vitamin malabsorption like biliopancreatic diversion. Many years of malabsorption are required to deplete vitamin E stores. Additional causes of vitamin E deficiency include chronic cholestasis and pancreatic insufficiency. Vitamin E deficiency is also seen with gastrointestinal diseases associated with malabsorption and due to inadequate supplementation in patients on total parenteral nutrition.

6.4.6.2 Physiologic Role of Vitamin E

In humans α-tocopherol is the active and most important biologic form of vitamin E. Vitamin E serves as an antioxidant and prevents the formation of toxic free radical products. It appears to protect cellular membranes from oxidative stress, and inhibits the peroxidation of polyunsaturated fatty acids of membrane phospholipids.

6.4.6.3 Clinical Manifestations of Vitamin E Deficiency

The neurological manifestations of vitamin E deficiency include a spinocerebellar syndrome with variable peripheral nerve involvement.[42,127] The phenotype is similar to that of Friedreich ataxia. The clinical features include cerebellar ataxia, hyporeflexia, proprioceptive, and vibratory loss, and an extensor plantar response. Cutaneous sensations may be affected to a lesser degree. Ophthalmoplegia, ptosis, and pigmentary retinopathy may be seen. An associated myopathy, at times with inflammatory infiltrates and rimmed vacuoles, has been described.[128] The neuropathy associated with vitamin E deficiency preferentially involves centrally directed fibers of large myelinated neurons. It is rare for vitamin E deficiency to present as an isolated neuropathy; isolated vitamin E deficiency with a demyelinating neuropathy has been reported.[129]

6.4.6.4 Diagnosis

Serum vitamin E levels are dependent on the concentrations of serum lipids, cholesterol, and very low density lipoproteins (VLDL). Hyperlipidemia or hypolipidemia can independently increase or decrease serum vitamin E without reflecting similar alterations in tissue levels of the vitamin.[130] Effective serum α-tocopherol concentrations are calculated by dividing the serum α-tocopherol by the sum of serum cholesterol and triglycerides. In patients with neurological manifestations due to vitamin E deficiency the serum vitamin E levels are frequently undetectable. Additional markers of fat malabsorption such as increased stool fat and decreased serum carotene levels may be present. Vitamin E determination can be done in adipose tissue.

Somatosensory evoked potential studies may show evidence of central delay, and nerve conduction studies may show evidence of an axonal neuropathy. With retinal pigmentary degeneration, abnormal electroretinograms may be seen. Spinal MRI in patients with vitamin E deficiency-related myeloneuropathy may show increased signal in the cervical cord dorsal column.[131]

6.4.6.5 Management

Early diagnosis and treatment of neurologic manifestations due to vitamin E deficiency may result in dramatic recovery.[108] The suggested supplementation in an asymptomatic postsurgical patient is a standard vitamin E containing a multivitamin-mineral preparation.

6.4.7 VITAMIN D

6.4.7.1 Vitamin D Deficiency and Bariatric Surgery

Vitamin D deficiency and reduced calcium and phosphorus intake have been reported following gastric bypass and partial gastrectomy.[7,69,132] Preoperative vitamin

D deficiency may be present.[39,133,134] Aches and pains occurring after 1 year of bypass surgery have been called bypass bone disease and are thought to be due to bone demineralization from impaired calcium absorption, often with concurrent vitamin D deficiency.[69] Bone mineral density may be significantly decreased after gastric bypass surgery.[135]

6.4.7.2 Physiologic Role of Vitamin D

Vitamin D exists in two forms: vitamin D_2 (ergocalciferol; produced by plants) and vitamin D_3 (cholecalciferol; derived from 7-dehydrocholesterol when exposed to ultraviolet light in the skin). Vitamin D functions more like a hormone than a vitamin. It acts intracellularly at high-affinity nuclear receptors that, when stimulated, alter gene transcription. Receptors in small bowel enterocytes enhance calcium and phosphorus absorption, and bone receptors stimulate mineralization of newly formed bone. Sun-stimulated skin synthesis can provide 100% of the daily requirement from 7-dehydrocholesterol in the absence of oral intake. In the liver vitamin D is hydroxylated to 25-hydroxy vitamin D. Further hydroxylation occurs in the kidney to 1,25-dihydroxy vitamin D, the active form. Vitamin D hydroxylation is increased by parathormone. With replete stores, 25-hydroxy vitamin D is hydroxylated to 24,25-dihydroxy vitamin D and is excreted in the bile and urine.

6.4.7.3 Clinical Manifestations of Vitamin D Deficiency

Vitamin D deficiency results in defective mineralization of newly formed bone. Vitamin D deficiency results in hypocalcemia with secondary hyperparathyroidism, which further impairs normal bone mineralization. This causes rickets in kids and osteomalacia in adults.

Vitamin D deficiency can cause a proximal myopathy, which often exists in association with osteomalacia, pathological fractures, and bone pain.[136,137] The pelvic and thigh musculature are involved more than the arms. A waddling gait may be present. Neck muscles may be involved; bulbar and ocular muscles are spared. Hypovitaminosis D has been associated with persistent, nonspecific musculoskeletal pain in some studies.[138] Proximal weakness, with or without myalgias, should prompt consideration of vitamin D deficiency. This objective muscle disease should be distinguished from a generalized sense of weakness that accompanies malnutrition. Severe hypocalcemia may result in tetany and may be associated with hypomagnesemia. Vitamin D deficiency has been reported to cause cutaneous hyperalgesia that is resistant to antidepressants and opiates but responds to vitamin D repletion.[139] Intermittent facial twitching and ophthalmoplegia in the setting of hypocalcemia have been reported years after gastric bypass surgery.[132] The relationship between multiple sclerosis and vitamin D deficiency has been the subject of recent research.[140] Vitamin D deficiency has been implicated in age-related cognitive dysfunction and dementia in some studies.[141,142]

6.4.7.4 Diagnosis

Vitamin D deficiency may be accompanied by decreased serum calcium and increased parathormone levels. Since 25-hydroxy vitamin D is hydroxylated to the active form, the level of 1,25-dihydroxy vitamin D may be normal, while its immediate precursor may be very low. Hence, vitamin D status is best assessed by 25-hydroxy vitamin D levels.[143] Other laboratory abnormalities may include raised alkaline phosphatase of bone origin, hypocalcemia, hypophosphatemia, raised parathormone, reduced urinary calcium excretion, and raised urinary hydroxyproline. Radiological changes of rickets or osteopenia may be present.

6.4.7.5 Management

Vitamin D can be given orally as vitamin D_2 or vitamin D_3. Four hundred IU of vitamin D per day is adequate to prevent deficiency in individuals with minimal sun exposure. With clinical deficiency, 50,000 IU weekly of vitamin D_2 or D_3 may be required for 6–8 weeks. This may be followed by 800–1000 U/day. Larger oral doses (or even parenteral administration) may also be required in the presence of malabsorption. Associated secondary hyperparathyroidism can cause hypercalcemia, hypercalciuria, and nephrolithiasis. This can be prevented by ensuring that there is adequate calcium repletion, and thus avoiding parathyroid stimulation. An inappropriately high phosphate level suggests secondary hyperparathyroidism. Laboratory monitoring is required with doses of 50,000 IU three times a week. Toxicity includes hypercalcemia, hypercalciuria, and renal failure. Serum and urine calcium and serum 25-hydroxy vitamin D should be monitored, and when urinary calcium excretion exceeds 100 mg/24 h, the vitamin D dose should be reduced. With liver dysfunction 25-hydroxy vitamin D (calciferol) can be used.

6.5 PREVENTION AND TREATMENT OF NEUROLOGIC COMPLICATIONS

Prevention, diagnosis, and treatment of neurologic disorders related to bariatric surgery are necessary parts of lifelong care after bariatric surgery.[16,69,88–90,144,145] Preoperative nutritional deficiencies need to be identified and treated. Patients who have been dieting may be at higher risk for postoperative deficiencies because of lower reserves.[16] Newer surgical techniques like purely restrictive procedures focus on increased satiety rather than malabsorption to influence weight loss. This is associated with a decreased incidence of neurologic complication. Malabsorptive procedures are associated with nutrient deficiencies and require lifelong monitoring and supplementation. Baseline preoperative data should be obtained to permit correction of deficiencies and to provide comparison values. The frequency of monitoring and amount of supplementation vary slightly in different guidelines and are related to the underlying procedure.[89,90,145] Malabsorptive procedures like Roux-en-Y gastric bypass and, in particular, biliopancreatic diversion with or without duodenal switch require a more aggressive approach than the adjustable gastric banding.

All bariatric surgery patients should have baseline laboratory studies that include complete blood count, electrolytes, glucose, creatinine, liver function tests, serum iron and ferritin, iron binding capacity, vitamin B_{12}, folate, vitamin D, calcium, intact parathormone, albumin and prealbumin, and bone density.[88–90] These parameters should be determined periodically thereafter, particularly so in patients undergoing malabsorptive procedures. In select cases thiamine, zinc, selenium, copper, vitamin

TABLE 6.5
Daily Mineral and Vitamin Supplementation Following Bariatric Surgery

B_{12}	350–500 µg of the oral crystalline form; some may need monthly intramuscular injections of 1000 µg
Folic acid	400–800 µg
Vitamin D	800–1200 units
Iron	65–130 mg
Calcium citrate	1200–2000 mg
Thiamine	50–100 mg
Copper	2 mg
Vitamin A	5000–1000 IU
Vitamin E	400 IU
Vitamin K	300 µg–1 mg

Note: Indefinite use of vitamin and mineral supplements is required after malabsorptive procedures like Roux-en-Y gastric bypass. Standard multivitamin and mineral preparations may be inadequate sources of iron and vitamin B_{12}. Supplementation with vitamins A, E, and K is required in patients who have undergone biliopancreatic diversion with duodenal switch. There are no formal recommendations regarding copper supplementation. Zinc supplementation may increase the risk of copper deficiency.

A, and vitamin E measurements may be indicated. The initial follow-up frequency of biochemical parameters may be every 3 months for the first year, every 6 months for the second year, and annually thereafter.

Standard multivitamin with mineral supplements may not prevent development of B_{12} or iron deficiency.[71,146,147] Table 6.5 summarizes suggested doses of daily supplements.[6,69,89,90,148,149] Much of this can be provided through a standard multivitamin-mineral preparation.

Long-term follow-up with dietary counseling is important. Following bariatric surgery, patients need to be on high-protein and low-fat diets in addition to vitamin supplementation. Increased consumption of fiber and complex carbohydrates is encouraged. Avoidance of simple sugars decreases gastrointestinal symptoms. Small frequent meals should be consumed without simultaneous consumption of liquids. Nutritional deficiencies may develop despite vitamin supplementation.

The management of neurologic complications related to a nutrient deficiency is discussed in the individual sections above. At times a specific nutrient deficiency as a cause for a specific neurologic manifestation is not identified. Multiple nutritional deficits may coexist. Correction of a particular deficiency may not result in reversal of the related neurologic manifestation. Gradual clinical improvement or stabilization may be seen. In a patient with gastric banding and severe nausea and vomiting, temporarily loosening the band may permit more food to pass and provide relief from these symptoms. In rare cases improvement may be seen only following surgical revision.[4,89]

REFERENCES

1. Abarbanel JM, Berginer VM, Osimani A, Solomon H, Charuzi I. Neurologic complications after gastric restriction surgery for morbid obesity. *Neurology* 1987;37:196–200.
2. Berger JR. The neurological complications of bariatric surgery. *Arch Neurol* 2004;61:1185–1189.
3. Koffman BM, Greenfield LJ, Ali II, Pirzada NA. Neurologic complications after surgery for obesity. *Muscle Nerve* 2006;33:166–176.
4. Juhasz-Pocsine K, Rudnicki SA, Archer RL, Harik SI. Neurologic complications of gastric bypass surgery for morbid obesity. *Neurology* 2007;68:1843–1850.
5. Kazemi A, Frazier T, Cave M. Micronutrient-related neurologic complications following bariatric surgery. *Curr Gastroenterol Rep* 2010;12:288–295.
6. Becker DA, Balcer LJ, Galetta SL. The neurological complications of nutritional deficiency following bariatric surgery. *J Obes* 2012;2012:608534.
7. Banerji NK, Hurwitz LJ. Nervous system manifestations after gastric surgery. *Acta Neurol Scand* 1971;47:485–513.
8. Hoffman PM, Brody JA. Neurological disorders in patients following surgery for peptic ulcer. *Neurology* 1972;22:450.
9. Feit H, Glasberg M, Ireton C, Rosenberg RN, Thal E. Peripheral neuropathy and starvation after gastric partitioning for morbid obesity. *Ann Intern Med* 1982;96:453–455.
10. Paulson GW, Martin EW, Mojzisik C, Carey LC. Neurologic complications of gastric partitioning. *Arch Neurol* 1985;42:675–677.
11. Chaves LC, Faintuch J, Kahwage S, de Assis Alencar F. A cluster of polyneuropathy and Wernicke-Korsakoff syndrome in a bariatric unit. *Obes Surg* 2002;12:328–334.
12. Thaisetthawatkul P, Collazo-Clavell ML, Sarr MG, Norell JE, Dyck PJ. A controlled study of peripheral neuropathy after bariatric surgery. *Neurology* 2004;63:1462–1470.
13. Chang CG, Adams-Huet B, Provost DA. Acute post-gastric reduction surgery (APGARS) neuropathy. *Obes Surg* 2004;14:182–189.
14. Singh S, Kumar A. Wernicke encephalopathy after obesity surgery. *Neurology* 2007;68:807–811.
15. Clark N. Neuropathy following bariatric surgery. *Semin Neurol* 2010;30:433–435.
16. Rudnicki SA. Prevention and treatment of peripheral neuropathy after bariatric surgery. *Curr Treat Options Neurol* 2010;12:29–36.
17. Chang CG, Helling TS, Black WE, Rymer MM. Weakness after gastric bypass. *Obes Surg* 2002;12:592–597.
18. Khurana RN, Baudendistel TE, Morgan EF, Rabkin RA, Elkin RB, Aalami OO. Postoperative rhabdomyolysis following laparoscopic gastric bypass in the morbidly obese. *Arch Surg* 2004;139:73–76.
19. Aasheim ET. Wernicke encephalopathy after bariatric surgery: a systematic review. *Ann Surg* 2008;248:714–720.
20. Aasheim ET, Bjorkman S, Sovik TT, et al. Vitamin status after bariatric surgery: a randomized study of gastric bypass and duodenal switch. *Am J Clin Nutr* 2009;90:15–22.
21. Ernst B, Thurnheer M, Schmid SM, Schultes B. Evidence for the necessity to systematically assess micronutrient status prior to bariatric surgery. *Obes Surg* 2009;19:66–73.
22. Halverson JD. Micronutrient deficiencies after gastric bypass for morbid obesity. *Am Surg* 1986;52:594–598.
23. Clements RH, Katasani VG, Palepu R, et al. Incidence of vitamin deficiency after laparoscopic Roux-en-Y gastric bypass in a university hospital setting. *Am Surg* 2006;72:1196–1202; discussion 1203–1194.
24. Malinowski SS. Nutritional and metabolic complications of bariatric surgery. *Am J Med Sci* 2006;331:219–225.

25. Elias WJ, Pouratian N, Oskouian RJ, Schirmer B, Burns T. Peroneal neuropathy following successful bariatric surgery. Case report and review of the literature. *J Neurosurg* 2006;105:631–635.
26. Macgregor AM, Thoburn EK. Meralgia paresthetica following bariatric surgery. *Obes Surg* 1999;9:364–368.
27. Salas-Salvado J, Garcia-Lorda P, Cuatrecasas G, et al. Wernicke's syndrome after bariatric surgery. *Clin Nutr* 2000;19:371–373.
28. Sola E, Morillas C, Garzon S, Ferrer JM, Martin J, Hernandez-Mijares A. Rapid onset of Wernicke's encephalopathy following gastric restrictive surgery. *Obes Surg* 2003;13:661–662.
29. Foster D, Falah M, Kadom N, Mandler R. Wernicke encephalopathy after bariatric surgery: losing more than just weight. *Neurology* 2005;65:1987; discussion 1847.
30. Sanchez-Crespo NE, Parker M. Wernicke's encephalopathy: a tragic complication of gastric bypass. *J Hosp Med* 2006;1(Suppl 2):72.
31. Al-Fahad T, Ismael A, Soliman MO, Khoursheed M. Very early onset of Wernicke's encephalopathy after gastric bypass. *Obes Surg* 2006;16:671–672.
32. Jiang W, Gagliardi JP, Raj YP, Silvertooth EJ, Christopher EJ, Krishnan KR. Acute psychotic disorder after gastric bypass surgery: differential diagnosis and treatment [see comment]. *Am J Psychiatry* 2006;163:15–19.
33. Worden RW, Allen HM. Wernicke's encephalopathy after gastric bypass that masqueraded as acute psychosis: a case report. *Curr Surg* 2006;63:114–116.
34. Longmuir R, Lee AG, Rouleau J. Visual loss due to Wernicke syndrome following gastric bypass. *Semin Ophthalmol* 2007;22:13–19.
35. Lakhani SV, Shah HN, Alexander K, Finelli FC, Kirkpatrick JR, Koch TR. Small intestinal bacterial overgrowth and thiamine deficiency after Roux-en-Y gastric bypass surgery in obese patients. *Nutr Res* 2008;28:293–298.
36. Iannelli A, Addeo P, Novellas S, Gugenheim J. Wernicke's encephalopathy after laparoscopic Roux-en-Y gastric bypass: a misdiagnosed complication. *Obes Surg* 2010;20:1594–1596.
37. Walker J, Kepner A. Wernicke's encephalopathy presenting as acute psychosis after gastric bypass. *J Emerg Med* 2012;43:811–814.
38. Carrodeguas L, Kaidar-Person O, Szomstein S, Antozzi P, Rosenthal R. Preoperative thiamine deficiency in obese population undergoing laparoscopic bariatric surgery. *Surg Obes Relat Dis* 2005;1:517–522.
39. Flancbaum L, Belsley S, Drake V, Colarusso T, Tayler E. Preoperative nutritional status of patients undergoing Roux-en-Y gastric bypass for morbid obesity. *J Gastrointest Surg* 2006;10:1033–1037.
40. Thomson AD, Marshall EJ. The natural history and pathophysiology of Wernicke's encephalopathy and Korsakoff's psychosis. *Alcohol Alcohol* 2006;41:151–158.
41. Sechi G, Serra A. Wernicke's encephalopathy: new clinical settings and recent advances in diagnosis and management. *Lancet Neurol* 2007;6:442–455.
42. Kumar N. Neurologic presentations of nutritional deficiencies. *Neurol Clin* 2010;28:107–170.
43. Kumar N. Acute and subacute encephalopathies: deficiency states (nutritional). *Semin Neurol* 2011;31:169–183.
44. Koike H, Ito S, Morozumi S, et al. Rapidly developing weakness mimicking Guillain–Barré; syndrome in beriberi neuropathy: two case reports. *Nutrition* 2008;24:776–780.
45. Murphy C, Bangash IH, Varma A. Dry beriberi mimicking the Guillain–Barre syndrome. *Pract Neurol* 2009;9:221–224.
46. Faigle R, Mohme M, Levy M. Dry beriberi mimicking Guillain–Barre syndrome as the first presenting sign of thiamine deficiency. *Eur J Neurol* 2012;19:e14–e15.
47. Gollobin C, Marcus WY. Bariatric beriberi. *Obes Surg* 2002;12:309–311.

48. Reuler JB, Girard DE, Cooney TG. Current concepts. Wernicke's encephalopathy. *N Engl J Med* 1985;312:1035–1039.

49. Harper CG, Giles M, Finlay-Jones R. Clinical signs in the Wernicke-Korsakoff complex: a retrospective analysis of 131 cases diagnosed at necropsy. *J Neurol Neurosurg Psychiatry* 1986;49:341–345.

50. Galvin R, Brathen G, Ivashynka A, et al. EFNS guidelines for diagnosis, therapy and prevention of Wernicke encephalopathy. *Eur J Neurol* 2010;17:1408–1418.

51. Lough ME. Wernicke's encephalopathy: expanding the diagnostic toolbox. *Neuropsychol Rev* 2012;22:181–194.

52. Kopelman MD. The Korsakoff syndrome. *Br J Psychiatry* 1995;166:154–173.

53. Cook CC, Hallwood PM, Thomson AD. B vitamin deficiency and neuropsychiatric syndromes in alcohol misuse. *Alcohol Alcohol* 1998;33:317–336.

54. Thomson AD, Cook CC, Touquet R, Henry JA, Royal College of Physicians London. The Royal College of Physicians report on alcohol: guidelines for managing Wernicke's encephalopathy in the accident and emergency department. *Alcohol Alcohol* 2002;37:513–521. Erratum appears in *Alcohol Alcohol* 2003;38(3):291.

55. Homewood J, Bond NW. Thiamin deficiency and Korsakoff's syndrome: failure to find memory impairments following nonalcoholic Wernicke's encephalopathy. *Alcohol* 1999;19:75–84.

56. Talwar D, Davidson H, Cooney J, O'Reilly St. JD. Vitamin B(1) status assessed by direct measurement of thiamin pyrophosphate in erythrocytes or whole blood by HPLC: comparison with erythrocyte transketolase activation assay [see comment]. *Clin Chem* 2000;46:704–710.

57. Donnino MW, Miller J, Garcia AJ, McKee E, Walsh M. Distinctive acid-base pattern in Wernicke's encephalopathy. *Ann Emerg Med* 2007;50:722–725.

58. Sriram K, Manzanares W, Joseph K. Thiamine in nutrition therapy. *Nutr Clin Pract* 2012;27:41–50.

59. Antunez E, Estruch R, Cardenal C, Nicolas JM, Fernandez-Sola J, Urbano-Marquez A. Usefulness of CT and MR imaging in the diagnosis of acute Wernicke's encephalopathy. *AJR Am J Roentgenol* 1998;171:1131–1137.

60. Fei GQ, Zhong C, Jin L, et al. Clinical characteristics and MR imaging features of nonalcoholic Wernicke encephalopathy. *AJNR Am J Neuroradiol* 2008;29:164–169.

61. Merola JF, Ghoroghchian PP, Samuels MA, Levy BD, Loscalzo J. Clinical problem-solving. At a loss. *N Engl J Med* 2012;367:67–72.

62. Zuccoli G, Motti L. Atypical Wernicke's encephalopathy showing lesions in the cranial nerve nuclei and cerebellum. *J Neuroimaging* 2008;18:194–197.

63. Schabelman E, Kuo D. Glucose before thiamine for Wernicke encephalopathy: a literature review. *J Emerg Med* 2012;42:488–494.

64. Thomson AD, Marshall EJ. The treatment of patients at risk of developing Wernicke's encephalopathy in the community. *Alcohol Alcohol* 2006;41:159–167.

65. Sechi G. Prognosis and therapy of Wernicke's encephalopathy after obesity surgery. *Am J Gastroenterol* 2008;103:3219.

66. Traviesa DC. Magnesium deficiency: a possible cause of thiamine refractoriness in Wernicke-Korsakoff encephalopathy. *J Neurol Neurosurg Psychiatry* 1974;37:959–962.

67. Harper C. Wernicke's encephalopathy: a more common disease than realised. A neuropathological study of 51 cases. *J Neurol Neurosurg Psychiatry* 1979;42:226–231.

68. Fried RT, Levy M, Leibowitz AB, Bronster DJ, Iberti TJ. Wernicke's encephalopathy in the intensive care patient. *Crit Care Med* 1990;18:779–780.

69. Crowley LV, Seay J, Mullin G. Late effects of gastric bypass for obesity. *Am J Gastroenterol* 1984;79:850–860.

70. Amaral JF, Thompson WR, Caldwell MD, Martin HF, Randall HT. Prospective hematologic evaluation of gastric exclusion surgery for morbid obesity. *Ann Surg* 1985;201:186–193.

71. Provenzale D, Reinhold RB, Golner B, et al. Evidence for diminished B_{12} absorption after gastric bypass: oral supplementation does not prevent low plasma B_{12} levels in bypass patients. *J Am Coll Nutr* 1992;11:29–35.

72. Vargas-Ruiz AG, Hernández-Rivera G, Herrera MF. Prevalence of iron, folate, and vitamin B_{12} deficiency anemia after laparoscopic Roux-en-Y gastric bypass. *Obes Surg* 2008;18:288–293.

73. Brolin RE, Gorman JH, Gorman RC, et al. Are vitamin B_{12} and folate deficiency clinically important after Roux-en-Y gastric bypass? *J Gastrointest Surg* 1998;2:436–442.

74. Green R, Kinsella LJ. Current concepts in the diagnosis of cobalamin deficiency [see comment]. *Neurology* 1995;45:1435–1440.

75. Tefferi A, Pruthi RK. The biochemical basis of cobalamin deficiency. *Mayo Clin Proc* 1994;69:181–186.

76. Lindenbaum J, Healton EB, Savage DG, et al. Neuropsychiatric disorders caused by cobalamin deficiency in the absence of anemia or macrocytosis. *N Engl J Med* 1988;318:1720–1728.

77. Healton EB, Savage DG, Brust JC, Garrett TJ, Lindenbaum J. Neurologic aspects of cobalamin deficiency. *Medicine (Baltimore)* 1991;70:229–245.

78. Carmel R. Current concepts in cobalamin deficiency. *Annu Rev Med* 2000;51:357–375.

79. Carmel R, Green R, Rosenblatt DS, Watkins D. Update on cobalamin, folate, and homocysteine. *Hematology* 2003:62–81.

80. Saperstein DS, Wolfe GI, Gronseth GS, et al. Challenges in the identification of cobalamin-deficiency polyneuropathy. *Arch Neurol* 2003;60:1296–1301.

81. Lindenbaum J, Savage DG, Stabler SP, Allen RH. Diagnosis of cobalamin deficiency. II. Relative sensitivities of serum cobalamin, methylmalonic acid, and total homocysteine concentrations. *Am J Hematol* 1990;34:99–107.

82. Stabler SP, Allen RH, Savage DG, Lindenbaum J. Clinical spectrum and diagnosis of cobalamin deficiency [see comment]. *Blood* 1990;76:871–881.

83. Savage DG, Lindenbaum J, Stabler SP, Allen RH. Sensitivity of serum methylmalonic acid and total homocysteine determinations for diagnosing cobalamin and folate deficiencies [see comment]. *Am J Med* 1994;96:239–246.

84. Snow CF. Laboratory diagnosis of vitamin B_{12} and folate deficiency: a guide for the primary care physician [see comment]. *Arch Intern Med* 1999;159:1289–1298.

85. Solomon LR. Cobalamin-responsive disorders in the ambulatory care setting: unreliability of cobalamin, methylmalonic acid, and homocysteine testing. *Blood* 2005;105:978–985.

86. Locatelli ER, Laureno R, Ballard P, Mark AS. MRI in vitamin B_{12} deficiency myelopathy. *Can J Neurol Sci* 1999;26:60–63.

87. Andres E, Fothergill H, Mecili M. Efficacy of oral cobalamin (vitamin B_{12}) therapy. *Exp Opin Pharmacother* 2010;11:249–256.

88. Allied Health Sciences Section Ad Hoc Nutrition Committee, Aills L, Blankenship J, Buffington C, Furtado M, Parrott J. ASMBS Allied Health nutritional guidelines for the surgical weight loss patient. *Surg Obes Relat Dis* 2008;4:S73–108.

89. Mechanick JI, Kushner RF, Sugerman HJ, et al. American Association of Clinical Endocrinologists, The Obesity Society, and American Society for Metabolic and bariatric surgery medical guidelines for clinical practice for the perioperative nutritional, metabolic, and nonsurgical support of the bariatric surgery patient. *Surg Obes Relat Dis* 2008;4:S109–S184.

90. Heber D, Greenway FL, Kaplan LM, et al. Endocrine and nutritional management of the post-bariatric surgery patient: an Endocrine Society clinical practice guideline. *J Clin Endocrinol Metab* 2010;95:4823–4843.

91. Schleper B, Stuerenburg HJ. Copper deficiency-associated myelopathy in a 46-year-old woman [see comment]. *J Neurol* 2001;248:705–706.

92. Kumar N, McEvoy KM, Ahlskog JE. Myelopathy due to copper deficiency following gastrointestinal surgery. *Arch Neurol* 2003;60:1782–1785.

93. Kumar N, Ahlskog JE, Gross JB Jr. Acquired hypocupremia after gastric surgery. *Clin Gastroenterol Hepatol* 2004;2:1074–1079.

94. Kumar N, Gross JB Jr, Ahlskog JE. Copper deficiency myelopathy produces a clinical picture like subacute combined degeneration. *Neurology* 2004;63:33–39.

95. Weihl CC, Lopate G. Motor neuron disease associated with copper deficiency. *Muscle Nerve* 2006;34:789–793.

96. Kumar N. Copper deficiency myelopathy: human swayback. *Mayo Clin Proc* 2006;81:1371–1384.

97. Prodan CI, Bottomley SS, Holland NR, Lind SE. Relapsing hypocupraemic myelopathy requiring high-dose oral copper replacement. *J Neurol Neurosurg Psychiatry* 2006;77:1092–1093.

98. Spinazzi M, De Lazzari F, Tavolato B, Angelini C, Manara R, Armani M. Myelo-optico-neuropathy in copper deficiency occurring after partial gastrectomy. Do small bowel bacterial overgrowth syndrome and occult zinc ingestion tip the balance? *J Neurol* 2007;254:1012–1017.

99. Halfdanarson T, Kumar N, Li C-Y, Phyliky R, Hogan WJ. Hematological manifestations of copper deficiency. *Eur J Hematol* 2008;80(6):523–531.

100. Shahidzadeh R, Sridhar S. Profound copper deficiency in a patient with gastric bypass. *Am J Gastroenterol* 2008;103:2660–2662.

101. Prodan CI, Bottomley SS, Vincent AS, et al. Copper deficiency after gastric surgery: a reason for caution. *Am J Med Sci* 2009;337:256–258.

102. Griffith DP, Liff DA, Ziegler TR, Esper GJ, Winton EF. Acquired copper deficiency: a potentially serious and preventable complication following gastric bypass surgery. *Obesity* 2009;17:827–831.

103. Jaiser SR, Winston GP. Copper deficiency myelopathy. *J Neurol* 2010;257:869–881.

104. Choi EH, Strum W. Hypocupremia-related myeloneuropathy following gastrojejunal bypass surgery. *Ann Nutr Metab* 2010;57:190–192.

105. Btaiche IF, Yeh AY, Wu IJ, Khalidi N. Neurologic dysfunction and pancytopenia secondary to acquired copper deficiency following duodenal switch: case report and review of the literature. *Nutr Clin Pract* 2011;26:583–592.

106. Nations SP, Boyer PJ, Love LA, et al. Denture cream: an unusual source of excess zinc, leading to hypocupremia and neurological disease. *Neurology* 2008;71:639–643.

107. Hedera P, Peltier A, Fink JK, Wilcock S, London Z, Brewer GJ. Myelopolyneuropathy and pancytopenia due to copper deficiency and high zinc levels of unknown origin II. The denture cream is a primary source of excessive zinc. *Neurotoxicology* 2009;30:996–999.

108. Henri-Bhargava A, Melmed C, Glikstein R, Schipper HM. Neurologic impairment due to vitamin E and copper deficiencies in celiac disease. *Neurology* 2008;71:860–861.

109. Kumar N, Elliott MA, Hoyer JD, Harper CM Jr, Ahlskog JE, Phyliky RL. "Myelodysplasia," myeloneuropathy, and copper deficiency. *Mayo Clin Proc* 2005;80:943–946.

110. Kumar N, Butz JA, Burritt MF. Clinical significance of the laboratory determination of low serum copper in adults. *Clin Chem Lab Med* 2007;45:1402–1410.

111. Goodman BP, Bosch EP, Ross MA, Hoffman-Snyder C, Dodick DD, Smith BE. Clinical and electrodiagnostic findings in copper deficiency myeloneuropathy. *J Neurol Neurosurg Psychiatry* 2009:524–527.

112. Kumar N, Ahlskog JE, Klein CJ, Port JD. Imaging features of copper deficiency myelopathy: a study of 25 cases. *Neuroradiology* 2006;48:78–83.
113. Ferrara JM, Skeen MB, Edwards NJ, Gray L, Massey EW. Subacute combined degeneration due to copper deficiency. *J Neuroimaging* 2007;17:375–377.
114. Kumar G, Goyal MK, Lucchese S, Dhand U. Copper deficiency myelopathy can also involve the brain stem. *AJNR Am J Neuroradiol* 2010;10.3174/ajnr.A2261.
115. Boylan LM, Sugerman HJ, Driskell JA. Vitamin E, vitamin B-6, vitamin B-12, and folate status of gastric bypass surgery patients. *J Am Diet Assoc* 1988;88:579–585.
116. Mallory GN, Macgregor AM. Folate status following gastric bypass surgery (the great folate mystery). *Obes Surg* 1991;1:69–72.
117. Dudeja PK, Kode A, Alnounou M, et al. Mechanism of folate transport across the human colonic basolateral membrane. *Am J Physiol Gastrointest Liver Physiol* 2001;281:G54–G60.
118. Machado JD, Campos CS, Lopes Dah Silva C, et al. Intestinal bacterial overgrowth after Roux-en-Y gastric bypass. *Obes Surg* 2008;18:139–143.
119. Shorvon SD, Carney MW, Chanarin I, Reynolds EH. The neuropsychiatry of megaloblastic anaemia. *Br Med J* 1980;281:1036–1038.
120. Reynolds EH. Benefits and risks of folic acid to the nervous system [see comment]. *J Neurol Neurosurg Psychiatry* 2002;72:567–571.
121. Green R, Miller JW. Folate deficiency beyond megaloblastic anemia: hyperhomocysteinemia and other manifestations of dysfunctional folate status. *Semin Hematol* 1999;36:47–64.
122. Diaz-Arrastia R. Homocysteine and neurologic disease. *Arch Neurol* 2000;57:1422–1427.
123. Lucock M, Yates Z. Measurement of red blood cell methylfolate [see comment]. *Lancet* 2002;360:1021–1022; author reply 1022.
124. Gunter EW, Bowman BA, Caudill SP, Twite DB, Adams MJ, Sampson EJ. Results of an international round robin for serum and whole-blood folate [see comment]. *Clin Chem* 1996;42:1689–1694.
125. Stabler SP, Marcell PD, Podell ER, Allen RH, Savage DG, Lindenbaum J. Elevation of total homocysteine in the serum of patients with cobalamin or folate deficiency detected by capillary gas chromatography-mass spectrometry. *J Clin Invest* 1988;81:466–474.
126. de Luis DA, Pacheco D, Izaola O, Terroba MC, Cuellar L, Martin T. Clinical results and nutritional consequences of biliopancreatic diversion: three years of follow-up. *Ann Nutr Metab* 2008;53:234–239.
127. Sokol RJ. Vitamin E deficiency and neurologic disease. *Annu Rev Nutr* 1988;8:351–373.
128. Kleopa KA, Kyriacou K, Zamba-Papanicolaou E, Kyriakides T. Reversible inflammatory and vacuolar myopathy with vitamin E deficiency in celiac disease. *Muscle Nerve* 2005;31:260–265.
129. Puri V, Chaudhry N, Tatke M, Prakash V. Isolated vitamin E deficiency with demyelinating neuropathy. *Muscle Nerve* 2005;32:230–235.
130. Sokol RJ, Heubi JE, Iannaccone ST, Bove KE, Balistreri WF. Vitamin E deficiency with normal serum vitamin E concentrations in children with chronic cholestasis. *N Engl J Med* 1984;310:1209–1212.
131. Vorgerd M, Tegenthoff M, Kuhne D, Malin JP. Spinal MRI in progressive myeloneuropathy associated with vitamin E deficiency. *Neuroradiology* 1996;38(Suppl 1):S111–S113.
132. Marinella MA. Ophthalmoplegia: an unusual manifestation of hypocalcemia. *Am J Emerg Med* 1999;17:105–106.
133. Carlin AM, Rao DS, Meslemani AM, et al. Prevalence of vitamin D depletion among morbidly obese patients seeking gastric bypass surgery. *Surg Obes Relat Dis* 2006;2:98–103; discussion 104.

134. Nelson ML, Bolduc LM, Toder ME, Clough DM, Sullivan SS. Correction of preoperative vitamin D deficiency after Roux-en-Y gastric bypass surgery. *Surg Obes Relat Dis* 2007;3:434–437.

135. Coates PS, Fernstrom JD, Fernstrom MH, Schauer PR, Greenspan SL. Gastric bypass surgery for morbid obesity leads to an increase in bone turnover and a decrease in bone mass. *J Clin Endocrinol Metab* 2004;89:1061–1065.

136. Russell JA. Osteomalacic myopathy [see comment]. *Muscle Nerve* 1994;17:578–580.

137. Pfeifer M, Begerow B, Minne HW. Vitamin D and muscle function. *Osteoporos Int* 2002;13:187–194.

138. Plotnikoff GA, Quigley JM. Prevalence of severe hypovitaminosis D in patients with persistent, nonspecific musculoskeletal pain [see comment]. *Mayo Clin Proc* 2003;78:1463–1470.

139. Gloth FM 3rd, Lindsay JM, Zelesnick LB, Greenough WB 3rd. Can vitamin D deficiency produce an unusual pain syndrome? [see comment]. *Arch Intern Med* 1991;151:1662–1664.

140. Ramagopalan SV, Maugeri NJ, Handunnetthi L, et al. Expression of the multiple sclerosis-associated MHC class II allele HLA-DRB1*1501 is regulated by vitamin D. *PLoS Genet* 2009;5:e1000369.

141. Annweiler C, Allali G, Allain P, et al. Vitamin D and cognitive performance in adults: a systematic review. *Eur J Neurol* 2009;16:1083–1089.

142. Miller JW. Vitamin D and cognitive function in older adults: are we concerned about vitamin D-mentia? *Neurology* 2010;74:13–15.

143. Seamans KM, Cashman KD. Existing and potentially novel functional markers of vitamin D status: a systematic review. *Am J Clin Nutr* 2009:2009.27230Dv27231.

144. Brolin RE. Gastric bypass. *Surg Clin North Am* 2001;81:1077–1095.

145. Mason ME, Jalagani H, Vinik AI. Metabolic complications of bariatric surgery: diagnosis and management issues. *Gastroenterol Clin North Am* 2005;34:25–33.

146. Brolin RE, Gorman RC, Milgrim LM, Kenler HA. Multivitamin prophylaxis in prevention of post-gastric bypass vitamin and mineral deficiencies. *Int J Obes* 1991;15:661–667.

147. Gasteyger C, Suter M, Gaillard RC, Giusti V. Nutritional deficiencies after Roux-en-Y gastric bypass for morbid obesity often cannot be prevented by standard multivitamin supplementation. *Am J Clin Nutr* 2008;87:1128–1133.

148. Malone M. Recommended nutritional supplements for bariatric surgery patients. *Ann Pharmacother* 2008;42:1851–1858.

149. Matrana MR, Davis WE. Vitamin deficiency after gastric bypass surgery: a review. *South Med J* 2009;102:1025–1031.

7 Selected Nutritional Deficiencies (Zinc, Selenium, Vitamins A, D, E, and K, and Niacin)

Yaniv Cozacov, Hira Ahmad, and Raul J. Rosenthal

CONTENTS

7.1 INTRODUCTION

Trace elements and vitamins play an essential role in homeostasis and biochemical processes needed for life, such as cellular utilization of oxygen, DNA reproduction, and maintaining cell membrane integrity. Deficiencies may present with specific syndromes, or a spectrum of clinical presentations, from malaise and loss of appetite to severe infections and heart failure.[1] While access to proper nutrition is necessary, also important are the amounts of the different nutrients ingested by food choices made, and that absorption proceeds in a suitable fashion.[2] There are few studies examining preoperative and postoperative nutritional status in morbidly obese patients opting for metabolic surgery, and the reported prevalence of nutritional deficiencies varies widely due to differences in definitions of deficiency, patient populations, surgical techniques, supplement protocols, and lengths and completion of patient follow-up.[3,4]

We have entered a new era in clinical gastroenterology, one in which malnutrition and malabsorption are by-products of metabolic surgery. Although much research has been done on short-term and long-term effects of bariatric surgery on weight loss, less is known about its long-term clinical and nutritional consequences of changes in the gastrointestinal anatomy and physiology. This also refers to the change in the quantity and quality of diet, which results in vitamin and mineral deficiencies.[3] The latency period of overt and subclinical symptoms differs, depending on the micronutrient in question, and we have to consider the relatively young age of some of our patients, as the postoperative course may take over a period of several decades.[5]

Malabsorptive bariatric procedures, such as Roux-en-Y gastric bypass (RYGB) and biliopancreatic diversion and duodenal switch (BPD-DS), produce a mild form of pancreatic insufficiency, resulting correspondingly in malabsorption of both proteins and fats.[5] Pancreatico-cibal asynchrony, a relative pancreatic insufficiency, also potentially contributes to the malabsorption as the intestinal reconstruction excludes the passage of food through the duodenum. Some have even reported adding pancreatic enzyme replacement therapy in order to reduce fat malabsorption.[6,7]

If previously thought that micronutrient deficiency was solely the result of metabolic surgery, today we know that malnourishment and poor quality of foods are major factors contributing to nutrient deficiency found in patients opting for bariatric surgery. These poor nutritional habits of morbidly obese patients make them more susceptible to lower levels of vitamins. Thus, morbid obesity should be considered a malnutritional state.

Various studies have shown that in RYGB, the magnitude of fat malabsorption is highly variable and correlates with the length of proximal jejunum used to create the biliopancreatic limb, but no correlation was found between the Roux limb length measurement and micronutrient serum concentrations. Biliopancreatic limbs of 40–50 cm had reduced fat absorption by an average of 10 g/day, whereas 70–75 cm biliopancreatic limbs reduced fat absorption by an average of 40 g/day.[8] Shortening of the common channel and increased delay of the delivery of the digestive secretions, while at the same time the pancreatic lipase is becoming less effective, are the main culprits of the reduced absorption. Also, longer biliopancreatic limbs predispose to bacterial overgrowth, which results in the deconjugation of bile acids, further retarding fat digestion and absorption of fat-soluble vitamins and minerals.[9–11]

The fat malabsorption described here does not occur in patients undergoing laparoscopic sleeve gastrectomy (LSG). In the postoperative course of LSG, there is no suggestion for vitamin supplementation, and evidence-based data on necessity of supplementation as a result of LSG do not exist in literature. In contrast, as mentioned here, preoperative existing deficits should be supplemented.[12] It should also be kept in mind that the nutritional deficiencies are a concern after any bariatric surgery procedure due to the oral restriction and not just malabsorption. When comparing nutritional deficiencies after LSG and RYGB, it was found that overall LSG had fewer incidences of nutrient deficiencies in the first 2 years after surgery than RYGB.[13]

Serum levels of selected vitamins and micronutrients might decrease despite the use of a vitamin-mineral supplement, and patients need a regular follow-up and individualized prescription of supplementation after the surgical procedure in order to prevent and treat early vitamin deficiencies.[14] It should always be remembered that for patients who have any evidence of protein-calorie malnutrition, deficient micronutrient levels are highly associated and should also be addressed.

7.2 VITAMIN A

7.2.1 INTRODUCTION

Vitamin A deficiency after metabolic surgery is an underreported complication that deserves critical attention in the ongoing medical management of our patients. Its well-known function is in rhodopsin formation and the prevention of night blindness. Vitamin A also plays a role in immune function, skin health, and antioxidant activity. Epithelial cells are highly dependent on vitamin A, which also elucidates its role in wound healing in patients on chronic steroids.

7.2.2 BIOCHEMISTRY

Vitamin A is a fat-soluble vitamin, referring to different retinols. Precursors of vitamin A are the carotenoids, β-carotene being the most common. The structure of the metabolites of retinols plays a role in their function. A covalent double bond is responsible for the unique role in vision processes. As oxidation and polymerization destroy retinoids, they must be protected from light, oxygen, and high temperature.[15]

7.2.3 ABSORPTION AND METABOLISM

Foods rarely have the active form of vitamin A, retinol. Precursors are found in foods of animal origin: egg yolks, liver, fish oil, whole milk, and butter. Carotenoid molecules vary greatly. They are red, yellow, and orange in color. Vitamin A is 70–90% absorbed in the small intestine by way of micelles across the brush border into the enterocyte, and then are packaged into chylomicrons.[16] The efficiency of this absorption is estimated to be 60–80% and is best in the proximal upper GI, but decreases lower in the gut. Within the enterocytes, carotenoids are converted to active forms of the vitamin.

Carotenoids circulate bound to retinol-binding protein (RBP), which is synthesized by the liver. In the liver they are further metabolized or stored. Fifty to eighty-five percent of the total body retinols are stored in the liver. The precursor, however, β-carotene, can be stored in adipose cells. The kidneys are mainly responsible for excretion of RBP and retinol via renal catabolism and glomerular filtration.[17]

7.2.4 ETIOLOGY OF DEFICIENCY

Normally the liver contains a 2-year storage of vitamin A,[18] but up to 80% of morbidly obese patients have inadequate stores[19]; therefore, in this adult patient population only a 4-week period might be given prior to deficiency ensuing when on a nutrient-deficient diet.[20] Vitamin A deficiency is shown to be present in patients preoperatively.[14] For patients undergoing RYGB, vitamin A deficiency prevalence was found in astonishing ranges from 10 to 69%—in many cases, despite supplementation.[21–23] A summary of the etiology, signs and symptoms, and treatment of deficiency is shown in Table 7.1.

Increased incidence of vitamin A deficiency is also found 3, 6, and 12 months postoperatively.[14,24] Different studies have used different postoperative time frames for follow-up measurements of vitamin A. Reports claim as much as 50% deficiency in patients 30 days postoperatively. Some studies have shown improvement at 1 year, but others did not. It has been reported that 69% of patients undergoing RYGB were deficient at 4 years postoperatively, signifying the underacknowledged status and chronicity of the deficiency.[22,23,25,26]

TABLE 7.1
Deficiencies and Treatment

Vitamin	Etiology of Deficiency	Signs/Symptoms	Treatment
Vitamin A	**Primary vitamin A deficiency** is usually caused by prolonged decreased dietary intake **Secondary vitamin A deficiency** may be due to decreased bioavailability of provitamin A carotenoids or interference with absorption, storage, or transport of vitamin A Deficiency is common in prolonged protein–energy insufficiency Vitamin A deficiency is more prevalent after malabsorptive bariatric surgery due to reduced intake of foods high in vitamin A and fat needed for fat-soluble vitamin absorption as well as malabsorption induced by bypassing the duodenum Longer biliopancreatic limbs predispose one to bacterial overgrowth resulting in deconjugation of bile acids and further reduced fat digestion and absorption of fat-soluble vitamin A	• Impaired wound healing • Night blindness • Bitot spots, conjunctival xerosis, xerophthalmia • Drying, scaling, and follicular thickening of the skin and respiratory infections can result	Dietary deficiency is traditionally treated with vitamin A palmitate in oil 60,000 IU po once/day for 2 days, followed by 4500 IU po once/day If vomiting or malabsorption is present or xerophthalmia is probable, a 200,000 IU dose should be given to an adult for 2 days, with a third dose at least 2 weeks later Without corneal changes: 10,000–25,000 IU/day vitamin A orally until clinical improvement (usually 1–2 weeks) With corneal changes: 50,000–100,000 IU vitamin A IM for 3 days followed by 50,000 IU/day IM for 2 weeks Evaluate for concurrent iron and copper deficiency, which can impair resolution of vitamin A deficiency

(Continued)

TABLE 7.1 (CONTINUED)
Deficiencies and Treatment

Vitamin	Etiology of Deficiency	Signs/Symptoms	Treatment
Vitamin D	**Reduced absorption:** Malabsorption can deprive the body of dietary vitamin D; only a small amount of 25(OH)D is recirculated enterohepatically Vitamin D deficiency is more prevalent after bariatric surgery, in part due to reduced intake of foods high in vitamin D and fat needed for fat-soluble vitamin absorption, but also to malabsorption induced by bypassing the duodenum Longer biliopancreatic limbs predispose one to bacterial overgrowth, resulting in deconjugation of bile acids and further reduced fat digestion and absorption of fat-soluble vitamin D **Inadequate exposure or intake:** Inadequate direct sunlight exposure or sunscreen use in combination with inadequate intake may result in clinical deficiency	• Muscle aches, muscle weakness, and bone pain • Hypocalcemia, which may cause tetany and paresthesias of the lips, tongue, and fingers, carpopedal and facial spasm, and if very severe, seizures • Osteomalacia, osteoporosis	To treat the deficiency, correct deficiencies of Ca and phosphate and give supplemental vitamin D; higher doses of vitamin D_2 (e.g., 25,000–50,000 IU every week or every month) are sometimes prescribed; because vitamin D_3 is more potent than vitamin D_2, it is now preferred 50,000 IU/week ergocalciferol (D_2) orally or intramuscularly, for 8 weeks

(Continued)

TABLE 7.1 (CONTINUED)
Deficiencies and Treatment

Vitamin	Etiology of Deficiency	Signs/Symptoms	Treatment
Vitamin E	Vitamin E deficiency may occur after bariatric surgery in part due to reduced intake of foods high in vitamin E and fat needed for fat-soluble vitamin absorption Malabsorption induced by bypassing the duodenum Longer biliopancreatic limbs predispose one to bacterial overgrowth resulting in deconjugation of bile acids and further reduced fat digestion and absorption of fat-soluble vitamin E	• The main symptoms are mild hemolytic anemia and nonspecific neurologic deficits—ataxia, weakness, and vision changes • Abetalipoproteinemia results in progressive neuropathy and retinopathy in the first two decades of life • In children, chronic cholestatic hepatobiliary disease or cystic fibrosis causes neurologic deficits, including spinocerebellar ataxia with loss of deep tendon reflexes, truncal and limb ataxia, loss of vibration and position senses, ophthalmoplegia, muscle weakness, ptosis, and dysarthria • In adults with malabsorption, vitamin E deficiency very rarely causes spinocerebellar ataxia because adults have large vitamin E stores in adipose tissue	If malabsorption causes clinically evident deficiency, α-tocopherol 15–25 mg/kg po once daily should be given; mixed tocopherols (200 to 400 IU) can be given However, larger doses of α-tocopherol given by injection are required to treat neuropathy during its early stages or to overcome the defect of absorption and transport in abetalipoproteinemia An optimal therapeutic dose of vitamin E has not been clearly defined; potential antioxidant benefits of vitamin E can be achieved with supplements of 100–400 IU/day

(Continued)

TABLE 7.1 (CONTINUED)
Deficiencies and Treatment

Vitamin	Etiology of Deficiency	Signs/Symptoms	Treatment
Vitamin K	Deficiency results from extremely inadequate oral intake, fat malabsorption, or use of warfarin Long-term antibiotic use may also precipitate vitamin K deficiency potentially due to changes in gut microflora lending to reduced vitamin K synthesis Deficiency may occur after bariatric surgery in part due to reduced intake of foods high in vitamin K and fat needed for fat-soluble vitamin absorption, but also to malabsorption induced by bypassing the duodenum Longer biliopancreatic limbs predispose one to bacterial overgrowth resulting in deconjugation of bile acids and further reduced fat digestion and absorption of fat-soluble vitamin K	• Easy bruisability and mucosal bleeding (especially epistaxis, GI hemorrhage, menorrhagia, and hematuria) can occur • Low levels of vitamin K have been found in those with osteoporosis; vitamin K is common therapy for osteoporosis in Japan and other countries	Phytonadione (USP generic name for vitamin K_1) should be given po or sc; the usual adult dose is 1–20 mg (rarely, even when it is correctly diluted and given slowly, IV replacement can result in anaphylaxis or anaphylactoid reactions) Parenteral dose of 10 mg For chronic malabsorption, 1–2 mg/day, orally, or 1–2 mg/week parenterally

This postoperative vitamin A deficiency may persist or develop despite daily supplementation.[14,22] Vitamin A deficiency potentially worsens after the RYGB procedure.[23,27,28] The increased prevalence of abnormal postoperative levels may be associated with lower intake of foods containing vitamin A and fats and due to malabsorption caused by the exclusion of the main absorption site.

Vitamin A directly correlates with prealbumin levels; thus, the more malnourished the patient is, the more likely he or she is to be vitamin A deficient.[24] On the other hand, interaction of retinol with carrier proteins determines the serum vitamin A concentration, and thus total body stores of vitamin A may not be truly deficient. The latter has been shown, whereby addressing the protein malnutrition, the micronutrient levels normalize.[29]

7.2.5 Signs and Symptoms of Deficiency

Surprisingly, despite the high incidence of low vitamin A levels, clinical manifestations of deficiency are scarce after gastric bypass and respond rapidly to vitamin A supplementation. For BPD, several case reports detailed ophthalmologic complications such as night blindness and corneal xerosis postoperatively.[30,31]

Vitamin A is also essential for the developing fetus. The eyes, heart, ears, and lungs depend on retinoic acid. Vitamin A plays a role in glycoprotein synthesis and signaling pathways, enhancing communication, recognition, adhesion, and aggregation at the cellular level.

Gestational night blindness is associated with complex fetal complications, such as increased risk of low birth weight, diarrhea, acute respiratory disease, poor growth, and microphthalmia.[32] A reported untreated mother who developed night blindness with undetectable serum vitamin A concentrations during the third trimester delivered an infant who proved to be vitamin A deficient as well. Also reported was a temporary neonatal blindness case in an infant born to a mother with vitamin A deficiency and nyctalopia from a previous bariatric surgery she had.[33]

This exemplifies the importance of treating nutrient deficiencies, to prevent offspring from experiencing consequences in female metabolic surgery patients.[33] To date, there is no recommendation for vitamin A supplementation for pregnant women who underwent bariatric surgery, but it should be considered. A daily dose of 10,000 IU of retinol acetate orally was shown to be the most suitable in a postoperative RYGB patient. This dose is safe for use by pregnant women with no risk of teratogenicity.[32]

Among all micronutrients, vitamin A is considered the micronutrient most closely associated with infectious diseases. The underlying mechanism is uncertain, although the importance of adequate vitamin A in maintaining epithelial "barrier" integrity and immune competence is suggestive. It has been shown that pregnant women having night blindness are at highly increased risk for morbidity and mortality from infectious causes, especially of the urinary, digestive, and respiratory systems.[34]

A low-fat diet, which potentially limits the absorption of fat-soluble vitamins, and higher levels of oxidative stress occurring after surgery are both potential culprits for vitamin A deficiency.[35] Liver disease, of any etiology, may exacerbate an underlying deficiency by reducing hepatic stores and the production of retinol-binding protein.[18]

A negative correlation between retinol, β-carotene, and BMI exists. The higher the BMI, the higher the risk there is of being vitamin A deficient. This was shown with no significant difference with regard to the dietary ingestion of sources for vitamin A. This implies that higher metabolic utilization against oxidative stress is present in morbidly obese patients.[22] Furthermore, these low concentrations of circulating antioxidants may contribute to an increased risk and to severity of atherosclerotic disease.

Decreased visual acuity over time could be attributed secondary to diabetic retinopathy, and one should be careful to rule out vitamin A deficiency as a cause, as early vitamin A replenishment can rapidly improve visual function, but if delayed, permanent damage can ensue.[36] Following metabolic surgery, up to 70% of patients have been reported to complain of decreased night vision and 33% noted the new onset of persistently dry eyes postoperatively. Furthermore, 39% of patients report a subjective decline in visual acuity in the postoperative period.[16]

Night blindness associated with vitamin A deficiency is probably more common after duodenal switch,[37,38] but it is also seen after gastric bypass surgery.[16,39] A patient with vitamin A deficiency after undergoing BPD surgery was reported to have visual deterioration up to the point of legal blindness 3 years postoperatively. The patient also failed to consume vitamin supplements 18 months prior to presentation.[26] After 6 months of treatment, the patient's visual acuity returned to 20/40 in both eyes.

It is important to become familiar with the earliest symptoms of vitamin A deficiency, including impaired dark adaptation, or simply night blindness. Later on, xerophthalmia, corneal xerosis, and corneal scarring develop. Keratomalacia and xerophthalmia are accompanied by Bitot signs (white spots on the conjunctiva due to the collection of corneal substances). Surgeons must recognize that the development and progression of these abnormalities occur insidiously over weeks, months, or years, especially for symptoms of optic neuropathy.

The vitamin A deficiency complication of xerosis was reported in up to 38% of patients, night vision changes for 68%, and 23% of patients report eye pain or foreign body sensation. Interestingly enough, some were not found to have low serum levels of vitamin A.[16] This highlights the importance of questioning any visual changes during the follow-up visits.

7.2.6 TREATMENT

The Recommended Dietary Allowance (RDA) of vitamin A is 1000 mg of retinol equivalents (RE) for men and 800 mg RE for women. One RE of vitamin A is equal to 3.33 IU of the vitamin. Rarely, symptoms of hypervitaminosis can occur, including anorexia, headache, bone and muscle pain, vomiting, alopecia, liver damage, and coma. These symptoms can often be reversed when vitamin A intake levels are reduced.

7.2.7 CONCLUSION

Perhaps all metabolic surgery patients should undergo vitamin A level determinations pre- and postoperatively on an annual basis, with appropriate referral for ophthalmologic evaluation for any patient with ocular complaints and vitamin A deficiency. It is prudent to ask the bariatric patient at any follow-up examination for night blindness, and it is imperative to take note of the potential of an epidemic syndrome of iatrogenic vitamin A deficiency, given the astonishing increase in worldwide obesity and metabolic surgery.

7.3 VITAMIN D

Vitamin D is a hormone regulating both skeletal and extraskeletal functions, including immune function, cancer prevention, and cardiovascular health.[40] It is well described that obese people are predisposed to vitamin D deficiency.[41,42] Some of the theories identified are hepatic feedback inhibition by increased serum $1,25(OH)_2D$ precursor,[43] sunlight underexposure,[44] and reduced bioavailability of vitamin D because of sequestration by adipose tissue.[45] Hyperparathyroidism has been observed in 25–48% in the morbidly obese presenting to bariatric surgery as well,[4,46,47] where some claim that hypovitaminosis D with secondary hyperparathyroidism should be added to the crowded list of sequelae of morbid obesity.

Metabolic bone disease, calcium, and vitamin D regulation are discussed in further detail elsewhere in this book.

7.4   VITAMIN E

7.4.1   INTRODUCTION AND BIOCHEMISTRY

Vitamin E refers to a group of eight fat-soluble compounds that include both tocopherols and tocotrienols. The attachment of different groups to the carbon ring determines whether the vitamin is alpha, beta, gamma, or delta. Most of the research is focused on the α-tocopherol form of vitamin E, as it is the most biologically active form[48]; thus, the two terms (*vitamin E* and *α-tocopherol*) are used interchangeably.

Vitamin E (α-tocopherol) is the main lipid-soluble antioxidant that protects against the lipid peroxidation of membranes.[49] It is a free radical scavenger, preventing lipid peroxidation within the cells and organelles. Vitamin E also has a role in red blood cells' flexibility as they make their way through the arterial network.

Plants synthesize vitamin E, and it is mainly found in vegetable oils, leafy vegetables, fruits, meats, and nuts. It is stored within fatty tissues of animals and humans due to its fat-soluble properties. Even though a diet that includes meat supplies vitamin E, the amount of vitamin E obtained from plant sources is a lot greater than that obtained from a meat-inclusive diet.[17]

7.4.2   ABSORPTION AND METABOLISM

The bioavailability of vitamin E is dependent on the fat content of food. Vitamin E bioavailability from fortified breakfast cereal is greater than that from encapsulated supplements.[50] Vitamin E absorption requires bile acids, fatty acids, and monoglycerides for micelle formation. The absorption of vitamin E is less than 50%. Once the micelle crosses the water layer and releases its contents into the enterocyte, vitamin E is packaged into chylomicrons and enters the circulation.

In terms of storage, 90% of vitamin E is found in adipose tissue.[51] It is unclear if a specific organ is responsible for storage and release of vitamin E as needed. Vitamin E is excreted mainly via bile, urine, feces, and the skin. It is first oxidized, and then conjugated to form glucoronate in the liver. It may undergo further degradation by the kidneys, to be excreted in the urine. However, the main route of vitamin E elimination is via feces.

7.4.3   ETIOLOGY OF DEFICIENCY

It has been suggested that increased adiposity contributes to the increased oxidative stress in obese patients.[52] Weight loss surgery might alleviate some of the damage by an indirect effect of lowering the total mass of adipose. But this effect could be counteracted by the decreased bioavailability of antioxidants, such as vitamin E, thus signifying again the importance of balanced nutrition.[49] In contrast, when evaluating oxidative stress after vertical-type banding, increased concentrations of vitamin E were reported after surgery; therefore, decreased weight seems to decrease oxidative stress, and when nutrient absorption is not disturbed, increased levels of antioxidants and vitamin E specifically are noted.

Because of the ubiquitous distribution of tocopherols in foods, symptomatic vitamin E deficiency virtually is never the consequence of a dietary inadequacy.[53] For patients undergoing metabolic surgery, up to 20% of patients showed vitamin E deficiency preoperatively, 26% at 6 months, 60% at 1 year, and 65.7% at 2 years after RYGB.[49,54] On the other hand, some report low concentrations of vitamin E tendency at baseline, rather than after RYGB. Some patients were reported to be deficient despite daily supplementation of 10 mg vitamin E per day.[39]

7.4.4 SIGNS AND SYMPTOMS OF DEFICIENCY

Symptomatic deficiency of vitamin E is uncommon. At 1–4 years after undergoing RYGB and BPD-DS, although 4–10% of subjects were found to be vitamin E deficient, no clinical manifestations were reported.[55–58]

In childhood, a deficiency could lead to spinocerebellar syndrome with peripheral nerve involvement, presenting similar to Friedreich's ataxia. An onset of ataxia, hyporeflexia, proprioceptive and vibratory loss, and ophthalmoplegia and ptosis in an adolescent patient should always prompt a metabolic surgeon to think about spinocerebellar syndrome.

In cases in which the deficiency is due to a malabsorptive procedure, regular supplementation doses may be inadequate, and large oral dosages or intramuscular administration of vitamin E should be used when replenishing body stores. If fat malabsorption is a complication of the bariatric patient, a water-miscible product is available and effective.[50] However, the majority of patients who consumed supplements of vitamin E near the RDA were found to maintain a normal vitamin status at 1 year after having RYGB.[55]

7.4.5 TREATMENT

One milligram of vitamin E is approximately 30–50% in the alpha form and therefore is readily absorbed. The other forms are not stored as efficiently and usually are therefore excreted. Consequently, the RDA of vitamin E is set based on the α-tocopherol form of the vitamin. Fifteen IU of α-tocopherol a day for both men and women is sufficient. Toxicity is not a major concern.

7.5 VITAMIN K

7.5.1 INTRODUCTION

Vitamin K refers to a group of related compounds. Each form serves as an essential nutrient required by the liver for posttranslational modifications of proteins. The major function of vitamin K is as a cofactor in the synthesis of clotting factors VII,

IX, and X and prothrombin, as well as proteins C and S. It also serves as a cofactor for some proteins in regulation of osteocalcin and bone formation.

7.5.2 BIOCHEMISTRY

The two main types for vitamin K are dietary vitamin K_1 (phylloquinone or phytonadione), found in green vegetables like spinach and broccoli, and vitamin K_2 (menaquinones), synthesized by gut flora. Vitamin K_2 has about 60% of the activity of vitamin K_1.

7.5.3 ABSORPTION AND METABOLISM

Sources of vitamin K are either diet or bacterial production in the colon, both of which are affected after metabolic surgery. Vitamin K_1 is synthesized by plants. Common sources of vitamin K_1 in diet are kale, spinach, collards, Swiss chard, mustard greens, turnips, broccoli, brussel sprouts, cabbage, and asparagus. Sources for vitamin K_2 include goose liver pate, hard and soft cheeses, egg yolk, butter, and chicken liver.[59]

For women, 90 µg/day, and 120 µg/day for men are considered to be adequate intakes.[60] Dietary intake provides about half of the requirement, and the intestinal bacteria produce the other half. Just two tablespoons of parsley contain 153% of the RDA of vitamin K.[60]

Dietary vitamin K is protein-bound and cleaved by pancreatic enzymes and solubilized by bile salts, aiding in absorption from the proximal intestine. The efficiency of this absorption is about 80%. Similar to other fat-soluble vitamins, vitamin K is incorporated into chylomicrons, secreted into the lymph, and it then enters the bloodstream.[60]

Vitamin K_2 is the main storage form of vitamin K. Bacteria in the colon convert K_1 to K_2, and in addition add various side chains to K_2 to produce its various types. However, vitamin K is not stored in the body to any significant degree. The liver stores 90% of vitamin K in its dietary form. But the stores are very labile, and concentrations drop to 25% just 3 days after dietary depletion. Other stores include, to a lesser degree, adipose tissue and bone.[61] Vitamin K is mainly excreted in feces via bile, and in small amounts in the urine.[60]

7.5.4 ETIOLOGY OF DEFICIENCY

As it is widely distributed in plants and produced by readily available gut flora, vitamin K deficiency in the United States is rare. Also, vitamin K is easily recycled within cells. Nonetheless, it is well known that a long-term antibiotic regimen may precipitate vitamin K deficiency. Also, similar to other micronutrients in complicated cases of metabolic surgery requiring additional hospitalization and the use of total parenteral nutrition, patients may require supplementation of vitamin K as well.

7.5.5 Signs and Symptoms of Deficiency

Clinical signs and symptoms of vitamin K deficiency include easy bruisability, mucosal bleeding, or any other sign of unexplained bleeding due to coagulation abnormality. Depending on the severity of vitamin K deficiency, only prothrombin time (PT) may be abnormally elevated in mild deficiency, but both PT and partial thromboplastin time (PTT) may be affected in severe deficiencies. Although elevated PT implies vitamin K deficiency, normal levels do not rule out a subclinical deficiency.

In the adult population, subjects with liver disease, cystic fibrosis, inflammatory bowel disease, or bulimia, or people on drugs such as salicylates or barbiturates, can develop vitamin K deficiency. There has also been a report of a patient treated for pneumococcal sepsis and purpura fulminans who had undergone RYGB. The significant and persistent reductions in proteins C and S related to depleted vitamin K were thought to precipitate the hypercoagulable state, resulting in disseminated intravascular coagulation (DIC) and subsequent intravascular hemolysis.[62]

Compared to adults, newborns are at increased risk for vitamin K deficiency.[63] There is a universal consensus for the need for vitamin K prophylaxis in newborns,[64] and probably the most important issue with vitamin K relates to pregnancy. Metabolic surgery has been reported to increase fertility in women[65] as well as to decrease overall maternal morbidity,[66] but not without risk. Severe complications resulting from maternal, and subsequently fetal, vitamin K deficiency have been reported. The main severe complication relates to intracranial bleeding of the newborn. The deficiency could also affect the mother, causing complications, such as postpartum haemorrhage.[67]

Another very severe complication, thought to be related to malabsorptive metabolic surgery (BDP-DS and RYGB) associated with extreme vitamin K depletion, is chondrodysplasia punctata.[68] It is a severe complication with extreme dysmorphia and multiple anomalies, which may eventually lead to the death of the newborn. There is a similarity between the pathophysiology of chondrodysplasia punctata and the teratogenicity seen with warfarin.

7.5.6 Conclusion

Young females undergoing metabolic surgery should be educated on vitamin supplementation and dietary choices so that they can understand the future consequences of the different deficiencies and complications associated with noncompliance. Patients should keep in mind that careful nutritional follow-up during pregnancy is mandatory, because nutritional deficiencies such as vitamin K deficiency can lead to life-threatening bleeding.[69] It is also important for the physician to know how to prevent the possible poor dramatic outcomes.

7.6 ZINC

7.6.1 INTRODUCTION

Zinc's role in human biology was defined in 1961, when it was speculated that Iranian males may have suffered from growth retardation and hypogonadism due to its deficiency.[70]

7.6.2 BIOCHEMISTRY

Zinc is needed for DNA synthesis, cell division, gene expression, activity of various enzymes, and wound healing. It is essential for normal development and function of cell-mediating innate immunity, neutrophils, and natural killer cells.[71] The latter was shown when zinc deficiency led to atrophy of the thymus and lymphoid tissue in experimental animals.[72] Zinc supplementation also has various benefits in humans, regardless of a deficiency, such as in treatment of common cold,[73] or when given in combination with INF-α, where it was found to be more effective against chronic hepatitis C than therapy with INF-α alone.[74] Zinc has also been shown to reduce the duration, severity, and incidence of diarrhea in children in developing countries.[75]

Correction of zinc deficiency improves the absorption of water and electrolytes by the intestine, leads to a faster regeneration of the gut epithelium, and increases the levels of enterocyte brush-border enzymes after an episode of acute gastritis. Treatment of *Helicobacter pylori* with polaprezinc (zinc-L-carnosine, an antiulcer drug) led to an improved cure rate in combination with antimicrobial triple therapy.[76]

7.6.3 ABSORPTION AND METABOLISM

Zinc is mainly found in red meat, poultry, and fortified breakfast cereal in the Western diet.[77] It is absorbed in the duodenum and proximal jejunum. Deficiencies of zinc (and copper) could be the result of accumulation of adipose tissue, which in turn increases the production of adipocytokines, causing a chronic inflammatory state. The latter induces the expression of proteins in hepatocytes, promoting metal accumulation in the liver and in fat cells, lowering zinc levels.[78]

7.6.4 ETIOLOGY OF DEFICIENCY

In patients opting for metabolic surgery, the prevalence of zinc deficiency was found to be at large. In the literature it has been reported that 14–75% of patients preoperatively were found to be zinc deficient. The prevalence changes postoperatively. Some reported improvement, while others found the contrary to be true. Nonetheless, low zinc plasma levels were found in 34–68% of the patients 2 months after RYGB procedure,[79] and at 50% prevalence 4 years postoperatively.[13,23,25,54,78,79]

7.6.5 Signs and Symptoms of Deficiency

Zinc deficiency could occur in all bariatric procedures, but more commonly in RYGB and BPD-DS. The most common complaint referenced to zinc deficiency is hair loss.[80] It is reported to occur in up to a third of patients after undergoing vertical banded gastroplasty. If frank hair loss is not observed, thinning of the hair has been reported, as well as sparsity of pubic and axillary hair.[81] Hair loss can be easily reversed by supplementation of 600 mg of zinc sulfate daily.

Probably due to the role of zinc in immunity and epithelial growth, enterocutaneous fistula and surgical wound infection complications have been reported to be associated with zinc-deficient patients. Acrodermatitis enterohepatica is characterized by periorificial (around the natural orifices) and acral dermatitis, alopecia (loss of hair), and diarrhea. Early skin signs include erythematous desquamative patterns and eczematous plaques, which may eventually evolve into vesiculobullous lesions. Nail abnormalities such as onychodystrophy and paronychia, as well as ocular findings and mucosal lesions such as stomatitis, angular cheilitis, blepharitis, conjunctivitis, and photophobia, are less common.[82]

7.6.6 Treatment

Supplementation of zinc is recommended at 60 mg.[83] Based on symptoms such as hair loss, immune deficiency, or dry skin, 220 mg per day or every other day is reasonable.[84] Zinc and calcium supplementation should be suggested to be taken at different times, because zinc reduces calcium absorption.[12] High zinc intake also reduces absorption of copper and iron and vice versa.[85]

7.6.7 Conclusion

It is imperative for caregivers to know how to recognize the specific skin and hair loss changes discussed above, and take zinc deficiency into consideration in the differential diagnosis of similar symptoms among patients who underwent metabolic surgery.

7.7 SELENIUM

7.7.1 Introduction

Selenium is an essential micronutrient in the diet. It has significant health benefits, and is becoming recognized as one of the more promising cancer chemopreventative agents. Selenium deficiency was described historically in endemic areas where the soil is deficient in this metal. The entity selenium-deficient dilated cardiomyopathy was first described in 1935 in the Keshan Province of China, where the disorder was reversed to an extent with selenium supplementation. Prophylactic use of selenium has eradicated this syndrome.[86]

7.7.2   BIOCHEMISTRY

Selenium functions in some selenoproteins, though its most important role is in the cellular antioxidant defense system, being a cofactor for glutathione peroxidase, which catalyzes reactions that remove reactive oxygen species. It also acts in various metabolic processes in the liver, kidney, heart, skeletal muscle, lens of the eye, and erythrocytes.[87]

In the thyroid gland, selenium serves as a cofactor for thyroid hormone deiodinases, which activate and deactivate thyroid hormones and their metabolites. Selenium was also found to have positive outcomes in treatment of Hashimoto's disease, reducing TPO antibody levels.[88]

7.7.3   ABSORPTION AND METABOLISM

Selenium-rich foods include Brazil nuts, sunflower seeds, fish, shellfish, meats, poultry, mushrooms, grains, and onions—all of which may be avoided early on in the period following metabolic surgery, as they are hard to pass through the narrowed lumens. As patients go into their first postoperative year, some may be able to partially tolerate these foods, though others may be persistently intolerant, reducing their selenium intake. Bread is also a common source of dietary selenium in the United States.

7.7.4   ETIOLOGY OF DEFICIENCY

Patients undergoing bariatric surgery can be considered at risk for selenium deficiency based on overall reduction in nutrient intake and the fact that the majority of selenium uptake occurs in the duodenum and proximal jejunum. Almost 100% of selenomethionin is absorbed from the duodenum. The presence of other antioxidants in nutritional intake after bariatric surgery, such as vitamins E and C, appears to enhance the absorption of selenium.[89]

Obese patients were shown to have lower selenium and glutathione peroxidase levels despite adequate intake of dietary selenium. This finding worsened with increasing features of the metabolic syndrome.[90,91] For patients opting for metabolic surgery, a third were shown to be selenium deficient preoperatively.[54] Some have reported the preoperative prevalence of low selenium levels to be 58% among the bariatric patient popplulation.[23]

Postoperatively, patients show a 25% drop in selenium levels 3 months after either metabolic procedure, despite adequate intake of selenium; thus, it is postulated that the surgery itself has an acute effect on selenium and glutathione peroxidase levels, possibly consuming antioxidants in the postoperative recovery period. The latter is supported by the fact that levels return to baseline within 1 year of the procedure, and only 3% of patients are found to be deficient, though some reported 14–22% deficiency.[23,80,89]

More importantly, in cases where metabolic surgery has undergone a complication, and the patient requires further hospitalization, and later might even rely on total parenteral nutrition (TPN) as his or her sole source of nutrition, dilated cardio-myopathy due to selenium deficiency poses a serious morbidity.

7.7.5 SIGNS AND SYMPTOMS OF DEFICIENCY

Roughly a dozen cases of cardiomyopathy have been ascribed to selenium deficiency resulting from chronic TPN use or GI disease, almost half resulting in death. The survivors experienced reversal of cardiomyopathy symptoms after selenium was added to their TPN solutions. Cardiomyopathy may be responsive in just a few days to selenium therapy, where patients significantly improve and can be sent home on maintenance intravenous selenium.

Another exemplification for the level of suspicion needed in a bariatric patient is described for a hypoalbumenic patient with symptoms of lethargy and weak-ness and found to be malnourished who received TPN in order to correct his or her nutritional status. But 2 weeks after initiation of TPN, the patient experienced chest tightness, breathlessness, anxiety, and symptoms of acute dilated congestive heart failure (peripheral edema, bilateral pleural effusions, and ascites), along with an abnormal ECG.[92] Troponin levels were drawn, and found to be within the nor-mal range. It is important to remember that TPN solutions lack selenium unless it is specifically added. Also, a patient with acute heart failure who underwent BPD was reported to have improved cardiac function 3 weeks after repletion with sele-nium supplementation.[21]

Additionally, severe deficiency can cause myopathy, arrhythmia, muscle wasting, impaired immunity, low thyroid function, loss of skin and hair pigmentation, whit-ened nail beds, and even progressive encephalopathy.[89]

7.7.6 TREATMENT

Some question selenium supplementation, based on the observation that postopera-tive deficiencies normalize on their own without supplementation, and an adequate, varied food intake seems to be sufficient.[12] Nonetheless, the Institute of Medicine lists the Recommended Dietary Allowance (RDA) for selenium to range from 20 to 55 μg/day for children and adults.[93] It has also been noted that certain populations such as the critically ill may need higher daily intakes.[89]

When supplementation is warranted, high blood levels of selenium (>100 μg/dl) can result in a condition called selenosis, comprising gastrointestinal upsets, hair loss, white blotch nails, garlic breath odor, fatigue, irritability, and nerve damage.[94]

7.7.7 CONCLUSION

There is insufficient evidence to support routine selenium screening or supplementa-tion after bariatric surgery. However, selenium levels should be checked in patients with a malabsorptive bariatric surgical procedure who have unexplained anemia or fatigue, persistent diarrhea, cardiomyopathy, or metabolic bone disease.[95]

7.8 NIACIN

7.8.1 INTRODUCTION AND BIOCHEMISTRY

Water-soluble vitamin deficiencies are more common after metabolic surgery that has a malabsorption component (RYGB and BPD), compared to fat-soluble vitamins.[21] Also, water-soluble vitamin deficiencies manifest early in the postoperative period, whereas the fat-soluble deficiencies develop more slowly, depending on the extent of fat malabsorption.[96]

Niacin, vitamin B3, nicotinic acid, and vitamin PP are all names of an organic compound that is an essential human nutrient. Niacin is converted into nicotinamide adenine dinucleotide (NAD) in the body. It exists within the redox-active coenzymes, NAD and its phosphate counterpart (NADP). It is required for nonredox reactions in DNA repair, calcium mobilization, and the synthesis of fatty acids and steroids, as well as in the oxidation of glucose-6-phosphate to ribose-5-phosphate in the pentose phosphate pathway.[97]

7.8.2 ABSORPTION AND METABOLISM

Most niacin intake comes from liver, meat, fish, poultry, enriched and whole grain bread and bread products, and fortified ready-to-eat cereals. It is also present in energy drinks, with more than twice the recommended daily intake for niacin. It can also be synthesized from tryptophan, an essential amino acid.

Niacin is absorbed through the stomach and proximal intestinal mucosa by simple diffusion, where about a third is protein-bound and the rest is in the free form. Small amounts can be stored in the liver, but most niacin is excreted in the urine easily due to its water solubility.[98]

7.8.3 ETIOLOGY OF DEFICIENCY

Classically, niacin deficiency is associated with endemic pellagra, where corn (lacking tryptophan) serves as the main source for carbohydrates, and nonendemic pellagra in alcoholics, and some is reported in Crohn's disease.[99] Carcinoid syndrome could also precipitate the condition, as tryptophan is converted mainly to serotonin, rather than niacin. Also, converting tryptophan to niacin requires other vitamins and minerals; thus, a deficiency could be secondary to vitamin B_6 depletion, for example.

In bariatric patients, regarding the prevalence of niacin deficiency, it was found that among patients opting for surgery, 5.6% of the subjects had niacin deficiency preoperatively.[54]

7.8.4 SIGNS AND SYMPTOMS OF DEFICIENCY

The classical hallmarks of pellagra are dermatitis, diarrhea, and dementia, and eventually death. The main signs are a rash and GI symptoms, such as anorexia and abdominal pain. The rash is described as hyperkeratotic, affecting mainly the face, chest, and dorsum of the hands and feet. The neurologic manifestations include peripheral neuropathy, but this is less specific to niacin deficiency and can arise from other deficiencies as well. Dementia or encephalopathy is the result of a severe deficiency.

Pellagra was reported to occur after just 3 months in a patient who underwent RYGB. The presentation included glossitis, angular cheilitis, and an erythematous, desquamative dermatitis on the neck, in sun-exposed areas, with photosensitivity causing a burning sensation on the arms as well.[100]

7.8.5 TREATMENT

Niacin is the oldest lipid-lowering drug being used for heart attack and stroke prevention. Recently, in the HPS2-THRIVE trial (randomized, placebo controlled, with over 26,000 patients, and an average follow-up of close to 4 years),[101] it was found that niacin's adverse side effects outweigh the benefits when used in combination with cholesterol-lowering statins, or that niacin showed no added benefit in terms of reductions in heart-related death, nonfatal heart attack, stroke, or the need for angioplasty or bypass procedures. Niacin was also found to increase the incidence of bleeding and infections, compared to placebo. The AIM-HIGH trial found similar results with no benefit to niacin treatment.[102] As caregivers to a morbidly obese population plagued with hypercholesterolemia routinely prescribed with niacin supplements following bariatric procedures, we must carefully review this treatment. Preventing deficiency, as well as avoiding adverse side effects, is of great importance.

The RDA of niacin is 2–12 mg for children, 14 mg for women, 16 mg for men, and 18 mg for pregnant or breast-feeding women. Tolerable upper limits of niacin to avoid flushing are considered to be 35 mg per day. Doses above that have been reported to cause hepatotoxity as well as dermatologic manifestations.[103] Flushing is the main side effect of niacin supplementation, and dosage should decrease or be stopped if this occurs. Other classic side effects include itching, rashes, indigestion, diarrhea, diabetes, and myopathy.

7.8.6 CONCLUSION

As the human liver stores small amounts of niacin, and it is readily metabolized in our body, deficiencies in patients undergoing metabolic surgery are of concern and postoperative supplementation is recommended; however, prescription to our patients should be carefully planned and followed. Side effects are common and must be well recognized and addressed promptly.

7.9 CONCLUSION

Iatrogenic epidemic of malnutrition should be prevented. This relies on several aspects, including the patient, the surgeon, and a comprehensive team of healthcare professionals inclusive of dietitians. Although deficiencies appear to be prevalent, luckily symptomatic deficiencies are not, and the majority of the literature on this matter rests on a few selected case reports.

The high prevalence of micronutrient deficiencies has been demonstrated in the morbidly obese seeking metabolic surgery. Performing a basal assessment of micronutrient status, including albumin, prealbumin, vitamin D, vitamin B_{12}, ferritin, and intact parathyroid hormone (iPTH), is valued. Copper, zinc, and selenium evaluation are warranted if specific findings arise. Beginning supplementation to alleviate the detected deficiencies prior to surgery could potentially improve the evolution of these patients and decrease postoperative nutritional complications.

Despite malabsorption and reduced intake, and thus expected deterioration of nutritional status, metabolic surgery overall brings morbidly obese patients' vitamin status closer to that of nonobese healthy individuals. Nonetheless, nutritional deficiencies are very common and occur despite supplementation with the standard multivitamin preparation. Therefore, careful postoperative follow-up is indicated to detect and treat those deficiencies,[104] and patients will require lifelong additional doses of prophylactic supplementation to maintain optimal micronutrient status.[5] Nutritional deficiency screening and treatment should vary depending on the chosen bariatric procedure.

Nutritional supplements offered should meet all needs. The given supplement is usually enough to avoid deficiencies, but studies are needed to determine whether there is vitamin and mineral dosages capable of preventing deficiency in all patients after metabolic procedures. The American Association of Clinical Endocrinologists, in conjunction with The Obesity Society and the American Society for Metabolic and Bariatric Surgery, published extensive guidelines for the nutritional support of the metabolic surgery patient, including pre- and postoperative monitoring and supplementation.[105]

Multiple institutes report the reason for fat-soluble vitamin deficiency is largely due to the noncompliance of patients to their recommended supplementation. This must be recognized and addressed, and patients must be educated on the significance and importance of compliance. Furthermore, patients can be educated on symptoms of the different deficiencies, so if a complication arises, early treatment can ensue.

As most individuals undergoing surgery for treatment of obesity are women, this makes preconception care critical. It is essential to screen and correct for nutritional deficiencies for this population at reproductive age, as increased sexual activity and significant improvement in fertility are reported. Supplementing accordingly to avoid any complications during the increased demand period by the fetus and mother of pregnancy is crucial. It would also be wise to send our patients for nutritional screening mid-pregnancy as well. Important supplementation for pregnant women who have undergone bariatric surgery includes iron, vitamin A, vitamin B_{12}, vitamin K, and folate, as deficiencies are associated with maternal and fetal complications, including severe anemia, congenital abnormalities, low birth weight, and failure to thrive.[21]

Another important aspect of care is reflected in the young. With the increasing prevalence of metabolic surgery in adolescents, extra care should be taken regarding many of the discussed essential vitamins and minerals that can be deficient, as these deficiencies can result in severed growth, delayed puberty, and developmental abnormalities.

We monitor micronutrient levels regularly to detect early nutritional deficiencies and to initiate appropriate therapies. Tests for micronutrients and vitamin levels are recommended to be performed preoperatively, then at 3- to 6-month intervals postoperatively for the first 2 years, and annually thereafter.[106]

It has been reported often in case reports that the road to diagnosing a nutrient deficiency involves several earlier stops, where the patient seeks comfort for the different symptoms with varied caregivers. Today, with the increasing knowledge and understanding of metabolic surgery, patients should be monitored carefully, and if signs and symptoms relevant to a specific deficiency or multitude of deficiencies arise, they should be addressed promptly and accurately.

Normalizing deficiencies must be sought for in all patients, as normalizing is possible with simple treatment, and rates of deficiency-free should be 100%. On the rare occasion where medical treatment does not compensate for the deficiencies, revisional surgery of the bariatric procedure may be warranted for reversal of the malabsorptive component. This chapter illustrates the necessity for lifelong vitamin supplementation and surveillance after metabolic surgery.

REFERENCES

1. Chan S, Gerson B, Subramaniam S. The role of copper, molybdenum, selenium, and zinc in nutrition and health. *Clin Lab Med* 1998;18(4):673–685.
2. Bradley EL 3rd, Isaacs J, Hersh T, Davidson ED, Millikan W. Nutritional consequences of total gastrectomy. *Ann Surg* 1975;182(4):415–429.
3. Kushner RF. Micronutrient deficiencies and bariatric surgery. *Curr Opin Endocrinol Diabetes* 2006;13(5):405–411. doi:10.1097/01.med.0000244220.53163.85.
4. Toh SY, Zarshenas N, Jorgensen J. Prevalence of nutrient deficiencies in bariatric patients. *Nutrition* 2009;25(11–12):1150–1156. doi:10.1016/j.nut.2009.03.012.
5. Hammer HF. Medical complications of bariatric surgery: focus on malabsorption and dumping syndrome. *Dig Dis* 2012;30(2):182–186.
6. Fujioka K. Follow-up of nutritional and metabolic problems after bariatric surgery. *Diabetes Care* 2005;28(2):481–484. doi:10.2337/diacare.28.2.481.
7. Rivero HG, Abdemur A, Rosenthal RJ. Diagnosis and treatment of dumping syndrome after gastric bypass for morbid obesity. In Thompson CC, ed., *Bariatric endoscopy.* New York, NY: Springer; 2013:161–169. Available at http://link.springer.com/10.1007/978-1-4419-1710-2_16 (accessed September 21, 2013).
8. Odstrcil EA, Martinez JG, Santa Ana CA, et al. The contribution of malabsorption to the reduction in net energy absorption after long-limb Roux-en-Y gastric bypass. *Am J Clin Nutr.* 2010;92(4):704–713. doi:10.3945/ajcn.2010.29870.
9. Layer P, Go VL, DiMagno EP. Fate of pancreatic enzymes during small intestinal aboral transit in humans. *Am J Physiol.* 1986;251(4 Pt 1):G475–G480.
10. Deh Carvalho Machado J, Campos CS, Lopes Dah Silva C, et al. Intestinal bacterial overgrowth after Roux-en-Y gastric bypass. *Obes Surg* 2007;18(1):139–143. doi:10.1007/s11695-007-9365-y.
11. Tabaqchali S, Hatzioannou J, Booth CC. Bile-salt deconjugation and steatorrhoea in patients with the stagnant-loop syndrome. *Lancet* 1968;2(7558):12–16.
12. Pech N, Meyer F, Lippert H, Manger T, Stroh C. Complications and nutrient deficiencies two years after sleeve gastrectomy. *BMC Surg* 2012;12(1):13.
13. Gehrer S, Kern B, Peters T, Christoffel-Courtin C, Peterli R. Fewer nutrient deficiencies after laparoscopic sleeve gastrectomy (LSG) than after laparoscopic Roux-Y-gastric bypass (LRYGB)—a prospective study. *Obes Surg* 2010;20(4):447–453.
14. Donadelli SP, Junqueira-Franco MVM, de Mattos Donadelli CA, et al. Daily vitamin supplementation and hypovitaminosis after obesity surgery. *Nutrition* 2011. Available at http://www.sciencedirect.com/science/article/pii/S0899900711002449 (accessed January 24, 2013).
15. Shils M, Olson J, Shike M, Ross C. Vitamin A. In *Modern nutrition in health and disease.* 9th ed. Baltimore: Williams & Wilkins; 1999:305–313.

16. Eckert MJ, Perry JT, Sohn VY, et al. Incidence of low vitamin A levels and ocular symptoms after Roux-en-Y gastric bypass. *Surg Obes Relat Dis* 2010;6(6):653–657.

17. Groff JL, Gropper SS, Hunt SM. The fat soluble vitamins. In *Advanced nutrition and human metabolism*. Minneapolis: West Publishing Company; 1995:284–324.

18. Chae T, Foroozan R. Vitamin A deficiency in patients with a remote history of intestinal surgery. *British J Ophthalmol* 2006;90(8):955–956.

19. Pereira SE, Saboya CJ, Saunders C, Ramalho A. Serum levels and liver store of retinol and their association with night blindness in individuals with class III obesity. *Obes Surg* 2012:1–7.

20. Trumbo P, Yates AA, Schlicker S, Poos M. Dietary Reference Intakes: vitamin A, vitamin K, arsenic, boron, chromium, copper, iodine, iron, manganese, molybdenum, nickel, silicon, vanadium, and zinc. *J Am Diet Assoc* 2001;101(3):294–301. doi:10.1016/S0002-8223(01)00078-5.

21. Shankar P, Boylan M, Sriram K. Micronutrient deficiencies after bariatric surgery. *Nutrition* 2010;26(11):1031–1037.

22. Pereira S, Saboya C, Chaves G, Ramalho A. Class III obesity and its relationship with the nutritional status of vitamin A in pre- and postoperative gastric bypass. *Obes Surg* 2009;19(6):738–744.

23. Madan AK, Orth WS, Tichansky DS, Ternovits CA. Vitamin and trace mineral levels after laparoscopic gastric bypass. *Obes Surg* 2006;16(5):603–606.

24. Zalesin KC, Miller WM, Franklin B, et al. Vitamin A deficiency after gastric bypass surgery: an underreported postoperative complication. *J Obes.* 2010;2011. Available at http://www.hindawi.com/journals/jobes/aip/760695/ (accessed January 24, 2013).

25. Slater GH, Ren CJ, Siegel N, et al. Serum fat-soluble vitamin deficiency and abnormal calcium metabolism after malabsorptive bariatric surgery. *J Gastrointest Surg* 2004;8(1):48–55; discussion 54–55.

26. Lee WB, Hamilton SM, Harris JP, Schwab IR. Ocular complications of hypovitaminosis A after bariatric surgery. *Ophthalmology* 2005;112(6):1031–1034.

27. Brolin RE, LaMarca LB, Kenler HA, Cody RP. Malabsorptive gastric bypass in patients with superobesity. *J Gastrointest Surg* 2002;6(2):195–203; discussion 204–205.

28. Clements RH, Katasani VG, Palepu R, et al. Incidence of vitamin deficiency after laparoscopic Roux-en-Y gastric bypass in a university hospital setting. *Am Surg* 2006;72(12):1196–1202; discussion 1203–1204.

29. Smith FR, Goodman DS, Zaklama MS, Gabr MK, el-Maraghy S, Patwardhan VN. Serum vitamin A, retinol-binding protein, and prealbumin concentrations in protein-calorie malnutrition. I. A functional defect in hepatic retinol release. *Am J Clin Nutr* 1973;26(9):973–981.

30. Quaranta L, Nascimbeni G, Semeraro F, Quaranta CA. Severe corneoconjunctival xerosis after biliopancreatic bypass for obesity (Scopinaro's operation). *Am J Ophthalmol* 1994;118(6):817–818.

31. Hatizifotis M, Dolan K, Newbury L, Fielding G. Symptomatic vitamin A deficiency following biliopancreatic diversion. *Obes Surg* 2003;13(4):655–657. doi:10.1381/096089203322190916.

32. Chagas CB, Saunders C, Pereira S, Silva J, Saboya C, Ramalho A. Vitamin A deficiency in pregnancy: perspectives after bariatric surgery. *Obes Surg* 2012. doi:10.1007/s11695-012-0822-x.

33. Huerta S, Rogers LM, Li Z, Heber D, Liu C, Livingston EH. Vitamin A deficiency in a newborn resulting from maternal hypovitaminosis A after biliopancreatic diversion for the treatment of morbid obesity. *Am J Clin Nutr* 2002;76(2):426–429.

34. Christian P, West KP Jr, Khatry SK, et al. Night blindness during pregnancy and subsequent mortality among women in Nepal: effects of vitamin A and beta-carotene supplementation. *Am J Epidemiol* 2000;152(6):542–547.

35. Chaves GV, Pereira SE, Saboya CJ, Ramalho A. Nutritional status of vitamin A in morbid obesity before and after Roux-en-Y gastric bypass. *Obes Surg* 2007;17(7):970–976.
36. De Salvo G, Maguire JI, Lotery AJ. Vitamin A deficiency-related retinopathy after bariatric surgery. *Graefe's Arch Clin Exp Ophthalmol* 2012;250(6):941–943.
37. Aasheim ET, Søvik TT, Bakke EF. Night blindness after duodenal switch. *Surg Obes Relat Dis* 2008;4(5):685–686. doi:10.1016/j.soard.2008.05.001.
38. Aasheim ET, Björkman S, Søvik TT, et al. Vitamin status after bariatric surgery: a randomized study of gastric bypass and duodenal switch. *Am J Clin Nutr* 2009;90(1):15–22.
39. Aasheim ET, Johnson LK, Hofsø D, Bøhmer T, Hjelmesæth J. Vitamin status after gastric bypass and lifestyle intervention: a comparative prospective study. *Surg Obes Relat Dis* 2012;8(2):169–175.
40. Khazai N, Judd SE, Tangpricha V. Calcium and vitamin D: skeletal and extraskeletal health. *Curr Rheumatol Rep* 2008;10(2):110–117.
41. Parikh SJ, Edelman M, Uwaifo GI, et al. The relationship between obesity and serum 1,25-dihydroxy vitamin D concentrations in healthy adults. *J Clin Endocrinol Metab* 2004;89(3):1196–1199.
42. Ybarra J, Sánchez-Hernández J, Pérez A. Hypovitaminosis D and morbid obesity. *Nurs Clin North Am* 2007;42(1):19–27, v. doi:10.1016/j.cnur.2006.12.001.
43. Bell NH, Epstein S, Greene A, Shary J, Oexmann MJ, Shaw S. Evidence for alteration of the vitamin D-endocrine system in obese subjects. *J Clin Invest* 1985;76(1):370–373. doi:10.1172/JCI111971.
44. Compston JE, Vedi S, Ledger JE, Webb A, Gazet JC, Pilkington TR. Vitamin D status and bone histomorphometry in gross obesity. *Am J Clin Nutr* 1981;34(11):2359–2363.
45. Wortsman J, Matsuoka LY, Chen TC, Lu Z, Holick MF. Decreased bioavailability of vitamin D in obesity. *Am J Clin Nutr* 2000;72(3):690–693.
46. Carlin AM, Rao DS, Meslemani AM, et al. Prevalence of vitamin D depletion among morbidly obese patients seeking gastric bypass surgery. *Surg Obes Relat Dis* 2006;2(2):98–103; discussion 104. doi:10.1016/j.soard.2005.12.001.
47. Hamoui N, Anthone G, Crookes PF. Calcium metabolism in the morbidly obese. *Obes Surg* 2004;14(1):9–12. doi:10.1381/096089204772787211.
48. Burton GW. Vitamin E: molecular and biological function. *Proc Nutr Soc* 1994;53(2):251–262.
49. Dadalt C, Fagundes RLM, Moreira EAM, et al. Oxidative stress markers in adults 2 years after Roux-en-Y gastric bypass. *Eur J Gastroenterol Hepatol* 2012. doi:10.1097/MEG.0b013e32835d0ae0.
50. Kumar N. Nutritional neuropathies. *Neurol Clin* 2007;25(1):209–255. doi:10.1016/j.ncl.2006.11.001.
51. Child R, Brown S, Day S, Donnelly A, Roper H, Saxton J. Changes in indices of antioxidant status, lipid peroxidation and inflammation in human skeletal muscle after eccentric muscle actions. *Clin Sci* 1999;96(1):105–115.
52. Gletsu-Miller N, Hansen JM, Jones DP, et al. Loss of total and visceral adipose tissue mass predicts decreases in oxidative stress after weight-loss surgery. *Obesity (Silver Spring)* 2009;17(3):439–446. doi:10.1038/oby.2008.542.
53. Steephen AC, Traber MG, Ito Y, Lewis LH, Kayden HJ, Shike M. Vitamin E status of patients receiving long-term parenteral nutrition: is vitamin E supplementation adequate? *JPEN J Parenter Enteral Nutr* 1991;15(6):647–652.
54. Ernst B, Thurnheer M, Schmid SM, Schultes B. Evidence for the necessity to systematically assess micronutrient status prior to bariatric surgery. *Obes Surg* 2009;19(1):66–73.
55. Boylan LM, Sugerman HJ, Driskell JA. Vitamin E, vitamin B-6, vitamin B-12, and folate status of gastric bypass surgery patients. *J Am Diet Assoc* 1988;88(5):579–585.
56. Schweitzer DH. Mineral metabolism and bone disease after bariatric surgery and ways to optimize bone health. *Obes Surg* 2007;17(11):1510–1516.

57. Dolan K, Hatzifotis M, Newbury L, Lowe N, Fielding G. A clinical and nutritional comparison of biliopancreatic diversion with and without duodenal switch. *Ann Surg* 2004;240(1):51–56.

58. Bunnell RH, De Ritter E, Rubin SH. Effect of feeding polyunsaturated fatty acids with a low vitamin E diet on blood levels of tocopherol in men performing hard physical labor. *Am J Clin Nutr* 1975;28(7):706–711.

59. Katsuyama H, Ideguchi S, Fukunaga M, Saijoh K, Sunami S. Usual dietary intake of fermented soybeans (Natto) is associated with bone mineral density in premenopausal women. *J Nutr Sci Vitaminol* 2002;48(3):207–215.

60. Shearer MJ, McBurney A, Barkhan P. Studies on the absorption and metabolism of phylloquinone (vitamin K_1) in man. *Vitam Horm* 1974;32:513–542.

61. Usui Y, Tanimura H, Nishimura N, Kobayashi N, Okanoue T, Ozawa K. Vitamin K concentrations in the plasma and liver of surgical patients. *Am J Clin Nutr* 1990;51(5):846–852.

62. Cone LA, Waterbor RB, Sofonio MV. Purpura fulminans due to *Streptococcus pneumoniae* sepsis following gastric bypass. *Obes Surg* 2004;14(5):690–694.

63. Shearer MJ. Vitamin K. *Lancet* 1995;345(8944):229–234.

64. Shearer MJ, Fu X, Booth SL. Vitamin K nutrition, metabolism, and requirements: current concepts and future research. *Adv Nutr* 2012;3(2):182–195. doi:10.3945/an.111.001800.

65. Bilenka B, Ben-Shlomo I, Cozacov C, Gold CH, Zohar S. Fertility, miscarriage and pregnancy after vertical banded gastroplasty operation for morbid obesity. *Acta Obstet Gynecol Scand* 1995;74(1):42–44.

66. Hezelgrave NL, Oteng-Ntim E. Pregnancy after bariatric surgery: a review. *J Obes* 2011;2011:501939. doi:10.1155/2011/501939.

67. Bersani I, Carolis MPD, Salvi S, Zecca E, Romagnoli C, De Carolis S. Maternal–neonatal vitamin K deficiency secondary to maternal biliopancreatic diversion. *Blood Coagul Fibrinolysis* 2011;22(4):334.

68. Kang L, Marty D, Pauli RM, Mendelsohn NJ, Prachand V, Waggoner D. Chondrodysplasia punctata associated with malabsorption from bariatric procedures. *Surg Obes Relat Dis* 2010;6(1):99–101. doi:10.1016/j.soard.2009.05.004.

69. Eerdekens A, Debeer A, Van Hoey G, et al. Maternal bariatric surgery: adverse outcomes in neonates. *Eur J Pediatr* 2010;169(2):191–196.

70. Prasad AS, Halsted JA, Nadimi M. Syndrome of iron deficiency anemia, hepatosplenomegaly, hypogonadism, dwarfism and geophagia. *Am J Med* 1961;31:532–546.

71. Shankar AH, Prasad AS. Zinc and immune function: the biological basis of altered resistance to infection. *Am J Clin Nutr* 1998;68(2 Suppl):447S–463S.

72. Fraker PJ, Haas SM, Luecke RW. Effect of zinc deficiency on the immune response of the young adult A/J mouse. *J Nutr* 1977;107(10):1889–1895.

73. Prasad AS, Beck FWJ, Bao B, Snell D, Fitzgerald JT. Duration and severity of symptoms and levels of plasma interleukin-1 receptor antagonist, soluble tumor necrosis factor receptor, and adhesion molecules in patients with common cold treated with zinc acetate. *J Infect Dis* 2008;197(6):795–802. doi:10.1086/528803.

74. Takagi H, Nagamine T, Abe T, et al. Zinc supplementation enhances the response to interferon therapy in patients with chronic hepatitis C. *J Viral Hepatol* 2001;8(5):367–371.

75. Hoque KM, Binder HJ. Zinc in the treatment of acute diarrhea: current status and assessment. *Gastroenterology* 2006;130(7):2201–2205. doi:10.1053/j.gastro.2006.02.062.

76. Kashimura H, Suzuki K, Hassan M, et al. Polaprezinc, a mucosal protective agent, in combination with lansoprazole, amoxycillin and clarithromycin increases the cure rate of *Helicobacter pylori* infection. *Aliment Pharmacol Ther* 1999;13(4):483–487.

77. Nutrient data products and services. Available at http://www.ars.usda.gov/Services/docs.htm?docid = 9673 (accessed March 27, 2013).

78. De Luis DA, Pacheco D, Izaola O, Terroba MC, Cuellar L, Cabezas G. Micronutrient status in morbidly obese women before bariatric surgery. *Surg Obes Relat Dis* 2011. Available at http://www.sciencedirect.com/science/article/pii/S1550728911006988 (accessed January 24, 2013).

79. Cominetti C, Garrido AB Jr, Cozzolino SMF. Zinc nutritional status of morbidly obese patients before and after Roux-en-Y gastric bypass: a preliminary report. *Obes Surg* 2006;16(4):448–453. doi:10.1381/096089206776327305.

80. Pech N, Meyer F, Lippert H, Manger T, Stroh C. Complications and nutrient deficiencies two years after sleeve gastrectomy. *Bmc Surg* 2012;12(1):13.

81. Walsh S, Benton EC. Think zinc: a further cause of deficiency to be remembered. *Clin Exp Dermatol* 2009;34(6):731–732. doi:10.1111/j.1365-2230.2008.03062.x.

82. Cunha SF de C, Gonçalves GAP, Marchini JS, Roselino AMF. Acrodermatitis due to zinc deficiency after combined vertical gastroplasty with jejunoileal bypass: case report. *Sao Paulo Med J* 2012;130(5):330–335.

83. Aills L, Blankenship J, Buffington C, Furtado M, Parrott J. ASMBS Allied Health nutritional guidelines for the surgical weight loss patient. *Surg Obes Relat Dis* 2008;4(5):S73–S108. doi:10.1016/j.soard.2008.03.002.

84. Davies DJ, Baxter JM, Baxter JN. Nutritional deficiencies after bariatric surgery. *Obes Surg* 2007;17(9):1150–1158.

85. Pech N, Meyer F, Lippert H, Manger T, Stroh C. Complications, reoperations, and nutrient deficiencies two years after sleeve gastrectomy. *J Obes* 2012;2012:828737. doi:10.1155/2012/828737.

86. Fryer MJ. Rationale for clinical trials of selenium as an antioxidant for the treatment of the cardiomyopathy of Friedreich's ataxia. *Med Hypotheses* 2002;58(2):127–132. doi:10.1054/mehy.2001.1474.

87. Brown KM, Arthur JR. Selenium, selenoproteins and human health: a review. *Public Health Nutr* 2001;4(2B):593–599.

88. Mazokopakis EE, Papadakis JA, Papadomanolaki MG, et al. Effects of 12 months treatment with L-selenomethionine on serum anti-TPO levels in patients with Hashimoto's thyroiditis. *Thyroid* 2007;17(7):609–612. doi:10.1089/thy.2007.0040.

89. Freeth A, Prajuabpansri P, Victory JM, Jenkins P. Assessment of selenium in Roux-en-Y gastric bypass and gastric banding surgery. *Obes Surg* 2012:1–6.

90. Kimmons JE, Blanck HM, Tohill BC, Zhang J, Khan LK. Associations between body mass index and the prevalence of low micronutrient levels among US adults. *MedGenMed* 2006;8(4):59.

91. Alasfar F, Ben-Nakhi M, Khoursheed M, Kehinde EO, Alsaleh M. Selenium is significantly depleted among morbidly obese female patients seeking bariatric surgery. *Obes Surg* 2011;21(11):1710–1713.

92. Boldery R, Fielding G, Rafter T, Pascoe AL, Scalia GM. Nutritional deficiency of selenium secondary to weight loss (bariatric) surgery associated with life-threatening cardiomyopathy. *Heart Lung Circulation* 2007;16(2):123–126.

93. Dietary Reference Intakes for vitamin C, vitamin E, selenium, and carotenoids. Available at http://www.nap.edu/catalog.php?record_id = 9810 (accessed April 17, 2013).

94. Goldhaber SB. Trace element risk assessment: essentiality vs. toxicity. *Regul Toxicol Pharmacol* 2003;38(2):232–242.

95. Mechanick JI, Youdim A, Jones DB, et al. Clinical practice guidelines for the perioperative nutritional, metabolic, and nonsurgical support of the bariatric surgery patient—2013 update: cosponsored by American Association of Clinical Endocrinologists, The Obesity Society, and American Society for Metabolic and Bariatric Surgery. *Obesity (Silver Spring)* 2013;21(Suppl 1):S1–27. doi:10.1002/oby.20461.

96. Schweitzer DH, Posthuma EF. Prevention of vitamin and mineral deficiencies after bariatric surgery: evidence and algorithms. *Obes Surg* 2008;18(11):1485–1488.

97. McCormick DB, Meyers RA. Co-enzymes, biochemistry of. In *Encyclopedia of molecular biology and molecular medicine*. Vol 1. Berlin: VCH; 1996:396–406.
98. Bechgaard H, Jespersen S. GI absorption of niacin in humans. *J Pharm Sci* 1977;66(6):871–872.
99. McCormick DB. Niacin. In *Modern nutrition in health and disease*. 6th ed. Philadelphia: Lea & Febiger; 1988:370–375.
100. Ashourian N, Mousdicas N. Images in clinical medicine. Pellagra-like dermatitis. *N Engl J Med*. 2006;354(15):1614. doi:10.1056/NEJMicm050641.
101. HPS2-THRIVE randomized placebo-controlled trial in 25 673 high-risk patients of ER niacin/laropiprant: trial design, pre-specified muscle and liver outcomes, and reasons for stopping study treatment. *Eur Heart J* 2013. doi:10.1093/eurheartj/eht055.
102. Boden WE, Probstfield JL, Anderson T, et al. Niacin in patients with low HDL cholesterol levels receiving intensive statin therapy. *N Engl J Med* 2011;365(24):2255–2267. doi:10.1056/NEJMoa1107579.
103. Dietary Reference Intakes for thiamin, riboflavin, niacin, vitamin B_6, folate, vitamin B_{12}, pantothenic acid, biotin, and choline. Available at http://www.nap.edu/catalog.php?record_id = 6015 (accessed April 16, 2013).
104. Gasteyger C, Suter M, Gaillard RC, Giusti V. Nutritional deficiencies after Roux-en-Y gastric bypass for morbid obesity often cannot be prevented by standard multivitamin supplementation. *Am J Clin Nutr* 2008;87(5):1128–1133.
105. Mechanick JI, Kushner RF, Sugerman HJ, et al. American Association of Clinical Endocrinologists, The Obesity Society, and American Society for Metabolic and Bariatric Surgery medical guidelines for clinical practice for the perioperative nutritional, metabolic, and nonsurgical support of the bariatric surgery patient. *Obesity (Silver Spring)* 2009;17(Suppl 1):S1–S70, v. doi:10.1038/oby.2009.28.
106. Malinowski SS. Nutritional and metabolic complications of bariatric surgery. *Am J Med Sci* 2006;331(4):219–225.

8 Pharmacology of Drugs and Nutritional Supplements

Margaret Malone

CONTENTS

The purpose of this chapter is to review the changes in drug and nutrient disposition that may occur after bariatric surgery. Although the published literature remains limited regarding drug dosing in obese individuals and bariatric patients, basic pharmacokinetic principles can generally be applied. These data from studies and case reports are used to guide modification of dosage regimens and pharmaceutical formulation choices. The impact of bariatric surgery on drug and nutrient absorption is determined by the type of surgery performed, which will be highlighted in this chapter. The effect of surgery on vitamin, mineral, and micronutrient status is primarily covered in the chapters devoted to those specific nutrients elsewhere in this text.

8.1 TYPES OF BARIATRIC PROCEDURES AND THEIR POTENTIAL IMPACT ON DRUG DISSOLUTION AND ABSORPTION

Bariatric procedures that are purely restrictive (gastric banding), restrictive with reduced contact with the gastric mucosa and digestive juices (sleeve gastrectomy), restrictive and malabsorptive (gastric bypass), and primarily malabsorptive (biliopancreatic diversion, jejunoileal bypass) have different effects on drug and nutrient absorption. Procedures associated with malabsorption are more likely to impair drug and nutrient absorption depending on the site of absorption and the bioavailability of the drug under normal circumstances. Since the majority of drugs are absorbed in the small intestine, the potential effect on drug absorption can be estimated by knowing the length of small bowel excluded (short limb versus long limb) and the potential for the drug to be absorbed more distally in the intestine.[1-3]

Changes in drug disposition are dependent on factors that affect absorption, distribution, metabolism, and excretion. When reviewing the medication regimen for a bariatric patient, the clinician should consider the usual pharmacokinetics of the drug and the release characteristics of the current formulation. There are several comprehensive reviews of the complexity of drug disposition for those requiring an in-depth discussion of this topic.[1-5] The primary clinical and pharmacokinetic effects on drug therapy as related to the bariatric surgery patient are reviewed below.

8.1.1 CHANGES IN DRUG DISSOLUTION

Drugs from a solid dosage form (tablets or capsules), when taken orally, need to first disintegrate and then dissolve into solution before the drug can cross the mucosal membrane. For some drugs this is the rate-limiting step for absorption and is most important when delayed release or pH-dependent release formulations are being considered.[2] Additionally, after bariatric surgery, gastric mixing, which normally enhances drug dissolution, is reduced. Possible solutions include using liquid formulations, opening capsule contents prior to ingestion, crushing or chewing the medication, or changing to a nonoral formulation, for example, transdermal, parenteral, rectal, or inhaled.

The availability of a drug or the amount of drug that is absorbed is also dependent on the rate at which the drug crosses the cell membrane. In general, drugs that are lipid soluble can more easily cross the cell membrane than water-soluble drugs. Most drugs are absorbed through passive diffusion; however, some drugs

TABLE 8.1

Biopharmaceutical Drug Disposition Classification System (BDDCS)

Classification	Characteristics	Drug Examples
Class I	High solubility–high permeability No role for active transport Hepatic metabolism	Enalapril, metoprolol, nifedipine

Class II	Low solubility–high permeability
	Efflux transporters
	Hepatic metabolism
		Amiodarone, atorvastatin, azithromycin,
		  carvedilol, glyburide, ibuprofen, naproxen,
		  lansoprazole, ketoconazole

Class III	High solubility–low permeability Influx transporters Renal and biliary excretion	Amoxicillin, atenolol, cimetidine, fexofenadine, lisinopril, ranitidine, valsartan
Class IV	Low solubility–low permeability Influx and efflux transporters Renal and biliary excretion	Acetazolamide, chlorothiazide, ciprofloxacin, furosemide, neomycin

have facilitated or active transport, which enhances movement of the drug across the membrane. Some drugs, notably anticancer drugs, are actively pumped back across the membrane, which acts as an opposing force to drug absorption and is a source of drug resistance. The P-glycoprotein pump is one of the commonly known efflux carrier mechanisms. There is a concentration gradient of P-glycoprotein activity from the proximal (higher) to the distal (lower) small intestine. The Food and Drug Administration (FDA) Biopharmaceutical Drug Disposition Classification System (BDDCS) was developed to address drug disposition and assigns drugs into one of four classes, as shown in Table 8.1.[4] Drugs are classified according to their solubility, their ability to cross the cell membrane (permeability), the role of active transporters, and the primary method of excretion. These effects are complex and difficult to predict in nonbariatric patients, and there is very limited data other than small trials and case reports in the bariatric literature. However, these factors need to be considered when selecting a drug and dosage regimen, especially for drugs known to develop resistance in normal individuals.

8.1.2   Intestinal pH and Effect on Absorption

The pKa of the drug and the pH of the intestinal milieu affect the absorption of the drug. Drugs are optimally absorbed in their nonionized state. Weak acids are better absorbed in an acidic environment such as the stomach, and weak bases are better absorbed in an alkaline environment like the small intestine. The small intestine has a much larger surface area or absorptive capacity than the stomach and is the primary site of absorption for many drugs. The clinical efficacy of the drug may be altered after bariatric surgery depending on the extent of drug absorption (i.e., the percent or fraction of drug absorbed), the permeability characteristics of the drug, and the amount of small intestine that is bypassed.[4] The clinician should evaluate whether the absorption site is bypassed and if the drug/nutrient or the type of formulation is being presented to a part of the intestine that has a different pH than the usual environment in a nonsurgery patient.

Gastric bypass and gastroplasty procedures create a pouch that has an increased pH and avoids the exposure of the drug to the remnant stomach, which contains the majority of acid-producing cells. In procedures such as sleeve gastrectomy and biliopancreatic diversion (BPD) this section of the stomach is removed. Since the stomach is not the major site of absorption, this effect is only of clinical significance when the drug or formulation requires a low pH for optimal absorption, for example, iron, rifampin, ketoconazole, and digoxin.

8.1.3 Delayed Gastric Emptying

Although there is delayed gastric emptying following gastric bypass and BPD, there are insufficient data in the bariatric population to make specific therapeutic recommendations. Based on nonbariatric studies where gastric emptying was delayed, there was an observed decrease in the rate but not the extent of drug absorption.[5] Clinically this would be of importance if a particular therapeutic concentration needed to be achieved for efficacy, for example, anti-infective agents.

8.1.4 Changes in Transit Time and Reduced Mucosal Exposure

When transit time is decreased due to shorter intestinal length (especially gastric bypass and BPD), there is reduced opportunity for absorption. The proximal ileum has a larger surface area and a potentially greater absorptive capacity than the distal ileum.[2] However, the transit time is slower in the distal ileum, allowing more time for a drug or nutrient to be absorbed. The combined impact of these factors after bariatric surgery is unknown. Whether intestinal adaptation that is observed in patients with short bowel syndrome occurs after bariatric surgery, potentially enhancing absorption in the early years after surgery, is also unknown.[1,2] In addition, cytochrome P enzyme activity is greater in the proximal small intestine that affects drugs that have a high first-pass metabolism within the epithelium. When the proximal ileum is bypassed an increase in the availability should be expected. These effects on absorption are more likely to be clinically significant for drugs with low availability and are erratically absorbed under usual circumstances, such as thyroxine, phenytoin, and tacrolimus. Formulations that are extended release are likely to have impaired absorption due to reduced time available for absorption to occur at the optimal section of the intestine. Those products that have pH-dependent release mechanisms may not be presented to the intended site of action, and the coat will not disintegrate and release the drug appropriately.

Drugs that are fat soluble may depend on the presence of bile acids to enhance their absorption through mixing with bile acids. Enterohepatic recycling may not occur or be significantly reduced if the proximal ileum is bypassed and may impact the availability of some drugs (e.g., oral contraceptives, rifampin, thyroxine, phenytoin, cyclosporine). This problem is more likely to occur after long-loop gastric bypass procedures and BPD where drugs are presented to the distal ileum.

8.2 PHARMACOKINETIC ALTERATIONS IN OVERWEIGHT AND OBESE PATIENTS

While there is limited information, there are some known principles in the following section that can be used for dose extrapolation. Obese patients have a greater lean and fat body mass. The lean body mass accounts for 20–40% of the excess weight. Estimating the distribution and blood flow into adipose tissue is difficult. There are also changes in protein binding of drugs, especially those that are highly bound to albumin. The obese patients have larger kidneys, which may translate into a higher than expected glomerular filtration rate. Liver function, while hard to estimate, may be impaired prior to surgery due to fatty liver or cirrhosis and improve after surgery with weight loss; however, there are very limited data on drug dosing changes due to liver function alterations.[6]

8.2.1 Dosing Strategies for Overweight and Obese Patients

Cheymol[6] recommended the application of several general pharmacokinetic principles when dosing overweight and obese individuals:

- Hydrophilic drugs that are water soluble should be dosed according to ideal body weight, such as cimetidine, ranitidine, verapamil, and methyl prednisone.
- For drugs that distribute into lean body mass and partially into fat mass, loading dose should be calculated on ideal body weight + 40%, e.g., aminoglycoside antibiotics.
- For drugs that distribute equally between lean body mass and fat mass, including highly lipophilic drugs, loading doses should be based on total body weight, for example, lorazepam, diazepam, midazolam, trazodone, and fentanyl.
- Maintenance doses depend on the patient's ability to eliminate the drug from the body or the clearance. When clearance is altered, maintenance doses should be decreased or increased accordingly.
- Where necessary, for drugs that have a narrow therapeutic index (i.e., a narrow range between therapeutic and toxic serum levels), monitoring of drug levels to ensure efficacy while avoiding toxicity is recommended, for example, aminoglycoside antibiotics, phenytoin, and digoxin.
- When drugs are dosed according to therapeutic efficacy, for example, blood pressure, blood glucose, and low-density lipoprotein (LDL) cholesterol, dosing should be titrated according to the desired therapeutic outcome.
- When an expected outcome is not achieved, inadequate drug dosing should be considered.
- When toxicity is observed, the possibility of excessive dosing should be evaluated and an alternative dosage regimen implemented.

8.2.2   Concerns Regarding Weight-Based Dosing
in Overweight and Obese Individuals

In a comprehensive review of the topic, drug dosing recommendations based on weight or body surface area (BSA) were evaluated. Four equations used to estimate BSA and four alternative weight descriptor equations (ideal body weight, adjusted body weight, fat-free weight, and lean body weight) were discussed.[7] The usual body weights used as a reference standard for adults are 75 kg for males and 65 kg for females (i.e., the average 70 kg individual). Since the average weight for a male is 89 kg and for a female is 75 kg in the United States, when the 70 kg standard for a "normal weight" individual is used, the patient receives a 5–25% underestimate of the dose. This problem is further compounded in those who are overweight or obese. Using actual weight alone tends to overestimate the required dose in obese subjects,[8] and using BSA as the basis for dose calculations tends to underestimate the dose needed.[9] These errors are based on the assumption that in obese subjects drug disposition (i.e., clearance and distribution throughout body tissues) increases proportionally with size, which is generally not the case for most drugs. The authors reviewed the 905 FDA-approved drugs and determined that 19.3% ($n = 175$) had a weight-based dosing recommendation and 7.2% ($n = 65$) had a BSA-based dosing adjustment; 50.9% ($n = 89$) of these drugs also require dosing adjustment for renal impairment.

All of these factors potentially affect drug efficacy in a clinically significant manner and are presented in the following section based on clinical studies, case series, and case reports. There are concerns over the quality of the literature in the overweight and obese, which include small patient numbers; older studies with bariatric procedures that are no longer performed, such as jejunoileal bypass and vertical banded gastroplasty (although those data may be extrapolated to BPD or sleeve gastrectomy, respectively); and few studies with currently used procedures and therapeutic agents. Phase 3 clinical studies employed during drug development often exclude patients at both extremes of weight, and many exclude patients with a BMI of >30 kg/m^2.

8.3   CLINICALLY SIGNIFICANT DRUG THERAPY IMPACTED
BY OBESITY AND BARIATRIC SURGERY

8.3.1   Anti-Infective Drug Therapy

Some limited data are available from studies in the 1980s regarding dosing of anti-infective agents in the obese individual. Blouin et al.[10] conducted a pharmacokinetic study of amikacin in eight normal weight volunteers and five patients undergoing gastric bypass (weight, 132 ± 21.5 kg). Amikacin clearance was significantly greater in the obese patients than in the controls (131.2 ± 19.6 versus 83.2 ± 12.5 ml/min). However, when standardized to a body surface area of 1.73 m^2, the difference was not significant. The volume of distribution at steady state was also increased to 20 ± 2.9 L in obese patients versus 11.6 ± 2.0 L in controls. The terminal half-life was similar in both groups. The proposed reasons for the observed differences were increased extracellular fluid and total body water and increased glomerular filtration rate in the obese individuals. The authors recommended that larger daily doses of amikacin were needed with close therapeutic drug level monitoring.

Erythromycin has been shown to have reduced absorption after bariatric surgery (six gastroplasty, one gastric bypass).[11] Seven adult patients were administered the erythromycin base 250 mg as a single dose before and after surgery. The time to reach the maximum serum concentration (T_{max}) was prolonged by 85%, and the maximum concentration (C_{max}) was reduced by 50%. Two patients had no detectable serum drug levels after surgery.

Amoxicillin and macrodantin (nitrofurantoin) have been reported to have reduced efficacy after gastric bypass. In that case report, the patient had a urinary tract infection that had documented sensitivity to both drugs, which did not respond to the therapy.[12]

Ampicillin (administered using the prodrug pivampicillin 750 mg single oral dose) 500 mg was reported to have a reduction in bioavailability from 109% to 41% in six patients who had undergone a JIB procedure.[13] Although absorption was affected, the clearance, volume of distribution, and half-life for ampicillin were unchanged.

The pharmacokinetics of ciprofloxacin in obese patients have been reported.[14] Seventeen obese individuals (mean BMI 36.4 ± 3.9 kg/m^2) received 400 mg of ciprofloxacin as a 1 h intravenous infusion. Compared to control subjects (mean BMI 23.2 ± 2.4 kg/m^2) the clearance was 29% higher, the volume of distribution was lower, and the half-life was unchanged. Based on these findings, the authors concluded that while ciprofloxacin did not distribute fully into adipose tissue, partial distribution did occur such that a dosage increase was needed. Increasing the weight used for dosing in obese subjects by adding 45% of excess weight to the ideal body weight was recommended.

Forse et al.[15] compared tissue and serum levels of cefazolin obtained after 1 versus 2 g dosing in 30 patients undergoing vertical banded gastroplasty (mean BMI 47 ± 5 kg/m^2). Concentrations greater than the minimum inhibitory concentration were only achieved with the 2 g dose. A 2 g intravenous dose was then used prospectively for a 4-month period, and the wound infection rate fell from 16.5% to 5.6%, demonstrating improved clinical efficacy.

Aminoglycosides dosed using total body weight have been reported to cause increased nephrotoxicity in obese subjects.[16] However, using ideal body weight tends to result in underdosing. Accordingly, an adjustment accounting for 40% of excess weight (known as adjusted body weight) is commonly used for dosing.[17] Similar reports of increased toxicity have been published with amphotericin B, colistin, vancomycin, and telavancin.[18–21] Using total body weight for the initial dosing of vancomycin with subsequent use of therapeutic drug monitoring would be the optimal approach to drug therapy with these agents.[22] Elevations in creatinine kinase have been reported in obese subjects treated with daptomycin.[23,24] Daptomycin is dosed using total body weight and should be reduced if the creatinine clearance is less than 30 ml/min due to the risk of muscle damage. Limited data have also been published regarding drug dosing in obese subjects using linezolid, quinupristin-dalfopristin, fluconazole, flucystosine, sulfisoxazole, and antituberculous therapy in small case series and case reports, but are inadequate to use for making dosing suggestions.[22]

8.3.2 CARDIOVASCULAR DRUG THERAPY

Very limited data are available regarding the need for dosage adjustment of cardio-vascular drugs in patients who have undergone bariatric surgery. However, it has been reported that hypertension resolved in 70% of patients after surgery, particularly in those who had a lower postoperative BMI.[25] Over 80% (37 of 45) of the patients were taking antihypertensive medication before surgery. After 12, 24, and 48 months, respectively, only 44, 32, and 28% were still taking medication.[25]

There were no changes in digoxin pharmacokinetics in seven patients who underwent jejunoileal bypass.[26] Digoxin absorption was unimpaired. However, digoxin absorption occurs primarily in the duodenum and upper jejunum, and to a lesser extent, in the colon. There are no data from patients undergoing other bariatric procedures; however, it is likely that gastric bypass patients would experience decreased absorption. Digoxin serum levels should be monitored, especially during periods of rapid weight loss after surgery. Careful supervision of potassium and magnesium status is needed to avoid potential digoxin toxicity. Hydrochlorothiazide has been shown to have significantly reduced bioavailability after JIB.[27]

Clinicians need to be vigilant regarding new toxicity that may occur after surgery when dose reductions may be required as the patient loses weight. For example, Bourron et al.[28] published a case report of hyperthyroidism that occurred in a gastric bypass patient taking amiodarone who experienced greater than expected weight loss (45% of his preoperative weight in 6 months). The authors hypothesized that as the patient lost weight and the fat mass decreased, the volume of distribution of amiodarone decreased, leading to iodine overload and increased free thyroxine levels.

Doses of cardiovascular drugs need to be monitored closely during the first postoperative year until the patient's weight begins to plateau.

8.3.3 CENTRAL NERVOUS SYSTEM AGENTS

Phenytoin has a narrow therapeutic range, and serum levels should be monitored closely in all patients regardless of their weight. Phenytoin absorption has been demonstrated to be reduced after JIB, leading to loss of efficacy.[29] Until recently there were no published case reports in gastric bypass patients. Pournaras et al.[30] reported an epileptic patient who had been well controlled prior to surgery on phenobarbitone 60 mg daily and seizure-free for 30 years. One year after his gastric bypass surgery he had a seizure. His phenobarbitone dose was doubled and phenytoin 300 mg daily was added. Two years later he had another seizure. His phenobarbitone level was subtherapeutic, and his phenytoin level was undetectable. The phenytoin level was increased to 500 mg daily but remained undetectable. The drug therapy was changed to lamotrigine, which was well absorbed and the patient had no further seizures.

Fuller et al.[31] described a patient with schizophrenia who was well controlled with haloperidol 20 mg daily who became psychotic 3 days after her gastric bypass surgery. Her haloperidol had been discontinued by the surgeon 14 days prior to the operation. The haloperidol dose was doubled and the psychosis resolved. The dose was reduced back to the original dose and plasma concentrations demonstrated extensive absorption. The authors were unable to establish why an increased dose was needed during the period after surgery. They suggested it was due to the 14-day period presurgery without medication. Once the levels were restored to a steady state, the patient remained symptom-free.

8.3.4 MEDICATIONS USED IN THE MANAGEMENT OF ENDOCRINE DISORDERS

After gastric bypass, type 2 diabetes mellitus resolves in 80% of severely obese individuals. There are no published data regarding changes in drug disposition of drugs used in the management of diabetes conducted in bariatric patients. However, a small study (n = 20) was conducted over a 12-week period that evaluated the pharmacokinetics and pharmacodynamics of glyburide in obese diabetic patients.[32] Twelve obese (BMI 36.2 ± 9.2 kg/m^2) patients and eight nonobese (BMI 24.5 ± 2.1 kg/m^2) controls were included. Obese patients appeared to be more sensitive to the drug as defined by needing a lower dose to achieve a similar blood glucose.

Two case reports describe increased dosage requirements for thyroxine after JIB.[33,34] The bioavailability of the antithyroid medication propylthiouracil was unaffected after JIB.[13] Oral contraceptives have also been reported to have reduced absorption after JIB.[35] The levels of levonorgestrel and norethisterone that were observed were similar to those after low-dose contraceptives are used in normal weight women. Low-dose contraceptives should be avoided after bariatric surgery due to the high potential for lack of efficacy.

8.3.5 TRANSPLANTATION AND ONCOLOGY THERAPY

There are reports of reduced cyclosporine A absorption leading to lack of efficacy and inadequate immunosuppression. In one case the patient had a JIB 14 years prior to needing a cardiac transplant for idiopathic cardiomyopathy. At the time of transplant the JIB was taken down. The oral bioavailability of cyclosporine A prior to the surgery with the JIB intact was 19% and postsurgery with the JIB reversed was 53%. In addition, cyclosporine was undetectable in the serum 16 h after ingestion and did not show significant enterohepatic recycling when the JIB was intact.[36] A similar experience was reported with tacrolimus where the absorption was improved when the JIB was reversed.[37] Chensu et al. reported that the amount of cyclosporine required in a JIB patient who required a liver transplant was double the typical dosage.[38]

There are very limited data to help guide the use of anticancer drugs in obese patients and no reports specifically in bariatric patients. Sparreboom et al.[39] described the complexity of drug dosing in the obese cancer patient. They calculated pharmacokinetic parameters for eight commonly used anticancer drugs in obese patients (BMI ≥ 30 kg/m^2). Cisplatin, paclitaxel, and troxitabine showed increased clearance; carboplatin, docetaxel, irniotecan, and topotecan showed no change in clearance; and doxorubicin showed decreased clearance in women but not in men. While individuals receiving chemotherapy are more frequently of lower weight due to their underlying disease, clinical trials for breast cancer and colorectal cancer have shown poorer outcomes in obese subjects.[40–42] This may be multifactorial, but could also be a result of underdosing obese patients, especially when doses are capped at a maximum body surface area.

8.3.6 ANTICOAGULATION

The American Society for Metabolic and Bariatric Surgery (ASBMS) issued a position statement in June 2007 regarding the use of prophylactic measures for bariatric patients to reduce the risk of venous thromboembolism (VTE) during the perioperative period.[43] In summary, prophylactic measures including the use of lower-extremity compression devices and anticoagulant therapy are recommended as routine unless there are significant contraindications. The choice of regimen is still controversial, and guidelines for a specific approach have not been developed. However, there are clinical practice recommendations for use of low molecular weight heparins (LMWHs) in obese subjects.[44] As previously discussed in the course of this chapter, the authors noted that many studies exclude patients at the extremes of weight, and even when obese patients are included, the weight cutoff is generally 150–190 kg. The available evidence in 2009 was reviewed, resulting in the following recommendations for dosage and monitoring in obese subjects:

- Increasing the VTE prophylactic LMWH dosage by 30% in patients with a BMI of $\geq 40 kg/m^2$ may be appropriate.
- LMWH dosage should be based on total body weight.
- VTE treatment dosing using once daily regimens with enoxaparin in patients with a BMI of $>27 kg/m^2$ should be avoided.
- VTE treatment single daily dosing strategies for dalteparin (200 IU/kg/day) and tinzaparin (175 IU/kg/day) appear to be appropriate.
- VTE treatment doses do not appear to need to be capped for weight.
- ACS treatment dose capping refers to the individual LMWH specific recommendations.
- Anti-Xa monitoring is not needed in patients up to 190 kg.
- Anti-Xa monitoring is recommended in patients of >190 kg using LMWH doses based on total body weight and adjusting doses according to anti-Xa levels. The authors developed a nomogram for suggested dosage adjustments based on clinical practice.
- Where anti-Xa monitoring is unavailable, doses should be empirically reduced if bleeding complications occur.

The PROBE study showed an increased risk of thrombolic events in bariatric surgery patients when prophylaxis was withheld until discharge, which supports the current practice of perioperative dosing regimens.[45] Other interesting findings from the PROBE study were an increase of VTE associated with smoking, and that extended thromboprophylaxis of up to 30 days postdischarge may be beneficial since all thrombolic events occurred after discharge when prophylaxis had stopped. A recent study[46] recommended a VTE prophylaxis protocol using twice daily BMI-based dosing of enoxaparin. The protocol included pneumatic compression devices placed prior to the induction of anesthesia, the first dose of enoxaparin given 1 h prior to incision and then twice daily thereafter, and early postoperative ambulation. None of the patients experienced clinically significant DVT or PE during their stay or up to 2 years of follow-up. A small percentage (2.9%) of patients required discontinuation of enoxaparin and blood transfusion for postoperative bleeding.

The use of oral anticoagulants after bariatric surgery is difficult due to altered dietary intake and erratic drug absorption. Warfarin is a weak acid and is usually well absorbed in the acidic environment of the stomach in its nonionized form. As discussed earlier, after surgery where the stomach is bypassed or removed, the absorption of warfarin is significantly impaired.[47] Warfarin therapy using higher doses than normal and with close international normalized ratio (INR) monitoring may be possible in some patients. A safer approach to avoid toxicity and ensure efficacy would be the use of low molecular weight heparin. There are no currently published studies regarding the use of direct thrombin inhibitors in the bariatric surgery population.

8.4 SUMMARY OF STRATEGIES TO ADDRESS MEDICATION MANAGEMENT ISSUES IN THE BARIATRIC POPULATION

There are very limited evidence-based data in the bariatric population; however, several reviews in the literature have addressed this topic and made recommendations based on types of pharmaceutical formulations available and possible monitoring parameters.[48–50]

When the drug has a narrow therapeutic index (a small range in serum concentrations between efficacy and toxicity), therapeutic serum monitoring should be used and the drug dosed according to the concentrations required. In some cases where lack of efficacy is observed but the patient is known to be adherent to his or her medication regimen, checking serum drug levels may help to confirm lack of absorption. If the drug is not being adequately absorbed, possible strategies include increasing the dose while monitoring serum levels to achieve the desired therapeutic outcome, changing the formulation to an immediate release or liquid product, changing to a nonoral formulation (for example, topical, rectal, transdermal) or changing the drug to another similar agent that has better oral availability. Drugs that are known to have poor availability in normal circumstances should be avoided. Some drug formulations are best avoided after bariatric surgery, such as slow release or extended release products and pH-dependent release formulations. Drugs that are dosed according to therapeutic outcome, for example, blood pressure and blood glucose, should be dosed as needed to achieve the desired effect without causing toxicity. Drugs that are known to cause intestinal mucosal damage should be avoided, for example, nonsteroidal anti-inflammatory agents, aspirin, and bisphosphonates. The ASBMS guidelines[51] recommend bisphosphonates for the management of osteoporosis, but these medications should be taken with a full glass of water, which is difficult to consume for a patient who has had a restrictive procedure. Consideration should be given to intravenous administration of alendronate or zoledronic acid as an alternative approach.

Other practical considerations include the size and number of tablets the patient may need to take during the day. Help should be provided in designing an individualized medication and supplement regimen that avoids an excessive pill burden, interactions between agents, and facilitates patient adherence. Calcium supplements are often large and might be better replaced with chewable or liquid products, although they tend to be more expensive. Common examples of products used are presented in Table 8.2.

TABLE 8.2
Comparison of Commonly Used Calcium Supplementation Products

Product	Strength (mg) per Pill/Tab/Chew	Salt	Elemental Calcium (mg)	Vitamin D (IU)	Price	Generic CVS Brand	Additional Information
Os-Cal[00]	1250	Carbonate	500 (3/day)	N/A	?	20¢/day	Coated caplet (can be crushed)
Os-Cal +D	1250	Carbonate	500 (3/day)	200 D₃	34¢/day	19¢/day	Coated caplet (can be crushed)
Os-Cal Chewable		Carbonate	500 mg (3/day)	400 D₃	42¢/day		Chewable (lemon)
Tums[00]	500	Carbonate	200 (7.5/day)	N/A	26¢/day	21¢/day	Chewable
Tums EX	750	Carbonate	300 (5/day)	N/A	28¢/day	22¢/day	Chewable
Tums Ultra	1000	Carbonate	400 (4/day)	N/A	29¢/day	23¢/day	Chewable
Viactiv[00]	1250	Carbonate	500 (3/day)	N/A			
Viactiv +D	1250	Carbonate	500 (3/day)	100 D₃	42¢/day	32¢/day	Chewable
Citracal[00] +D	1500	Citrate	315 (5/day)	200 D₃	50¢/day		
Citracal Chews		Citrate	500 (3/day)	200 D₃	80¢/day		
Citracal Liquitabs	2736	Citrate	500 (3/day)				
Caltrate[00]	1500	Carbonate	600 (3/day)		27¢/day		Can be crushed
Caltrate+D	1500	Carbonate	600 (3/day)	400 D₃	33¢/day		Can be crushed
Oyster Shell		Carbonate	500				
Oyster Shell +D		Carbonate	500	200 D₂	9¢/day		
VitaFusion™ Calcium Gummy	500	Citrate		1000	24¢/day		Gummies—chewable, fruit flavors
Adora[00]	500	Carbonate		250 D₃	66¢/day		Milk chocolate, gluten-free
Calcet[00] Calcium Creamy Bites	500	Citrate		400 D₃	93¢/day		Creamy bites, chocolate fudge
Nature's Way Alive![00] Calcium	1000	Citrate		1000 D₃	49¢/day		Tablets (can be crushed)
Mason Natural[00] Calcium + D	600	Carbonate	600 (3/day)	400 D₃	14¢/day		Chewable tablets, coffee mocha flavor

Product	Elemental Calcium (mg)	Form	Serving	Vitamin D	Price	Notes
L'il Critters® Calcium Gummy Bears	200	Citrate	200 (2/day)	200 D$_3$	25¢/day	Gummies, gluten-free, wheat-free
Solgar® Calcium Citrate with Vitamin D	250	Citrate		150 D$_3$	48¢/day	
Solgar Chewable Calcium Wafer	500	Carbonate		N/A	19¢/day	
Solgar Chelated Calcium Tablets	167	Glycinate amino acid chelate, carbonate		N/A	56¢/day	
Caltrate Gummy Bites	250	Citrate	250 (2 tablets twice daily)	400 D$_3$	$1.09/day 83¢/day	Strawberry, lemon, and cherry gummies
Celebrate® Bariatric Calcium Plus	167	Citrate		133 D$_3$	50¢/day	Includes vitamin K, copper, and zinc
Celebrate Bariatric Calcium Plus Chewable	250	Citrate		250 D$_3$	53¢/day	Strawberry crème, hot cocoa flavors
Celebrate Bariatric Calcium Plus 500	500	Citrate			$1.43/day	Orange burst, cherry tart flavors
Celebrate Bariatric Soft Chews	250	Citrate		250 D$_3$	$1.18/day	Chocolate, caramel, berry flavors
Calcium Bites™ for Good Bone Health	500	Carbonate	500 (2/day)	500 D$_3$	$1.24/day	Chocolate caramel chews, gluten-free, 30 calories

Note: Price is based on meeting the daily requirement of 1500 mg of elemental calcium.

Prior to surgery the patient's medication regimen should be evaluated and a plan developed for appropriate management of chronic medications that will be required postoperatively and new supplements or medications that will be needed for weeks or lifelong after surgery.

8.5 SUGGESTIONS FOR MANAGING PREDICTABLE DRUG-INDUCED WEIGHT GAIN

There are many medications and drug classes associated with clinically significant weight gain; where possible, these drugs should be avoided. Weight gain should be considered an adverse effect in any patient, but especially in the bariatric patient before and after surgery. Although type 2 diabetes mellitus improves substantially after bariatric surgery such that medications are either discontinued or dosages are reduced, clinicians should be aware of weight gain associated with the use of insulin, sulfonylureas (glipizide, glyburide, glimepiride) thiazolidinediones (pioglitazone, rosiglitazone), and meglitinides (repaglinide, nateglinide). Many medications used to treat psychiatric and neurologic disease are associated with weight gain via a variety of proposed mechanisms[52–57] (Table 8.3). The amount and rate of weight gain vary widely between drugs and individual patient responses. The approximate weight gain for some commonly used medications is presented in Table 8.4. It is beyond the scope of this chapter to extensively review this topic in detail, but it is addressed elsewhere.[56,57] Weight gain with medication should be considered along with other adverse effects when designing a therapeutic regimen for individual patients. Alternative therapies, which are weight neutral, should be selected for individuals who are predisposed to overweight and obesity. The medication regimen should be evaluated before and after surgery to ensure that the best possible therapy is delivered with the lowest required dose and the most appropriate choice of therapy. Patients who require medications known to cause weight gain should proactively reduce their caloric intake at the start of treatment and increase their energy expenditure to avoid the anticipated gain. In some cases weight loss medication may be an appropriate addition to their regimen.

TABLE 8.3

Drug-Induced Weight Gain Associated with Medication Used in the Treatment of Psychiatric Disorders

Mechanism Leading to Increased Weight	Medication Class or Drug
Decreased metabolic rate of ~300 kcal/day	Tricyclic antidepressants, selective serotonin reuptake inhibitors, monoamine oxidase inhibitors, clozapine
Changes in insulin sensitivity, raised prolactin, gonadal dysfunction	Clozapine, olanzapine, risperidone
Interaction with dopamine d2, $5HT_{2A}$, $5HT_{2C}$, or histamine H_1 receptors	Clozapine, olanzapine, risperidone, quetiapine
Genetic polymorphism	Risperidone

TABLE 8.4

Typical Weight Gain Expected with Commonly Used Medications for the Treatment of Type 2 Diabetes Mellitus and Psychiatric or Neurologic Disorders[52–57]

Medication Used in the Management of Diabetes Mellitus	Approximate Weight Gain
Insulin	4 kg
Sulfonylureas	2 kg
Thiazolidinediones	3–4.6 kg
Meglitinides	0.7–1.8 kg
Medication used in the management of psychiatric and neurologic disorders[52]	
Clozapine	1.7 kg/month
Olanzapine	2.3 kg/month
Risperidone	1.0 kg/month
Imipramine	3–4 kg total
Amitriptyline	2 kg total
Lithium	10 kg or greater
Valproate	0–15 kg
Carbamazepine	0–15 kg
Gabapentin	Up to 15% (dose related)
Selective serotonin reuptake inhibitors	Varies with drug, duration, and individual response

8.6 DRUG–NUTRIENT INTERACTIONS AND OTHER CONSIDERATIONS

The absorption and disposition for individual nutrients and the daily requirements to meet the needs of post-bariatric surgery patients are covered in the nutrient-specific chapters in this text. Nutrients that many patients find difficult to take due to gastrointestinal intolerance include iron, zinc, potassium, and magnesium replacement. Possible strategies include using more frequent lower individual doses; however, this approach increases the number of tablets the patient needs to take and contributes to nonadherence. Intravenous iron infusions may be necessary to restore iron stores in some patients, although there are no specific guidelines available regarding the dose regimen and indication for therapy.

There are a wide variety of calcium formulation supplements available with different salt forms, contents, and costs. Common examples of available products are presented in Table 8.2. Calcium citrate has been shown to have better absorption after gastric bypass and is the preferred salt form.[51] However, calcium carbonate products tend to be less expensive.

The cost of nutritional supplements primarily needed is around $40/month, which may lead to nonadherence and should be discussed as a potential issue with patients.

TABLE 8.5

Summary: Key Points for the Practicing Health Care Provider Managing Medication and Nutritional Supplement Regimens for Post-Bariatric Surgery Patients

Prior to surgery review chronic medications that will be required after surgery and ensure that they will still be effective, and if not, select an alternative dosage form, route of administration, or drug

Pharmacokinetics of a drug may alter after surgery

Pharmacokinetics of a drug may be altered in obese individuals

Therapeutic drug monitoring should be used for drugs with a narrow therapeutic index

Serum level monitoring should be done when lack of efficacy is suspected due to inadequate response, especially when good adherence is documented

Absorption of a drug or specific formulation may be reduced or absent after surgery

Avoid slow release and pH-dependent release drug formulations if malabsorption is a factor

Consider drug-induced weight gain as an adverse effect and select a weight-neutral alternative

Monitor for weight gain, especially after weight has reached a plateau postoperatively, and review and address factors contributing to weight regain of >5%

Ensure patients understand the need for lifelong nutritional supplements and the risks associated with nonadherence

Address the cost of required medications and supplements before surgery to ensure that this is not a potential contributing factor to nonadherence after surgery

Design a therapeutic regimen including drugs and supplements that the patient can reasonably follow on a daily basis; consider the use of alternative regimens, e.g., weekly or alternate day therapy, to minimize the pill burden each day

Avoid orally administered drugs if they cause gastrointestinal irritation: Nonsteroidal anti-inflammatory drugs (NSAIDs), aspirin, bisphosphonates, iron, potassium

Consider the effect of food on drug absorption and dose the medication accordingly in relation to meals

Where common drug food interactions exist under usual circumstances, these need to be especially considered in the bariatric patient. For example, divalent cations (calcium, iron, magnesium) interact with quinolone (ciprofloxacin, norfloxacin) antibiotics and tetracyclines; these regimens should be designed to separate the drug from the supplements even if this requires withholding supplements during a short course of antibiotic therapy. Thyroxine is poorly absorbed and should be separated from calcium and iron supplements. Iron can also impair the absorption of angiotensin-converting inhibitors and levopa/carbidopa.

Lastly, some drugs are better taken on an empty stomach to improve absorption (examples include bisphosphonates, captopril, cefaclor, digoxin, diltiazem, furosemide, proton pump inhibitors, zafirlukast, warfarin), while other drugs are better absorbed with food (examples include carbamazepine, fenofibrate, labetalol, metoprolol, tamsulosin, nitrofurantoin (Macrobid formulation)). Timing of medications in relation to food intake is difficult to achieve when patients are taking many medications and supplements and have a restriction on the amount that can be consumed at one time.

TABLE 8.6

Commonly Used Medications and Supplements Requiring Special Attention in the Post-Bariatric Surgery Patient

Medication or Supplement	Reason for Review
Iron, zinc, potassium, magnesium	Gastrointestinal intolerance, interactions with medications
Calcium supplements	Large size of some tablets that are hard to take, interactions with medications
Multivitamins	Ensure selected product contains the range of multivitamins and minerals that are needed for the bariatric patient
Aminoglycoside antibiotics	Monitor serum levels to ensure efficacy and avoid toxicity
Phenytoin	Poorly absorbed, monitor serum levels, change drug therapy to an alternative agent if needed
Thyroxine	Monitor for efficacy due to poor absorption
Warfarin	Monitor INR very closely, use low molecular weight heparin as first choice
Bisphosphonates	Consider nonoral dosing to avoid GI irritation
Antidiabetic, antihypertensive, and cholesterol-lowering medications	Dose according to desired outcome, monitor and reduce doses with weight loss as needed, especially in the first year postsurgery
Oral contraceptives	Low-dose formulations are likely to be ineffective
Ulcerogenic drugs and supplements	Consider the potential risk of mucosal damage to the gastric pouch

8.7 CONCLUSION

In conclusion, drug dosing in overweight and obese subjects is a poorly studied area. Data in bariatric surgery patients in particular are very sparse. Since it is unlikely that studies in obese subjects for drugs that are already marketed will be conducted, clinicians will need to apply some of the concepts discussed in this chapter. Providers and patients need to be vigilant for unanticipated changes in efficacy and toxicity for drugs and nutritional supplements. Tables 8.5 and 8.6 provide a summary of key points for providers to consider, and those drugs and nutrients that require special attention in the bariatric patient. Pharmacists should contribute to patient care through the provision of pharmacokinetic consultations, advice regarding formulation characteristics and selection, and medication therapy management services to optimize medication and nutritional supplement regimens.

REFERENCES

1. Padwal R, Brocks D, Sharma AM. 2010. A systematic review of drug absorption following bariatric surgery and its theoretical implications. *Obes Rev* 11:41–50.
2. Gubbins PO, Bertch KE. 1991. Drug absorption in gastrointestinal disease and surgery. *Clin Pharmacokinet* 21:431–447.
3. Andari Sawaya R, Jaffe J, Friedenberg L, Friedenberg FK. 2012. Vitamin, mineral and drug absorption following bariatric surgery. *Curr Drug Metab* 13(9):1345–55.

4. Chen ML, Amidon GL, Benet LZ, Lennernas H, Yu LX. 2011. The BCS, BDDCS and regulatory guidances. *Pharm Res.* DOI 10.1007/s11095-011-0438-1.
5. Gubbins PO, Bertch KE. 1991. Drug absorption in gastrointestinal disease and surgery. *Clin Pharmacokinet* 21:431–447.
6. Cheymol G. 1993. Clinical pharmacokinetics of drugs in obesity. *Clin Pharmacokinet* 25:103–114.
7. Pai MP. 2012. Drug dosing based on weight and body surface area: mathematical assumptions and limitations in obese adults. *Pharmacotherapy* 32(9):856–868.
8. Moorish GA, Pai MP, Green B. 2011. The effects of obesity on drug pharmacokinetics in humans. *Exp Opin Drug Metab Toxicol* 7:697–706.
9. Hunter RJ, Navo MA, Thaker PH, Bodurka DC, Wolf JK, Smith JA. 2009. Dosing chemotherapy in obese patients: actual versus assigned body surface area (BSA). *Cancer Treat Rev* 35:69–78.
10. Blouin RA, Brouwer KL, Record KE, et al. 1985. Amikacin pharmacokinetics in morbidly obese patients undergoing gastric bypass surgery. *Clin Pharmacol Ther* 4:70–72.
11. Prince RE, Pincheira JC, Mason EE, Printon KJ. 1984. Influence of bariatric surgery on erythromycin absorption. *J Clin Pharmacol* 24:523–527.
12. Magee SR, Shih G, Hume A. 2007. Malabsorption of oral antibiotics in pregnancy after gastric bypass. *J Am Board Fam Med* 20:310–313.
13. Kampmann JP, Klein H, Lumholtz B, Molholm JE. 1984. Ampicillin and propylthiouracil pharmacokinetics in intestinal bypass patients followed up to a year after operation. *Clin Pharmacokinet* 9:168–176.
14. Allard S, Kinzig M, Boivin G, et al. 1993. Intravenous ciprofloxacin disposition in obesity. *Clin Pharmacol Ther* 54:368–373.
15. Forse RA, Karam B, MacLean LD, et al. 1989. Antibiotic prophylaxis in morbidly obese patients. *Surgery* 106:750–757.
16. Corcoran GB, Salazar DE, Schentag JJ. 1988. Excessive aminoglycoside nephrotoxicity in obese subjects. *Am J Med* 85:279.
17. Traynor AM, Nafziger AN, Bertino JS. 1995. Aminoglycoside dosing weight correction factors for patients of various body sizes. *Antimicrob Agents Chemother* 39:545–548.
18. Harbath S, Pestonik SL, Lloyd JF, Burke JP, Samore MH. 2001. The epidemiology of nephrotoxicity associated with conventional amphotericin B therapy. *Am J Med* 111:528–534.
19. Deryke CA, Crawford AJ, Uddin N, Wallace MR. 2010. Colistin dosing and nephrotoxicity in a large community teaching hospital. *Antimicrob Agents Chemother* 54:4503–4505.
20. Lodise TP, Patel N, Lomaestro BM, Rodvold KA, Drusano GL. 2009. Relationship between initial vancomycin concentration time profile and nephrotoxicity among hospitalized patients. *Clin Infect Dis* 49:507–514.
21. Slover CM, Nkechi A, Barriere SL, Lu Q. Telavancin for treatment of complicated skin and skin structure infections in obese patients Chicago, IL: Interscience Conference on Antimicrobial Agents and Chemotherapy; 2011.
22. Pai MP, Bearden D. 2007. Antimicrobial dosing considerations in obese adult patients. *Pharmacotherapy* 27(8):1081–1091.
23. Figueroa DA, Mangini E, Amodio-Groton M, et al. 2009. Safety of high dose intravenous daptomycin treatment: three year cumulative experience in a clinical program. *Clin Infect Dis* 49:177–180.
24. Bhavnani SM, Rubino CM, Ambrose PG, Drusano GL. 2010. Daptomycin exposure and the probability of elevations in the creatinine phosphokinase level: data from a randomized trial of patients with bacteremia and endocarditis. *Clin Infect Dis* 50:1568–1574.
25. Carson JL, Ruddy ME, Duff AE, et al. 1994. The effect of gastric bypass on hypertension in morbidly obese patients. *Arch Intern Med* 154:193–200.

26. Beerman B, Hellstrom K, Rosen A. 1973. The gastrointestinal absorption of digoxin in seven patients with gastric or small intestinal reconstructions. *Acta Med Scand* 193:293–297.
27. Backman L, Beerman B, Groschinsky-Grind M, Halberg D. 1979. Malabsorption of hydrochlorothiazde following intestinal shunt surgery. *Clin Pharmacokinet* 4:63–68.
28. Bourron O, Ciangure C, Bouillot JL, Massias L, Poitou C, Oppert JM. 2007. Amiodarone induced hyperthyroidisim during massive weight loss following gastric bypass. *Obes Surg* 17:1525–1528.
29. Kennedy MC, Wade DN. 1979. Phenytoin absorption in patients with ileojejunal bypass. *Br J Clin Pharmacol* 7:515–518.
30. Pournaras DJ, Footitt D, Mahon D, Welbourn R. 2011. Reduced phenytoin levels in an epileptic patient following Roux-en-Y gastric bypass for obesity. *Obes Surg* 21:684–685.
31. Fuller AK, Tingle D, DeVane L, Scott JA, Stewart RB. 1986. Haloperidol pharmacokinetics following gastric bypass surgery. *J Clin Psychopharmacol* 6:376–377.
32. Jaber LA, Antal EJ, Slaughter RL, Welshman IR. 1993. The pharmacokinetics and pharmacodynamics of 12 weeks of glyburide therapy in obese diabetics. *Eur J Clin Pharmacol* 45:459–463.
33. Azizi F, Belur R, Albano J. 1979. Malabsorption of thyroid hormones after jejunoileal bypass for obesity. *Ann Intern Med* 90:941–942.
34. Bevan JS, Munro JF. 1986. Thyroxine malabsorption following intestinal bypass surgery. *Int J Obes* 10:245–246.
35. Victor A, Odlind V, Kral JG. 1987. Oral contraceptive absorption and sex hormone binding globulins in obese women: effects of jejunoileal bypass. *Gastroenterol Clin North Am* 16:483–491.
36. Knight GC, Macris MP, Duncan JM, Frazier OH, Cooley DA. 1988. Cyclosporine A pharmacokinetics in a cardiac allograft recipient with a jejuno-ileal bypass. *Transplant Proc* 20:351–355.
37. Kelley M, Jain A, Kashyap R, et al. 2005. Change in oral absorption of tacrolimus in a liver transplant recipient after reversal of jejunoileal bypass: a case report. *Transplant Proc* 37:3165–3167.
38. Chensu RY, Wu Y, Katz D, Rayhill S. 2003. Dose adjusted cyclosporine C2 in a patient with jejunoileal bypass as compared to seven other liver transplant recipients. *Ther Drug Monit* 25:665–670.
39. Sparreboom A, Wolff AC, Mathijssen RHJ, et al. 2007. Evaluation of alternate size descriptors for dose calculation of anticancer drugs in the obese. *J Clin Oncol* 25:4707–4713.
40. Meyerhardt JA, Tepper JE, Niedzwiecki D, et al. 2004. Impact of body mass index on outcomes and treatment related toxicity in patients with stage 2 and 3 rectal cancer: findings from Intergroup Trial 0114. *J Clin Oncol* 22:648–657.
41. Chambers P, Daniels SH, Thompson LC, Stephens RJ. 2012. Chemotherapy dose reductions in obese patients with colorectal cancer. *Ann Oncol* 23:748–753.
42. Protani M, Coory M, Martin JH. 2010. Effect of obesity on survival of women with breast cancer: systematic review and meta analysis. *Breast Cancer Res Treat* 123:627–635.
43. ASBMS position statement on prophylactic measures to reduce the risk of venous thromboembolism in bariatric surgery patients June 2007. www.asbs.org/resources (accessed December 7, 2012).
44. Nutescu ED, Spinler SA, Wittowsky A, Dager WE. 2009. Low molecular weight heparins in renal impairment and obesity: available evidence and clinical practice recommendations across medical and surgical settings. *Ann Pharmacother* 43:1064–1083. DOI 10.1345/aph.1L194.

45. Hamad GG, Choban PS. 2005. Enoxaparin for thromboprophylaxis in morbidly obese patients undergoing bariatric surgery: findings of the prophylaxis against VTE outcomes in bariatric surgery patients receiving enoxaparin (PROBE) study. *Obes Surg* 15:1368–1374.

46. Singh K, Podolsky ER, Um S, et al. 2011. Evaluating the safety and efficacy of BMI based preoperative administration of low molecular weight heparin in morbidly obese patients undergoing Roux-en-Y gastric bypass surgery. *Obes Surg.* DOI 10.1007/s11695-011-0397-y.

47. Sobieraj DM, Wang F, Kirton OC. 2008. Warfarin resistance after total gastrectomy and Roux-en-Y esophagojejunostomy. *Pharmacotherapy* 28(12):1537–1541.

48. Malone M. 2003. Altered drug disposition in obesity and after bariatric surgery. *Nutr Clin Pract* 18:131–135.

49. Lizer MH, Papageorgeon H, Glembot TM. 2010. Nutritional and pharmacologic challenges in the bariatric patient. *Obes Surg* 20:1654–1659.

50. Miller AD, Smith KM. 2006. Medication and nutrient administration considerations after bariatric surgery. *Am J Health-Syst Pharm* 63:1852–1857.

51. AACE/TOS/ASBMS. 2009. Medical guidelines for clinical practice for the perioperative nutritional, metabolic and nonsurgical support of the bariatric surgery patient. *Obesity* 17(Suppl).

52. Jensen GL. 2008. Drug induced hyperphagia: what can we learn from psychiatric medications? *J Parenter Enteral Nutr* 32(5):578–581. DOI 10.1177/0148607108321708.

53. Brixner DI, Said Q, Corey-Lisle PK, et al. 2006. Naturalistic impact of second generation antipsychotics on weight gain. *Ann Pharmacother* 40(4):626–632.

54. Purnell JQ, Weyer C. Weight effect of current and experimental drugs for diabetes mellitus. *Treat Endocrinol* 2003;2(1):33–47.

55. Krentz AJ, Bailey CJ. Oral antidiabetic agents. *Drugs* 2005;(3):385–411.

56. Cheskin LJ, Bartlett SJ, Zayas R, Twilley CH, Allison DB, Contoreggi C. 1999. Prescription medications: a modifiable contributor to obesity. *S Med J* 92:898–904.

57. Malone M. 2005. Medications associated with weight gain. *Ann Pharmacother* 39:2048–2055.

9 Macronutrient Concerns
Protein–Energy Malnutrition

Pornpoj Pramyothin and Caroline M. Apovian

CONTENTS

9.1 INTRODUCTION

Protein–energy malnutrition (PEM) is one of the most serious complications of bariatric surgery. With contemporary restrictive bariatric procedures such as laparoscopic adjustable gastric banding (LAGB) and laparoscopic sleeve gastrectomy (LSG), or a combined restrictive-malabsorptive procedure such as standard Roux-en-Y gastric bypass (RYGB), PEM is rarely encountered unless in the presence of significant surgical complications or in patients who are noncompliant with postoperative dietary modifications.[1,2] For malabsorptive bariatric procedures, however, PEM remains a concern. The history and development of malabsorptive surgical procedures are closely related to PEM, as it is often the reason leading to modification of existing procedures or development of new approaches in hopes of avoiding this dreadful complication.[3] This chapter will briefly describe clinical characteristics of PEM in bariatric patients, and will discuss PEM in the context of historical and contemporary malabsorptive surgical procedures, including jejunoileal bypass (JIB), biliopancreatic diversion (BPD), and its variation, biliopancreatic diversion with duodenal switch (BPD/DS), long-limb Roux-en-Y gastric bypass (LL-RYGB), and distal Roux-en-Y gastric bypass (D-RYGB).

9.2 CLINICAL CHARACTERISTICS OF PROTEIN–ENERGY MALNUTRITION IN BARIATRIC PATIENTS

In the general population, PEM is defined as "decline in lean body mass with the potential for functional impairment at molecular, physiologic, and/or gross motor levels,"[4–6] which is usually accompanied by weight loss and decreased dietary intake (starvation). However, it has been shown that the decline in lean body mass, particularly during acute or chronic illness, is also a function of inflammation, which often coexists with starvation in these circumstances.[4] Nutritional intervention will fully reverse loss of lean body mass that occurs during pure starvation, while its success in patients who are both inflamed and starved is limited by the extent and duration of the ongoing inflammation.[4]

The American Society for Parenteral and Enteral Nutrition (ASPEN) and the Academy of Nutrition and Dietetics have published a consensus statement that outlines an etiology-based classification of adult PEM that takes into account the significance of inflammation in various disease states. The classification consists of three categories as follows[6]:

1. Starvation-related malnutrition is characterized by chronic starvation without inflammation, consistent with the clinical syndrome of marasmus previously described in the literature. Anorexia nervosa is an example.
2. Chronic disease-related malnutrition is characterized by loss of lean body mass that occurs as a result of persistent mild to moderate inflammation. Its pathophysiology resembles that of the syndrome cachexia. Examples include pancreatic cancer, rheumatoid arthritis, chronic heart failure, chronic renal insufficiency, and chronic liver diseases.
3. Acute disease or injury-related malnutrition occurs during severe inflammation as observed in acutely ill patients with severe infection, burns, trauma, and major surgery.

Clinical characteristics of inflammation include increased extracellular fluid (e.g., edema, pleural effusion, and ascites) and a decline in levels of visceral proteins (e.g., albumin and prealbumin).[5] These features are observed in patients with acute disease- or chronic disease-related malnutrition, but not in those with starvation-related malnutrition. Low serum levels of albumin and prealbumin have traditionally been associated with malnutrition. However, recent literature suggests that serum albumin and prealbumin levels do not accurately reflect nutritional status, but rather are indicators of severity of illness and inflammation.[7] As previously discussed, inflammation is known to have a significant impact on the nutritional status of an individual patient. Therefore, patients who develop severe hypoalbuminemia during acute illness are not necessarily malnourished, but are under severe stress and should promptly receive nutritional intervention when indicated.[4]

The intent of all bariatric procedures is to produce weight loss by reducing food intake, which is consistent with an iatrogenic form of starvation-related malnutrition. On the other hand, inflammation associated with acute illness is not an anticipated consequence of bariatric surgery, except during the immediate postoperative period and when severe surgical or medical complications develop (e.g., wound infection, anastomotic leakage, or venous thromboembolism). Therefore, unless otherwise noted, the term *PEM* will be used interchangeably with starvation-related malnutrition in the following sections of this chapter. Other findings that have been associated with PEM after bariatric surgery include asthenia, alopecia, and anemia.[1,2]

As starvation and weight loss are expected outcomes of bariatric surgery, concerns are not usually raised unless these changes deviate from usual clinical courses. At present, consensus is lacking to define what degree of changes should be considered excessive and problematic. However, the following characteristics may assist in identifying bariatric patients with or at risk for PEM:

1. Excessive weight loss. The typical course of weight loss after bariatric surgery is a function of the type of procedure performed. In most patients, postoperative weight loss does not continue beyond 12–18 months. Those who continue to lose weight after this period or lose more weight than expected for a particular procedure should be carefully evaluated for PEM.
2. Nonadherence with dietary recommendations. Dietary intake is dramatically altered after bariatric surgery, particularly over the first 6–12 months, with restrictions to only liquid and soft diet in the first month, and gradual progression to a more complex diet over the ensuing months.[8,9] Patients are asked to eat slowly in small portions and to chew thoroughly. Those who do not follow these recommendations may develop dysphagia, nausea, or vomiting, which may result in inadequate food intake.[10] In addition, food intake may also be affected by selective food aversion, particularly to red meat and sweets,[11–13] in which case poultry, eggs, fish, and dairy products are recommended. Published guidelines recommend an intake of 60–120 g of protein per day in the postoperative period,[14,15] which may not be achievable in some patients unless protein supplements are used.
3. Surgical complications. Postprandial vomiting and abdominal pain may occur as a consequence of surgical complications such as stomal stenosis or stricture, internal hernia, small bowel obstruction, marginal ulcers, or gastric band erosions in the case of LAGB. In addition, anastomotic leakage, intra-abdominal collection, and wound infection may also occur. These complications not only limit dietary intake, but also result in inflammation and acute disease-related malnutrition that favors further loss of lean body mass.[4]
4. Micronutrient deficiencies. Deficiencies of thiamine, vitamin B_{12}, vitamin D, calcium, iron, and other micronutrients after bariatric surgery may be attributable to inadequate absorption or supplementation, but may also stem from maladaptive eating behaviors. Evaluation for PEM should occur in conjunction with diagnosis and treatment of other micronutrient deficiencies.

Anatomical and physiological changes that occur after bariatric surgery vary widely depending on the distinct characteristics of each procedure. The remaining sections in this chapter will discuss the pathophysiology, clinical findings, and management of PEM, which complicates each of the malabsorptive operations, both historical and contemporary, including JIB, BPD, BPD/DS, LL-RYGB, and D-RYGB. As purely restrictive procedures rarely lead to PEM except when surgical complications occur, these procedures will not be discussed here.

9.3   JEJUNOILEAL BYPASS AND PROTEIN–ENERGY MALNUTRITION

JIB was the most widely performed bariatric procedure in the 1960s and 1970s. By anastomosing the proximal jejunum to the distal ileum, only 40–60 cm of small bowel was left in continuity, while a very long segment was bypassed (Figure 9.1),[16] resulting in significant malabsorption and excellent weight loss of up to 30–40% of the initial weight.[17,18] However, this procedure was abandoned by most in the 1980s due to an unacceptably high incidence of complications. Among these complications were excessive weight loss and weakness consistent with PEM, persistent diarrhea, and steatorrhea from fat malabsorption.[18,19] In one series, 15% of patients lost more than 50% of their initial weight, necessitating reversal of the procedure in a third of this subgroup, with one death in a cachectic patient who refused reversal of the procedure.[17] Other complications of JIB include hepatic failure, cirrhosis, bacterial overgrowth syndrome, fluid and electrolyte imbalances, oxalate renal stones, and micronutrient deficiencies, including vitamin B_{12}, iron, and calcium. JIB is no longer considered an appropriate surgical option for weight loss.

9.4   BILIOPANCREATIC DIVERSION AND PROTEIN–ENERGY MALNUTRITION

BPD is among the most effective bariatric procedures still in use today. However, the procedure is utilized by only a limited number of surgeons, as BPD or BPD/DS constitutes only 0.89% of all bariatric surgeries in the United States[20] and 2.2% of all bariatric surgeries worldwide.[21] This is probably a result of the perceived complexity of the procedure and concerns for late complications, such as PEM.[22] Scopinaro and colleagues from Genoa, Italy, were the first to perform BPD in 1976.[23,24] The procedure involves a distal partial gastrectomy, which reduces the volume of the gastric pouch to 200–500 ml, and a long Roux-en-Y reconstruction where the "alimentary limb" or "Roux limb" length (from gastroenterostomy to enteroenterostomy) varies between 250 and 350 cm and the common channel (from enteroenterostomy to ileocecal valve) length is 50 cm (Figure 9.2).[16]

With BPD, many of the serious complications of JIB are avoided because no blind small bowel loop is present. It is believed that the mechanism by which BPD results in long-term weight maintenance involves limitation of carbohydrate and fat absorption, and thus energy absorption, to a certain maximum threshold. As a result, energy

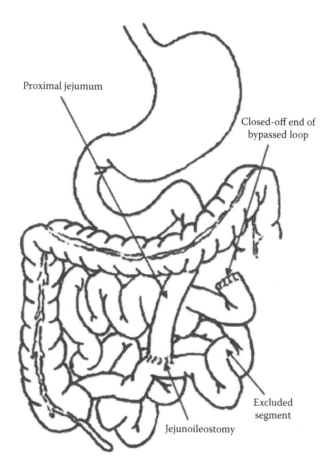

Proximal jejumum

Closed-off end of
bypassed loop

Excluded
segment

Jejunoileostomy

FIGURE 9.1   Jejunoileal bypass (JIB). (Reprinted with permission from Kim, D. W., and Apovian, C. M., in Rippe and Angelopoulos, eds., *Obesity: Prevention and Treatment*, CRC Press, Boca Raton, Florida, 2012, p. 194.)

absorption would not exceed this threshold despite overfeeding of carbohydrate and fat.[25] In contrast, protein absorption is a function of dietary intake, and approximately 70% of dietary protein is absorbed.[26] Scopinaro and colleagues assessed protein absorption in 15 patients who had undergone BPD 24–36 months earlier by administering I[125] albumin orally and demonstrated that approximately 73% of the administered amount was absorbed, while 27% of the radiolabeled albumin (equivalent to 7.4 g of nitrogen) was lost in the stool.[25] At the same time, total fecal nitrogen content was found to be 12.3 g in these patients, suggesting that the additional 4.9 g of fecal nitrogen represented gastrointestinal loss of endogenous nitrogen, which was significantly greater than what would be expected in normal physiology. It was postulated that this increased loss of endogenous nitrogen may play a significant role in the development of PEM after BPD, particularly during the early postoperative period when the ability of the patient to increase protein intake remains limited.[26]

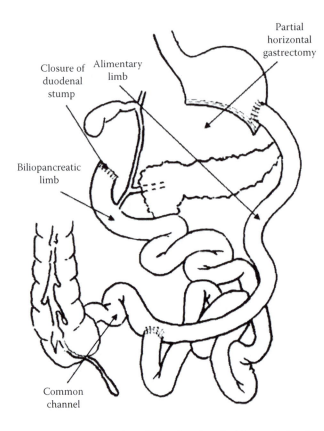

FIGURE 9.2   Biliopancreatic diversion (BPD). (Reprinted with permission from Kim, D. W., and Apovian, C. M., in Rippe and Angelopoulos, eds., *Obesity: Prevention and Treatment*, CRC Press, Boca Raton, Florida, 2012, p. 194.)

Hence, adequate protein intake is of paramount importance, and it has been suggested that up to 90 g of protein daily is required to prevent PEM after BPD.[27]

The original intent of the procedure was to produce malabsorption by delaying the mixing of food and biliopancreatic secretions so that pancreatic digestion would only occur in the common channel. However, subsequent physiologic studies demonstrated that almost none of the pancreatic enzymes reach the common limb, and that brush border intestinal enzymes are responsible for almost all of the carbohydrate and protein digestion that occurs after BPD.[28] For this reason, the length of the small bowel where digestion of protein and carbohydrate occurs (between the gastroenterostomy and the ileocecal valve, which is equal to the length of the alimentary limb plus the common channel) becomes the primary determinant of malabsorption severity, and thus of weight loss success and risk of PEM after BPD.[26,27] Gastric pouch volume in BPD is another determinant of malabsorption severity and PEM risk, as immediately after surgery small pouch sizes reduce appetite and cause dumping syndrome, leading to limited amount of food intake. In the long term, small gastric volumes result in rapid gastric emptying, decreased intestinal transit time, and decreased absorption of ingested nutrients.[25,26] Decreasing the size of the gastric pouch increases weight loss success but also increases the risk of PEM.

Scopinaro and colleagues have made modifications to the procedure over the years in an attempt to maximize weight loss success and minimize complications, particularly PEM. In their initial series, a very small gastric volume of 150 ml was chosen that was associated with an excellent 90% excess weight loss (EWL); however, it had a 30% incidence of PEM, with 10% of patients experiencing recurrent episodes of PEM.[29] It was observed that the patients who developed PEM had significantly smaller gastric volumes than those who did not.[27] In 1984, the group adopted an approach where gastric volume was selected according to patient characteristics, including age, sex, eating habits, and compliance, an approach known as ad hoc stomach BPD (AHS BPD). With this approach they were able to preserve excellent weight loss results, an average of 75% EWL, while decreasing PEM incidence to 11% with a PEM recurrence rate of 4.3%.[27] In order to further decrease PEM incidence, in 1992 the group made modifications to both the alimentary limb length and the stomach volume according to patient characteristics, also known as the ad hoc stomach ad hoc alimentary limb BPD (AHS-AHAL BPD) procedure. In patients at increased risk for PEM, a larger gastric pouch would be utilized and alimentary limb lengths would be increased from 200–250 cm to 300–350 cm. They were able to decrease PEM incidence further to 1%, with a 1% procedure reversal rate and an average of 71% of EWL.[27] Larrad-Jimenez and colleagues have described results of a modified BPD procedure involving an increased alimentary limb length of >300 cm and a gastric volume of 150–200 ml.[30] They were able to achieve 78% EWL in the morbid obesity group (BMI < 50 kg/m^2) and 63% EWL in the superobesity group (BMI ≥ 50 kg/m^2) at 10 years with an incidence of PEM of only 0.29%.

In cases where PEM did not resolve with nutrition support and reversal of the procedure was indicated, the Scopinaro group recommended increasing the length of the alimentary limb from 250 cm to 400 cm, which was usually accompanied by 25% regain of excess weight.[27] Revision of the 50 cm common channel to 200 cm has also been shown to correct the hypoalbuminemia and excessive weight loss after BPD.[31]

In contrast to protein and carbohydrate digestion, which occurs throughout the length of the alimentary limb and common channel, fat digestion can only occur within the common channel, as mixing of food with bile salts from biliopancreatic secretions is necessary.[28] A short common channel leads to disruption of enterohepatic circulation and wasting of bile salts, which causes a distinct reduction in serum cholesterol levels as synthesis of bile acids increases and the cholesterol pool is depleted.[26] However, this positive effect on cholesterol levels occurs at the expense of fat malabsorption, steatorrhea, and possible deficiencies of fat-soluble vitamins.[22] Occasionally, a paradoxical rise in triglyceride levels may be observed after BPD, as the hepatic very low density lipoprotein (VLDL) output increases to compensate for loss of cholesterol, resulting in a rise in serum triglyceride levels.[32] Increasing the common channel length from 50 cm to 75 or 100 cm has been shown to decrease the occurrence of this phenomenon.[26]

9.5 BILIOPANCREATIC DIVERSION WITH DUODENAL SWITCH AND PROTEIN–ENERGY MALNUTRITION

BPD/DS was first performed in 1988 by Hess and Hess,[33] then in 1993 by Marceau,[34–36] with subsequent development for laparoscopy by Ren,[37] as a modification of the original Scopinaro BPD in an attempt to reduce complications of the original BPD procedure by preserving the pylorus, maintaining control of gastric emptying, and thus preventing postgastrectomy symptoms, including diarrhea, dumping syndrome, and marginal ulcers.[34] The main difference between the original BPD and BPD/DS is the part of the stomach resection, with BPD/DS involving a sleeve gastrectomy in contrast to a distal partial gastrectomy in the original BPD procedure[22] (Figures 9.2 and 9.3).[16] It is believed that reduced parietal cell mass with sleeve gastrectomy and preservation of Brunner's glands in the duodenum, which neutralizes gastric acid load, likely contribute to a decreased risk of marginal ulcers after BPD/DS.[22] When compared with the original Scopinaro procedure, similar alimentary limb length (250–300 cm, or 40% of distance from ileocecal valve to ligament of Treitz) and stomach capacity (250 ml) were used, while a slightly longer common channel length

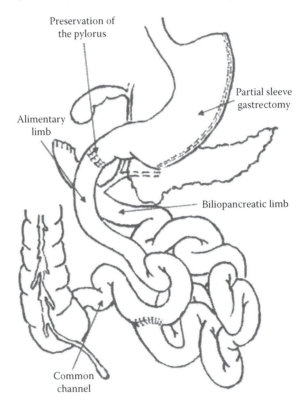

FIGURE 9.3 Biliopancreatic diversion with duodenal switch (BPD/DS). (Reprinted with permission from Kim, D. W., and Apovian, C. M., in Rippe and Angelopoulos, eds., *Obesity: Prevention and Treatment*, CRC Press, Boca Raton, Florida, 2012, p. 193.)

of 75–100 cm was chosen (compared with 50 cm in the original BPD). Like the original BPD, BPD/DS does not involve the presence of a blind small bowel loop. BPD/DS is the more commonly performed variation of the procedure in North America.[22]

Overall, PEM rarely occurs after BPD/DS at centers specialized in the procedure. Marceau and colleagues reported a 73% EWL after BPD/DS, with a 0.7% rate of PEM, which requires procedure revision or reversal over a 15-year period.[38] A third of the patients with PEM underwent complete reversal of the procedure, while the rest had their alimentary and common channels lengthened.[38] Comparing results of BPD/DS with the original BPD over a 10-year period at their center, Marceau et al. observed a 25% greater weight loss with BPD/DS in conjunction with a lower reversal rate for severe diarrhea and PEM (0.5% vs. 2.7%).[39] Over a period of 15 years, Hess and colleagues[40] reported an average of 75% EWL after BPD/DS with a 0.61% reversal rate for excessive weight loss, PEM, or severe diarrhea. Dorman et al.[41] reported on a cohort of patients who underwent BPD/DS over a course of 5 years and demonstrated a similar weight loss when compared with RYGB (30–35% of initial body weight) without any patients requiring revision surgery due to PEM.[41] Anthone and colleagues[42] reported an average of 66% EWL at 5 years and a 4.7% revision rate, with PEM and persistent diarrhea as the primary reasons for revision procedures.[43] The higher incidence of PEM after BPD/DS at this institution may be attributable to a smaller gastric pouch volume (100 ml) chosen for the procedure, which, as previously described, is associated with greater weight loss at the expense of increased risk for PEM.[26]

9.6 ROUX-EN-Y GASTRIC BYPASS AND PROTEIN–ENERGY MALNUTRITION

The gastric bypass operation was first developed by Mason and Ito[44] and subsequently underwent numerous modifications[45,46] until it became the RYGB procedure, which remains the most commonly performed bariatric procedure in the United States. Creation of a small gastric pouch (<30 ml) provides the restrictive component of the procedure.[47] The malabsorptive component is achieved as the jejunum is divided with the distal portion anastomosed to the stomach, forming the alimentary limb or Roux limb of the Roux-en-Y configuration, while the distal stomach and proximal small intestine (the biliopancreatic limb) is anastomosed to the ileum, forming the common channel where biliopancreatic secretions are mixed with partially digested food (Figure 9.4).[16] In contrast with BPD and BPD/DS, RYGB almost never leads to PEM or persistent diarrhea, but results in a smaller weight loss and a greater risk of weight regain. As the pylorus is sacrificed with RYGB, marginal ulcers and dumping syndrome occasionally occur after the procedure.[48]

In the early days of RYGB, the alimentary limb length typically used was between 50 and 75 cm.[49] Subsequently, it was evident that weight loss failure occurred in a significant number of the heaviest patients, particularly those with a BMI of ≥50 kg/m^2, so-called superobesity.[50,51] In order to address this problem, it was proposed that increasing alimentary limb length and decreasing common channel length, and thus increasing malabsorption, might allow more patients to meet weight loss goals after RYGB.[51] Variations of RYGB have been devised and used in some institutions either as

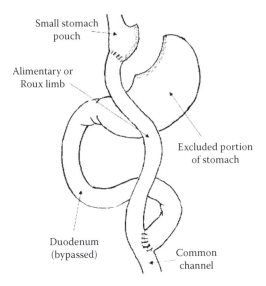

Small stomach
pouch

Alimentary or
Roux limb

Excluded portion
of stomach

Duodenum
(bypassed)

Common
channel

FIGURE 9.4   Roux-en-Y gastric bypass (RYGB). (Reprinted with permission from Kim, D. W., and Apovian, C. M., in Rippe and Angelopoulos, eds., *Obesity: Prevention and Treatment*, CRC Press, Boca Raton, Florida, 2012, p. 188.)

a primary procedure for superobese patients or as a revision procedure in patients who have not met weight loss goals after a traditional proximal or short Roux limb RYGB (RYGB with Roux limb length of <100 cm) among whom the restrictive component of the procedure, i.e., the gastric pouch and gastrojejunostomy, remained intact.[48,51] These procedures include LL-RYGB, which is defined as RYGB with an alimentary limb length of >100–150 cm, and D-RYGB, which is defined as RYGB with a short common channel length of <150 cm, both of which will be discussed in the following section.

9.7   LONG-LIMB ROUX-EN-Y GASTRIC BYPASS AND PROTEIN–ENERGY MALNUTRITION

In 1992 Brolin et al.[52] compared weight loss outcomes in superobese patients (defined as those who are ≥200 pounds overweight) who underwent RYGB with either a 75 cm (standard) or a 150 cm alimentary limb length (LL-RYGB) in a randomized-controlled trial, and demonstrated that those with a 150 cm alimentary limb had greater weight loss (64% vs. 50% EWL) without any incidence of PEM. Choban et al.[53] reported in 2002 results of a prospective randomized trial comparing RYGB with Roux limb lengths of 75 vs. 150 cm in 133 patients with BMI of <50 kg/m^2 and 150 vs. 250 cm in 64 superobese patients with BMI of ≥50 kg/m^2. The number of patients achieving >50% EWL was greater in superobese patients with a 250 cm Roux limb compared with those with a shorter Roux limb. In contrast, among patients with BMI of <50 kg/m^2 weight loss outcomes were similar between the two groups.[53] No PEM or significant metabolic complications were observed. Inabnet et al.[54] performed a prospective randomized trial comparing RYGB with short (alimentary limb length

100 cm and biliopancreatic limb length 50 cm) and long (alimentary limb length 150 cm and biliopancreatic limb length 100 cm) limb lengths in patients with BMI of <50 kg/m². The weight loss outcomes were similar between groups (70–75% EWL at 12 months). Again, none of the patients developed PEM or micronutrient deficiencies. However, internal hernias occurred more commonly in the long-limb group.

In 2001 MacLean et al.[55] retrospectively compared results of 242 obese patients who underwent RYGB with either a standard RYGB (40 cm alimentary limb and 10 cm biliopancreatic limb) or an LL-RYGB (100 cm alimentary limb and 100 cm biliopancreatic limb) and showed that superobese patients (those with a BMI of ≥50 kg/m²) benefit from longer alimentary limbs, while morbidly obese patients with a BMI of <50 kg/m² did not. The authors did not encounter PEM in any of the patients. In 2006, the same group reported long-term results from patients who were followed for >10 years[56] and demonstrated that at 5 and 10 years, neither those with a BMI of <50 kg/m² nor those with a BMI of ≥50 kg/m² benefited from longer limb lengths.

Overall, results of these studies are consistent with findings from a systematic review by Orci et al.,[57] which concluded that LL-RYGB may be effective at improving weight loss outcomes in the superobese population (BMI ≥50 kg/m²) but not in those with a BMI of <50 kg/m², and that incidence of PEM, micronutrient deficiencies, or severe malabsorption after LL-RYGB did not differ from that of conventional RYGB.[57]

9.8 DISTAL ROUX-EN-Y GASTRIC BYPASS AND PROTEIN–ENERGY MALNUTRITION

In 1997 Sugerman and colleagues[58] reported on superobese patients who underwent D-RYGB as a revision surgery due to weight loss failure after conventional RYGB. The procedure involved lengthening of the Roux limb to 140 cm and shortening of the common channel to 50 cm in the first 5 patients and to 150 cm in the last 22 patients. All five patients with a 50 cm common channel developed severe PEM and required conversion to a 150 to 200 cm common channel, and two patients died as a result of hepatic failure. Three of the 22 patients with a 150 cm common channel developed PEM and underwent reoperation to lengthen the common channel, and 4 patients required enteral or parenteral nutrition support. The rest of the patients had an excellent EWL of 69%. These findings support the notion that for patients undergoing a RYGB, a common channel length of at least 50–75 cm is required to prevent PEM and severe malabsorption.[48]

In 2001 Fobi and colleagues[59] retrospectively reported on results from 65 superobese patients with weight loss failure after standard RYGB who underwent D-RYGB as a revision procedure. The Roux limb was moved halfway down to decrease the common channel length by approximately 50%. The revision resulted in approximately a 20 kg additional weight loss. PEM occurred in 15 patients (23%), with 8 patients requiring enteral nutrition through a percutaneous gastrostomy tube, 5 patients requiring parenteral nutrition, and 6 patients (9.2%) requiring reversal of the procedure to standard RYGB.

Brolin et al.[60] made an observation that weight regain was common in patients who have undergone LL-RYGB after 4–5 years, which led the group to perform D-RYGB with a 75–100 cm common channel length as an attempt to improve weight loss among patients who were superobese. Surgical outcomes were retrospectively reported in 2002.[60] They observed the greatest weight loss with D-RYGB (64% EWL, $N = 47$) compared with LL-RYGB (61% EWL, $N = 152$) and standard RYGB (56% EWL, $N = 99$). Weight regain occurred less commonly in the D-RYGB group than with the LL-RYGB and conventional RYGB groups. None of the patients required a revision procedure; however, two patients in the D-RYGB group required parenteral nutrition support for PEM. The incidence of anemia was greatest after D-RYGB, while occurrence metabolic complications did not differ between the LL-RYGB and the standard RYGB group.[60]

In 2007 Brolin and Cody reported results of 54 patients who underwent D-RYGB as a revision procedure after failure to lose weight with either a standard RYGB, a LL-RYGB, or a pure gastric restrictive procedure.[61] Superobese patients comprised 38.9% of this group. In all patients whose primary procedure was RYGB, the gastrojejunostomy was revised. Mean EWL was 47.9% after 1 year. PEM developed in four patients (7.4%), including one patient who responded to a course of home parenteral nutrition, two who required lengthening of the common channel, and another patient who developed hypocalcemia and pathologic rib fractures after a 3-year hiatus without follow-up. This patient underwent surgical reversal of the procedure to a normal anatomy.[61]

In 2011, Kellum et al. reported on long-term results from 49 superobese patients who had undergone D-RYGB 20–25 years earlier,[62] demonstrating that 13 out of 23 patients (56.5%) with a 50 cm common channel required a revision procedure to lengthen the common channel compared with 8 out of 25 patients (32%) who had a common channel length of ≥ 100 cm. Among the other patients who were available for follow-up (~70% of the cohort), the average EWL was 66.8%. When compared with patients who underwent LL-RYGB (with a 150 cm alimentary limb and a 75 cm biliopancreatic limb) at the same center, those who underwent D-RYGB had greater weight loss at 5 years but were found to have lower serum albumin, hemoglobin, and iron levels.

In summary, while D-RYGB offered superior weight loss compared with standard RYGB or LL-RYGB, PEM and other metabolic complications occurred more commonly. For this reason, D-RYGB should not be considered as a first-line surgical option for obese patients and should be reserved only for superobese patients with significant obesity-related comorbidities who are committed to long-term follow-up and have no other significant risk factors for nutritional problems.[60]

9.9 CONCLUSION

PEM is one of the most feared complications of bariatric surgery and should be looked for in patients who develop excessive weight loss, maladaptive eating behaviors, postoperative mechanical complications, or micronutrient deficiencies. PEM is occasionally diagnosed after malabsorptive bariatric procedures, namely, BPD, BPD/DS, and D-RYGB. For these procedures, risk of PEM is increased with the smaller gastric pouch size and shorter common channel. LSG, LAGB, and conventional RYGB almost never result in PEM unless surgical complications occur. Among superobese patients with BMI of ≥ 50 kg/m^2, LL-RYGB may confer better weight loss outcomes than standard RYGB without increasing PEM risk. General recommendations in regard to intake of energy, protein, carbohydrate, fat, and fluids for bariatric patients in the postoperative period are summarized in Table 9.1.

TABLE 9.1
General Recommendations on Energy, Protein, Carbohydrate, Fat, and Fluids Intake after Bariatric Surgery

Category	Recommendations	Comments
Energy	• The energy intake that optimizes postoperative weight loss has not been defined.[63] • Caloric intake should be individualized according to the patient's physical activity, age, and sex.[63,64] • Energy expenditure can be determined using indirect calorimetry or predictive equations, such as the Mifflin–St. Jeor equation utilizing the patient's actual body weight.[65,66]	• Negative energy balance is an important determinant of postoperative weight loss success.[67,68] • Caloric intake usually increases with postoperative dietary progression, from 300–500 kcal/day in the first few months to 1,000–1,400 kcal/day at the end of the first year, and 2,000 kcal/day or greater afterwards.[8,12,68–70]
Protein	• Requirements: 1.0–1.5 g/kg/day ideal body weight.[64] Higher amounts of up to 2.1 g/kg/day ideal body weight may be considered in some patients.[15] Minimal requirements: 90 g/day[27,29] for BPD and 60–80 g/day[63] for other bariatric procedures. • U.S. DRI: Acceptable macronutrient distribution range for protein is 10–35%.[71] • During a meal, protein should be consumed first.[73] Encourage low-fat, soft, moist, or ground foods such as eggs, fish, ground turkey, legumes, cereals, cheese, and tofu.[63] Delay or avoid red meat and other tough and dry meat (such as pork or poultry), which is often poorly tolerated by bariatric patients.[64] Unsweetened dairy products should be slowly introduced into the diet, as lactose intolerance may develop after bariatric surgery.[73] • Protein intake is often inadequate after bariatric surgery, particularly during diet progression or as a result of food intolerances.[15,69] Modular protein supplements made from high-quality protein sources should be used as they provide adequate amounts of indispensable amino acids (IAAs). Such protein sources include milk, whey, casein, egg whites, and soy.[64]	• Protein requirement after bariatric surgery is increased. RDA of protein for the general population is 0.8 g/kg/day.[71] After BPD, the gastrointestinal loss of endogenous nitrogen is significantly increased, raising the minimal protein requirements in order to prevent PEM in this setting.[27,29] • Adequate protein intake is associated with a reduction in loss of lean body mass during rapid weight loss after surgery.[15] • Protein digestibility corrected amino acid (PDCAAS) score can be used to evaluate protein quality by comparing the IAA content of a protein against the daily requirement (EAR) for each IAA. High-quality proteins such as egg whites, milk, casein, whey, and soy have a PDCAA score of 100.[64]

(Continued)

TABLE 9.1 (CONTINUED)
General Recommendations on Energy, Protein, Carbohydrate, Fat, and Fluids Intake after Bariatric Surgery

Category	Recommendations	Comments
Carbohydrate	• U.S. DRI: RDA of carbohydrate is 130 g/day.[71] Acceptable macronutrient distribution range of carbohydrate is 45–65%.[71] AI of dietary fiber is 14 g/1,000 kcal of required energy.[71] • After the patient has an adequate protein intake, fresh fruits, vegetables, and complex carbohydrates (e.g., unsweetened cereals, potatoes) may be introduced.[63] Vegetables with high fibrous consistency such as celery stalks, corn, and artichokes should be consumed well cooked or pureed.[72] • Avoid simple sugar-containing foods (e.g., candy, cookies, pastries, cakes), fruit juice, and concentrated sweets, as they may cause dumping syndrome and can adversely affect weight loss.[63,64]	• Studies showed that most bariatric patients receive approximately 45% of their energy from carbohydrates.[63]

Fat	• U.S. DRI for total fat: RDA is not determined. Acceptable macronutrient distribution range is 20–35%.[71]
	• U.S. DRI for essential fatty acids[71]:
	  • Linoleic acid: AI 14–17 g/day in males and 11–12 g/day in females. Acceptable macronutrient distribution range is 5–10%.
	  • α-Linolenic acid: AI 1.6 g/day in males and 1.1 g/day in females. Acceptable macronutrient distribution range is 0.6–1.2%.
	• Encourage food choices that are low in fat and less energy dense.[63] Avoid fried foods. Choose mono- and polyunsaturated fatty acids over saturated fat. Fish oil is the source for n-3 fatty acids. Examples of oils that will provide a significant amount of essential fatty acids include olive oil, canola oil, soybean oil, and linseed oil.[63] Avoid foods high in trans fat (e.g., cookies, pastries, cakes, chips, margarines).[63]
		• Studies showed that after bariatric surgery most patients receive 30.2–41.7% of their energy from fat.[63]
		• After malabsorptive procedures, particularly BPD and BPD/DS, patients may develop fat malabsorption resulting in steatorrhea and diarrhea. These patients are at risk for deficiencies of fat-soluble vitamins.[22]

(Continued)

TABLE 9.1 (CONTINUED)
General Recommendations on Energy, Protein, Carbohydrate, Fat, and Fluids Intake after Bariatric Surgery

Category	Recommendations	Comments
Fluids	• Patients should drink at least 1.8 L[63] or 48–64 fl oz[72] of noncarbonated, calorie-free, caffeine-free clear liquids daily to prevent dehydration.	• Vomiting and diarrhea may exacerbate dehydration. • Dehydration may increase risk of gallstones.

Note: DRI = Dietary Reference Intake, RDA = Recommended Dietary Allowance, EAR = estimated average requirement, AI = adequate intake, IAA = indispensible amino acid.

REFERENCES

1. Kushner R. Managing the obese patient after bariatric surgery: a case report of severe malnutrition and review of the literature. *JPEN J Parenter Enteral Nutr* 2000;24:126–32.
2. Fujioka K, DiBaise JK, Martindale RG. Nutrition and metabolic complications after bariatric surgery and their treatment. *JPEN J Parenter Enteral Nutr* 2011;35:52S–59S.
3. Baker MT. The history and evolution of bariatric surgical procedures. *Surg Clin North Am* 2011;91:1181–201, viii.
4. Jensen GL, Bistrian B, Roubenoff R, Heimburger DC. Malnutrition syndromes: a conundrum vs continuum. *JPEN J Parenter Enteral Nutr* 2009;33:710–16.
5. Jensen GL, Mirtallo J, Compher C, Dhaliwal R, Forbes A, Grijalba RF, et al. Adult starvation and disease-related malnutrition: a proposal for etiology-based diagnosis in the clinical practice setting from the International Consensus Guideline Committee. *JPEN J Parenter Enteral Nutr* 2010;34:156–59.
6. White JV, Guenter P, Jensen G, Malone A, Schofield M. Consensus statement: Academy of Nutrition and Dietetics and American Society for Parenteral and Enteral Nutrition: characteristics recommended for the identification and documentation of adult malnutrition (undernutrition). *JPEN J Parenter Enteral Nutr* 2012;36:275–83.
7. Fuhrman MP, Charney P, Mueller CM. Hepatic proteins and nutrition assessment. *J Am Diet Assoc* 2004;104:1258–64.
8. Coughlin K, Bell RM, Bivins BA, Wrobel S, Griffen WO Jr. Preoperative and postoperative assessment of nutrient intakes in patients who have undergone gastric bypass surgery. *Arch Surg* 1983;118:813–16.
9. Avinoah E, Ovnat A, Charuzi I. Nutritional status seven years after Roux-en-Y gastric bypass surgery. *Surgery* 1992;111:137–42.
10. Andersen T, Pedersen BH, Henriksen JH, Uhrenholdt A. Food intake in relation to pouch volume, stoma diameter, and pouch emptying after gastroplasty for morbid obesity. *Scand J Gastroenterol* 1988;23:1057–62.
11. Kenler HA, Brolin RE, Cody RP. Changes in eating behavior after horizontal gastroplasty and Roux-en-Y gastric bypass. *Am J Clin Nutr* 1990;52:87–92.
12. Brolin RE, Robertson LB, Kenler HA, Cody RP. Weight loss and dietary intake after vertical banded gastroplasty and Roux-en-Y gastric bypass. *Ann Surg* 1994;220:782–90.
13. Burge JC, Schaumburg JZ, Choban PS, DiSilvestro RA, Flancbaum L. Changes in patients' taste acuity after Roux-en-Y gastric bypass for clinically severe obesity. *J Am Diet Assoc* 1995;95:666–70.

14. Heber D, Greenway FL, Kaplan LM, Livingston E, Salvador J, Still C, et al. Endocrine and nutritional management of the post-bariatric surgery patient: an Endocrine Society clinical practice guideline. *J Clin Endocrinol Metab* 2010;95:4823–43.

15. Mechanick JI, Youdim A, Jones DB, Garvey WT, Hurley DL, McMahon MM, et al. Clinical practice guidelines for the perioperative nutritional, metabolic, and nonsurgical support of the bariatric surgery patient—2013 update: cosponsored by American Association of Clinical Endocrinologists, The Obesity Society, and American Society for Metabolic and Bariatric Surgery. *Endocr Pract* 2013;19:337–72.

16. Kim DW, Apovian CM. Surgical treatment of obesity. In Rippe JM, Angelopoulos TJ, eds., *Obesity: prevention and treatment*. Boca Raton, FL: CRC Press; 2012:183–209.

17. Halverson JD, Wise L, Wazna MF, Ballinger WF. Jejunoileal bypass for morbid obesity. A critical appraisal. *Am J Med* 1978;64:461–75.

18. Hocking MP, Duerson MC, O'Leary JP, Woodward ER. Jejunoileal bypass for morbid obesity. Late follow-up in 100 cases. *N Engl J Med* 1983;308:995–99.

19. Byrne TK. Complications of surgery for obesity. *Surg Clin North Am* 2001;81:1181–93, vii–viii.

20. DeMaria EJ, Pate V, Warthen M, Winegar DA. Baseline data from American Society for Metabolic and Bariatric Surgery-designated Bariatric Surgery Centers of Excellence using the Bariatric Outcomes Longitudinal Database. *Surg Obes Relat Dis* 2010;6:347–55.

21. Buchwald H, Oien DM. Metabolic/bariatric surgery worldwide 2011. *Obes Surg* 2013;23:427–36.

22. Sudan R, Jacobs DO. Biliopancreatic diversion with duodenal switch. *Surg Clin North Am* 2011;91:1281–93, ix.

23. Scopinaro N, Gianetta E, Civalleri D, Bonalumi U, Bachi V. Bilio-pancreatic bypass for obesity. II. Initial experience in man. *Br J Surg* 1979;66:618–20.

24. Scopinaro N, Gianetta E, Adami GF, Friedman D, Traverso E, Marinari GM, et al. Biliopancreatic diversion for obesity at eighteen years. *Surgery* 1996;119:261–68.

25. Scopinaro N, Marinari GM, Pretolesi F, Papadia F, Murelli F, Marini P, et al. Energy and nitrogen absorption after biliopancreatic diversion. *Obes Surg* 2000;10:436–41.

26. Scopinaro N. Thirty-five years of biliopancreatic diversion: notes on gastrointestinal physiology to complete the published information useful for a better understanding and clinical use of the operation. *Obes Surg* 2012;22:427–32.

27. Scopinaro N. Biliopancreatic diversion: mechanisms of action and long-term results. *Obes Surg* 2006;16:683–89.

28. Scopinaro N, Marinari G, Gianetta E. The respective importance of the alimentary limb (AL) and the common limb (CL) in protein absorption (PA) after BPD [abstract 26]. *Obes Surg* 1977;7:108.

29. Scopinaro N, Adami GF, Marinari GM, Gianetta E, Traverso E, Friedman D, et al. Biliopancreatic diversion. *World J Surg* 1998;22:936–46.

30. Larrad-Jimenez A, Diaz-Guerra CS, de Cuadros Borrajo P, Lesmes IB, Esteban BM. Short-, mid- and long-term results of Larrad biliopancreatic diversion. *Obes Surg* 2007;17:202–10.

31. Vanuytsel JL, Nobels FR, Van Gaal LF, De Leeuw IH. A case of malnutrition after biliopancreatic diversion for morbid obesity. *Surg Obes Relat Dis* 1993;17:425–26.

32. Scopinaro N, Adami GF, Papadia FS, Camerini G, Carlini F, Fried M, et al. Effects of biliopanceratic diversion on type 2 diabetes in patients with BMI 25 to 35. *Ann Surg* 2011;253:699–703.

33. Hess DS, Hess DW. Biliopancreatic diversion with a duodenal switch. *Obes Surg* 1998;8:267–82.

34. Marceau P, Biron S, Bourque RA, Potvin M, Hould FS, Simard S. Biliopancreatic diversion with a new type of gastrectomy. *Obes Surg* 1993;3:29–35.

35. Lagace M, Marceau P, Marceau S, Hould FS, Potvin M, Bourque RA, et al. Biliopancreatic diversion with a new type of gastrectomy: some previous conclusions revisited. *Obes Surg* 1995;5:411–18.
36. Marceau P, Hould FS, Simard S, Lebel S, Bourque RA, Potvin M, et al. Biliopancreatic diversion with duodenal switch. *World J Surg* 1998;22:947–54.
37. Ren CJ, Patterson E, Gagner M. Early results of laparoscopic biliopancreatic diversion with duodenal switch: a case series of 40 consecutive patients. *Obes Surg* 2000;10:514–23; discussion 524.
38. Marceau P, Biron S, Hould FS, Lebel S, Marceau S, Lescelleur O, et al. Duodenal switch: long-term results. *Obes Surg* 2007;17:1421–30.
39. Marceau P, Biron S, Hould FS, Lebel S, Marceau S, Lescelleur O, et al. Duodenal switch improved standard biliopancreatic diversion: a retrospective study. *Surg Obes Relat Dis* 2009;5:43–47.
40. Hess DS, Hess DW, Oakley RS. The biliopancreatic diversion with the duodenal switch: results beyond 10 years. *Obes Surg* 2005;15:408–16.
41. Dorman RB, Rasmus NF, al-Haddad BJ, Serrot FJ, Slusarek BM, Sampson BK, et al. Benefits and complications of the duodenal switch/biliopancreatic diversion compared to the Roux-en-Y gastric bypass. *Surgery* 2012;152:758–65; discussion 765–67.
42. Anthone GJ, Lord RV, DeMeester TR, Crookes PF. The duodenal switch operation for the treatment of morbid obesity. *Ann Surg* 2003;238:618–27; discussion 627–28.
43. Hamoui N, Chock B, Anthone GJ, Crookes PF. Revision of the duodenal switch: indications, technique, and outcomes. *J Am Coll Surg* 2007;204:603–8.
44. Mason EE, Ito C. Gastric bypass in obesity. *Surg Clin North Am* 1967;47:1345–51.
45. Griffen WO Jr, Young VL, Stevenson CC. A prospective comparison of gastric and jejunoileal bypass procedures for morbid obesity. *Ann Surg* 1977;186:500–9.
46. Torres JC, Oca CF, Garrison RN. Gastric bypass: Roux-en-Y gastrojejunostomy from the lesser curvature. *South Med J* 1983;76:1217–21.
47. Alder RL, Terry BE. Measurement and standardization of the gastric pouch in gastric bypass. *Surg Gynecol Obstet* 1977;144:762–63.
48. Kellogg TA. Revisional bariatric surgery. *Surg Clin North Am* 2011;91:1353–71, x.
49. Pories WJ, Flickinger EG, Meelheim D, Van Rij AM, Thomas FT. The effectiveness of gastric bypass over gastric partition in morbid obesity: consequence of distal gastric and duodenal exclusion. *Ann Surg* 1982;196:389–99.
50. Bloomston M, Zervos EE, Camps MA, Goode SE, Rosemurgy AS. Outcome following bariatric surgery in super versus morbidly obese patients: does weight matter? *Obes Surg* 1997;7:414–19.
51. Brolin RE. Long limb Roux en Y gastric bypass revisited. *Surg Clin North Am* 2005;85:807–17, vii.
52. Brolin RE, Kenler HA, Gorman JH, Cody RP. Long-limb gastric bypass in the super obese. A prospective randomized study. *Ann Surg* 1992;215(4):387–95.
53. Choban PS, Flancbaum L. The effect of Roux limb lengths on outcome after Roux-en-Y gastric bypass: a prospective, randomized clinical trial. *Obes Surg* 2002;12:540–45.
54. Inabnet WB, Quinn T, Gagner M, Urban M, Pomp A. Laparoscopic Roux-en-Y gastric bypass in patients with BMI <50: a prospective randomized trial comparing short and long limb lengths. *Obes Surg* 2005;15:51–57.
55. MacLean LD, Rhode BM, Nohr CW. Long- or short-limb gastric bypass? *J Gastrointest Surg* 2001;5(5):525–30.
56. Christou NV, Look D, Maclean LD. Weight gain after short- and long-limb gastric bypass in patients followed for longer than 10 years. *Ann Surg* 2006;244:734–40.

57. Orci L, Chilcott M, Huber O. Short versus long Roux-limb length in Roux-en-Y gastric bypass surgery for the treatment of morbid and super obesity: a systematic review of the literature. *Obes Surg* 2011;21:797–804.
58. Sugerman HJ, Kellum JM, DeMaria EJ. Conversion of proximal to distal gastric bypass for failed gastric bypass for superobesity. *J Gastrointest Surg* 1997;1:517–24; discussion 524–26.
59. Fobi MA, Lee H, Igwe D Jr, Felahy B, James E, Stanczyk M, et al. Revision of failed gastric bypass to distal Roux-en-Y gastric bypass: a review of 65 cases. *Obes Surg* 2001;11:190–95.
60. Brolin RE, LaMarca LB, Kenler HA, Cody RP. Malabsorptive gastric bypass in patients with superobesity. *J Gastrointest Surg* 2002;6:195–203; discussion 204–5.
61. Brolin RE, Cody RP. Adding malabsorption for weight loss failure after gastric bypass. *Surg Endosc* 2007;21:1924–26.
62. Kellum JM, Chikunguwo SM, Maher JW, Wolfe LG, Sugerman HJ. Long-term results of malabsorptive distal Roux-en-Y gastric bypass in superobese patients. *Surg Obes Relat Dis* 2011;7:189–93.
63. Moize VL, Pi-Sunyer X, Mochari H, Vidal J. Nutritional pyramid for post-gastric bypass patients. *Obes Surg* 2010;20:1133–41.
64. Aills L, Blankenship J, Buffington C, Furtado M, Parrott J. ASMBS Allied Health nutritional guidelines for the surgical weight loss patient. *Surg Obes Relat Dis* 2008;4:S73–S108.
65. Academy of Nutrition and Dietetics Evidence Analysis Library. Adult weight management (AWM) determination of resting metabolic rate. http://andevidencelibrary.com (accessed June 20, 2013).
66. Snyder-Marlow G, Taylor D, Lenhard MJ. Nutrition care for patients undergoing laparoscopic sleeve gastrectomy for weight loss. *J Am Diet Assoc* 2010;110:600–7.
67. Warde-Kamar J, Rogers M, Flancbaum L, Laferrere B. Calorie intake and meal patterns up to 4 years after Roux-en-Y gastric bypass surgery. *Obes Surg* 2004;14:1070–79.
68. Bobbioni-Harsch E, Huber O, Morel P, Chassot G, Lehmann T, Volery M, et al. Factors influencing energy intake and body weight loss after gastric bypass. *Eur J Clin Nutr* 2002;56:551–56.
69. Moize V, Geliebter A, Gluck ME, Yahav E, Lorence M, Colarusso T, et al. Obese patients have inadequate protein intake related to protein intolerance up to 1 year following Roux-en-Y gastric bypass. *Obes Surg* 2003;13:23–28.
70. Bavaresco M, Paganini S, Lima TP, Salgado W Jr, Ceneviva R, Dos Santos JE, et al. Nutritional course of patients submitted to bariatric surgery. *Obes Surg* 2010;20:716–21.
71. Food and Nutrition Board, Institute of Medicine. *Dietary reference intakes for energy, carbohydrate, fiber, fat, fatty acids, cholesterol, protein, and amino acids.* Washington, DC: National Academies Press; 2005.
72. Kulick D, Hark L, Deen D. The bariatric surgery patient: a growing role for registered dietitians. *J Am Diet Assoc* 2010;110:593–99.
73. Bock MA. Roux-en-Y gastric bypass: the dietitian's and patient's perspectives. *Nutr Clin Pract* 2003;18:141–44.

10 Special Populations
Adolescents

Kathleen B. Hrovat, Linda M. Kollar,
and Thomas H. Inge

CONTENTS

10.1 INTRODUCTION

During the last three decades in the United States the prevalence and severity of obesity in adolescents has dramatically increased. Between 1980 and 2008 the percentage of adolescents aged 12–19 years who are obese increased from 5% to 18%. Additionally, approximately 4% of youth meet criteria for severe obesity (BMI ≥

99th percentile).[1,2] Severe obesity in adolescents is typically defined as a BMI of ≥120% of the 95th percentile or ≥35 kg/m².

Studies conclusively show that an overwhelming majority of children and adolescents with obesity will become obese adults, thus increasing their risk of developing serious and debilitating health conditions.[3] There are both immediate and long-term consequences of obesity to health and well-being in the adolescent population: type 2 diabetes mellitus, nonalcoholic fatty liver disease, obstructive sleep apnea, metabolic syndrome, hypertension, dyslipidemia, polycystic ovary syndrome, and degenerative joint disease are increasingly diagnosed. In addition, severely obese adolescents and children experience psychological sequelae, including depression and low self-esteem.[4]

Behavioral modification is typically the first line of treatment aimed at decreasing caloric intake and increasing physical activity. Long-term studies have failed to show significant sustained weight loss with conventional treatment of severe obesity in the adolescent population. Indeed, a recently published 3-year study included 643 children (ages 6–16 years) who met regularly with a multidisciplinary team for reinforcement of a lifestyle intervention for obesity. Treatment effects were substantially better for the younger children, but the older the participants were, the less effective the attempts at dietary and physical activity changes were. Adolescents with moderate obesity responded modestly, but 98% of teenagers with severe obesity had no demonstrable effect on weight over 3 years.[5] These findings, along with the fact that weight loss surgery (WLS) is successful for reversing obesity and obesity-related comorbidities in the majority of severely obese adults, are the clinical foundations upon which persuasive arguments to provide WLS to severely obese adolescents are increasingly made.[6]

Nationally representative data estimate that approximately 1,000 bariatric procedures are performed annually on adolescents. This rate of surgeries has remained stable since 2003.[7] The most common procedures performed in adolescents include Roux-en-Y gastric bypass (RYGB), vertical sleeve gastrectomy (VSG), and laparoscopic adjustable gastric band (LAGB). The LAGB has not been approved by the Food and Drug Administration for use in minors and is thus considered investigational. A number of evidence-based guidelines are now available for clinicians treating obese children and adolescents supporting the use of WLS in adolescents.[8,9]

10.2 WEIGHT LOSS SURGERY IN ADOLESCENTS

In the absence of age-specific predictors of outcomes, most specialists engaged in adolescent bariatric surgery advise that candidates for surgery should be referred to centers with multidisciplinary teams experienced in meeting the distinct physical and psychological needs of adolescents.[10,11] The multidisciplinary team should comprise the surgeon(s), physician (pediatric specialist), clinical nurse practitioner, nurse, psychologist(s), and registered dietitian (RD). Ideally the team would also include a social worker and an exercise specialist. Additionally, consulting team members in adolescent medicine and a cardiologist should be included.

It takes time to establish rapport and build trust with teens. It is ideal for the teen to have at least one consistent member of the interdisciplinary team that he or she sees at every visit. The parameters of the treatment plan process should be clearly explained so that the adolescent and family understand what will be required to meet the team expectations for readiness for surgery. Each visit should begin with a description of what will happen that day, including whom the teen will meet with and how long the visit should take to complete.

Careful assessment of the decisional capacity of the adolescent is required to assess the ability to understand the risks and benefits of an invasive, nonreversible, elective surgical procedure. Comprehensive psychological evaluation of the adolescent and the primary caregiver aids in the assessment of the family unit, with special attention to coping skills, psychosocial comorbidities, and strength of family function. The timing of surgery must be weighed against the patient's individual characteristics and family circumstances that could influence adherence to nutritional and physical activity recommendations, as well as long-term medical surveillance. Presently there are no data to suggest that prolonged preoperative weight management programs provide benefit for adolescents who undergo bariatric surgery.[12]

10.3 ELIGIBILITY CRITERIA

Widely adopted recommendations for patient selection[8] suggest that adolescent candidates for surgery have a BMI of ≥ 35 kg/m^2 and severe, weight-related comorbidities (e.g., type 2 diabetes, obstructive sleep apnea, benign intracranial hypertension, moderate nonalcoholic steatohepatitis) or a BMI of ≥ 40 kg/m^2 with less serious weight-related comorbidities.

10.3.1 CRITERIA FOR ADOLESCENTS BEING CONSIDERED FOR BARIATRIC SURGERY

- Have experienced failure of at least 6 months of organized weight loss attempts
- Demonstrated commitment to comprehensive medical and psychological evaluations before and after weight loss surgery
- Possess decisional capacity
- Have a supportive family environment
- Achieve physical maturity prior to WLS (typically at >13 years of age for females and >15 years of age for males, but objectively the assessment can be based on Tanner stages 4–5 or radiographically closed epiphyses of the hand/wrist)
- Have a supportive family environment

10.3.2 CONTRAINDICATIONS FOR SURGICAL TREATMENT OF OBESITY

- Pregnancy or breastfeeding
- Active substance abuse
- Inadequate social/family support
- Medically correctable causes of obesity

10.4 PREOPERATIVE NUTRITIONAL ASSESSMENT

Preoperative laboratory assessment will identify any micronutrient deficits due in part to nutrient-poor food choices, lack of dairy, low fruit and vegetable consumption, and low intake of whole grains. A daily multivitamin is recommended preoperatively for all surgical candidates to facilitate correction of preexisting micronutrient deficiencies.

The registered dietitian (RD) assessing the food consumption and eating patterns might benefit and glean more knowledge by administering a food frequency or eating behavior questionnaire. It is important to identify previous weight management attempts and the time periods they were used. Allow the adolescent or family member to describe "in their own words" why these previous efforts were discontinued. Information on the family environment and family as defined by the adolescent will aid in identifying the key players and the educational needs of the adolescent/family. The caloric needs of the patient based on height, ideal body weight, and age should be determined. The preoperative diet regimen supports a healthy, portion-controlled meal pattern that consists of adequate protein (1.0–1.5 g of protein/kg of ideal body weight), fruits, vegetables, and whole grains to achieve weight loss or, at a minimum, weight stability; typically, this plan should result in an intake of 15 kcal/kg of ideal body weight. During the preoperative period, an assessment of the adolescent's understanding and knowledge surrounding mindful eating, assessing hunger/fullness, and emotional eating will lead to healthier eating patterns and behaviors postoperatively.

The materials used for educating the adolescent should be offered in written, visual, and electronic form to accommodate different learning styles. Standardized materials assure that all patients are receiving the same information: healthy food choices, meal planning, label reading, measuring portions, vitamin/mineral supplementation, and protein sources.

Motivational interviewing is a scientifically tested method of counseling that is beneficial in facilitating modification of targeted dietary habits. This method, which relies on goal setting, is effective in helping the adolescent work on his or her targeted behavior change.[13] Goal setting with the adolescent is very different from goal setting with an adult. These goals may completely restructure the adolescent's routine, and therefore should be lower than normative goals. Allowing the adolescent and family to have input into what the goal will entail is important. The clinician should work on goals that are reasonable for the family and adolescent. An example: I will eat breakfast 3/5 days before school and my breakfast will include a protein.

During the preoperative period the patient is encouraged to maintain some method of self-monitoring. This exercise can include not only the recording of food/fluid intake, but also screen time and physical activity. This will help the patient develop and practice the behaviors that are widely believed to contribute to success postoperatively. There are many electronic apps that can be used, online systems, and paper-and-pencil methods. Emailing, texting, or journaling food records is often used. Willingness of the team and RD in particular to be open to a variety of systems allows adolescents to take ownership of the tracking that works best for them.

The preoperative period, typically 3–6 months, allows the multidisciplinary team to assess commitment, motivation, expectations, family support, and understanding of the WLS goals.

10.4.1 Suggested Topics to Address during This Period (3–6 Months Prior to Surgery)

- Correct any identified nutritional deficiencies via counseling or supplementation to assure the patient is replete at the time of surgery.
- Review healthy food choices, meal planning, measuring portions, label reading, eating from small (e.g., 8 in.) plates, using small utensils.
- Review dietary modifications specific to the proposed procedure.
- Set nutritional goals (measurable/attainable) with the patient at each visit that reinforce postoperative eating patterns.
- Have patient practice mindful eating, assessment of hunger/fullness.
- Have patient track or journal his or her daily intake.
- Have patient taste-test high-protein drinks (both commercially available products and those prepared with milk, sugar-free instant breakfast, and protein powder) and choose products/flavors that they will use during the 2-week preop liquid diet and postsurgically.
- Set water and sugar-free fluid goals.
- Set exercise/activity goals.

10.5 PREOPERATIVE WEIGHT LOSS

Preoperative weight loss is associated with fewer surgical complications.[14] There are various approaches used and criteria will differ by institution. Some programs require a percentage of weight loss based on initial body weight, while others use a preop liquid diet regimen. Typically the liquid diet is recommended for a 2-week period prior to surgery. Adolescents are capable of following an individualized meal plan provided by the RD.[15] Fluid goals and vitamin/mineral supplementation are also tracked during this preoperative liquid diet.

Sample of Preop Liquid Diet Regimen

1,000–1,200 calories

60 g protein

25 g fiber

Meals 1, 2, 3—protein shake: Either ready to drink or made with skim or 1% milk

Meal 4—not to exceed 400 calories

Water and sugar-free fluids = 64 oz

10.6 POSTOPERATIVE DIETARY PROGRESSION

The postop dietary advancement for the various surgeries will vary by the number of meals and the consistency, texture, and progression of the amount of food consumed at a meal. The diet is designed to restrict caloric intake in order to produce the desired weight loss (Table 10.1). The adolescent patient typically progresses at his or her own pace using the skills of assessing fullness practiced during the preoperative period. Programs may differ in their recommended advancement of the postoperative dietary regimen. Close monitoring with frequent phone calls, especially in the first 2 weeks after surgery, provides support and guidance for the adolescent patient during this challenging transitional time period.

It is normal for the postoperative patient to experience food intolerances and taste changes during the first 3–6 months after surgery. The RD's encouragement and creativity in suggesting various options for flavors and types of foods to try helps with adherence. Adding sugar-free flavors to the vanilla shake, freezing the shake and eating it with a spoon, and using lactaid milk or yogurt in a shake to increase tolerance are all useful tips.

Another dietary challenge that those having RYGB surgery (and to some extent, even after VSG) may experience is dumping syndrome. Sugar and concentrated sweets can cause dumping syndrome. Dumping is discomfort that occurs episodically following a meal. It is a behavior-induced syndrome that often follows bariatric procedures in which the pyloric sphincter is bypassed and the pouch is small, as in the RYGB procedure. Dumping is thought to result from rapid and increased stretching of the intestine that results from an undigested food bolus entering through the new gastric outlet, a path that is no longer regulated by a physiologic sphincter. Dumping syndrome is characterized by a set of symptoms, including cramping, sweating, heart racing, vomiting, and diarrhea. Patients who tend to eat quickly and who drink fluids with meals are at high risk for dumping. Those that experience dumping syndrome learn very quickly to avoid foods that are high in sugar. That said, some patients report never experiencing this syndrome despite ingestion of candy, ice cream, and regular soda.

All simple sugars in concentrated form should be omitted from the postsurgery diet regimen. Refined sugars rapidly absorb water from the body, causing symptoms. One hundred percent juice, typically consumed in large quantities preoperatively by the adolescent patient, is very hyperosmolar and has a higher concentration of sugar than most soft drinks. Also, adolescents are instructed to avoid condiments that are high in sugar, such as ketchup, honey mustard, sweet and sour sauce, and barbecue sauces, to avoid experiencing dumping syndrome.

Dumping symptoms may also occur after eating or drinking products that contain milk or milk products. Two considerations of milk consumption are the fat content and lactose content of milk. The natural sugar in milk, lactose, can cause bloating and gas in lactose-deficient patients. The malabsorptive procedure (RYGB) can result in inadequate lactose production, resulting in diarrhea, bloating, and gas after milk consumption. Soy milk, which is lactose-free, or lactaid treated milk can be substituted in these patients.

Late dumping syndrome can occur 1–3 h after eating. The symptoms of this late phase, weakness, sweating, and dizziness, may occur due to a rapid rise and fall in

TABLE 10.1
Postoperative Dietary Staging

	Stage 1 Ice Chips, Water, Sugar-Free Clear Liquids	Stage 2 Full Liquids High Protein	Stage 3 Smooth-Consistency Foods and Liquids	Stage 4 Soft Foods	Stage 5 All Textures Healthy Foods
RYGB	1 oz/h × 24–48 h, then ad lib × 3–7 days	Weeks 2–4	Weeks 4–6	Weeks 7–9	Week 9 for life
LAGB	1 oz/h × 24–48 h	Weeks 0–2	Weeks 3–4	Weeks 5–6	Week 7 for life
LSG	1 oz/h × 24–48 h, then ad lib × 3–7 days	Weeks 1–5	Weeks 5–8	Weeks 9–12	Week 13 for life
Goals	48–64 oz/day Acceptable sugar-free clear liquids include water, clear broth, sugar-free gelatin, sugar-free fruit-flavored drinks, sugar-free popsicles No carbonation, caffeine, or red dye	Calories: 500–600 kcal Protein: 50–60 g Fluid: 80–90 oz New foods: Skim or 1% milk, low-fat soy or lactaid milk, high-protein drinks, light plain or vanilla yogurt	Calories: 500–700 kcal Protein: 60 g Fluid: 80–90 oz New foods: Scrambled eggs, blenderized/minced turkey, chicken, flaked fish, or mashed tofu, tuna, melted low-fat cheese, small curd low-fat cottage cheese, low-fat ricotta cheese Try new foods every 2–3 days	Calories: 700–800 kcal Protein: 60 g Fluid: 80–90 oz New foods: Shaved deli meats, low-fat cheese, lean pork, cooked beans, soft or canned fruit in own juice, no skin, soft cooked or canned vegetables, toast, low-sugar cereal, crackers, oatmeal, rice, pasta, mashed potatoes Choose whole grain foods	Calories: 800–900 kcal Protein: 60 g Fluid: 80–90 oz New foods: All healthy food choices
Meal pattern	Continuous sipping	3–6 meals/day Volume: ½ cup/meal	3–4 meals/day Volume: ½ cup solid or 5–6 oz protein drink/meal	3–6 meals/day Volume: ½–1 cup solid or 8 oz protein drink	3–6 meals/day Volume: up to ¾–1½ cups/meal

Source: Fullmer, M.A. et al., *J. Pediatr. Gastroenterol. Nutr.*, 54(1), 2012, 125–35.

blood sugar levels. This type of hypoglycemia is referred to as alimentary hypoglycemia. The cause of this rapid swing in blood sugars may be due to eating sweets or
other simple carbohydrates. Recommended treatments include changes in eating habits. Patients are encouraged to eat a small meal that includes a complex carbohydrate
and a protein, avoid simple sugars, and avoid eating and drinking at the same time.

10.6.1   Additional Postoperative Dietary Recommendations

- Have a high-quality protein source at each meal.
- Meals should be eaten in 15–20 min. Do not eat in between meals.
- Stop eating at the first sign of fullness.
- Sip fluids continuously between meals to avoid dehydration.
- Do not drink fluids for 30 min after a meal.
- Eat slowly, taking small bites. Make sure that food is cut into small pieces.
  Food should be no larger than the size of a pea.
- Avoid foods that may cause dumping syndrome.

10.7   VITAMINS

Following surgery the adolescent must adhere not only to a prescribed dietary regimen but also to multivitamin therapy. Table 10.2 outlines the suggested supplementation after WLS. Little is known about multivitamin adherence following adolescent
bariatric surgery. Recent literature suggests a high rate of nonadherence in adolescents following WLS. Forgetting and difficulty swallowing multivitamins were the
two primary barriers identified in this study.[16]

The providers should encourage parents to assist in monitoring the vitamin intake,
especially in the early stages postoperatively. This will help with adherence. Other
helpful tips are putting notes on the bathroom mirror as a reminder and putting their
vitamins in a visible place, like next to their toothbrush or on the kitchen counter.
They can text themselves or have their parents text them a reminder to their phone or
put an alarm reminder on their phone.

TABLE 10.2
Postoperative Supplementation Recommendations

Supplement	Dose
Multivitamin or prenatal vitamin	1 tablet twice a day
Calcium citrate	500 mg tablet 3 times a day
Vitamin B_{12} (cobalamin)	500 μg/day or
	1,000 μg by injection over 4–6 weeks
Vitamin B_1 (thiamin)	50 mg/day
Vitamin D_3	3,000 IU

Source: Mechanick, J.I. et al., *Obesity (Silver Spring)*, 21(Suppl 1), S1–S27, 2013.

10.7.1 IRON

Iron deficiency is common in both males and females postsurgically. This is due, in part, to decreased intake of heme iron. Additionally, the decreased acid in the pouch does not allow the ferrous iron to be converted to the more absorbable form of ferric iron. Another complicating factor is that iron is absorbed in the duodenum, which is bypassed in the RYGB procedure. The literature recommends iron supplementation with 45–60 mg of iron per day, for those with deficiency.[17] Most programs recommend a prenatal vitamin supplementation for menstruating females.

10.7.2 MENSTRUAL CHANGES AND ANEMIA

Adolescent females with obesity are twice as likely to have early menarche and 40% more likely to have menstrual dysfunction. This menstrual dysfunction may be in the form of amenorrhea, both primary and secondary, or irregular menses with heavy bleeding.[18] These menstrual changes place the young woman at higher risk for anemia. Young women with anemia should have a gynecological evaluation and treatment of the menstrual dysfunction in addition to iron supplementation to achieve resolution of anemia prior to surgery.

10.7.3 FOLATE

Folate deficiency can occur due to decreased intake of folate-rich foods. The bypassed duodenum is the primary site of folate absorption. However, folate absorption can take place along the entire length of the small bowel with adaptation after surgery. The recommended intake is 800–1,000 mg of folate per day. This is the dose most commonly found in over-the-counter multivitamins and prescription prenatal vitamins.

10.7.4 VITAMIN B_{12} (COBALAMIN)

Food sources rich in B_{12} are typically consumed in small quantities following bariatric surgery. Given the less acidic environment in the pouch, compared to the normal stomach, after RYGB surgery, it is difficult to release the protein-bound B_{12} from foods ingested. After RYGB surgery it is more difficult for the unbound B_{12} to pair up with intrinsic factor (IF) to form IF/B_{12} complexes for absorption in the ileum. Consequently, after RYGB surgery the IF/B_{12} complex cannot form, and therefore little absorption takes place.

The literature recommends the use of sublingual B_{12} in an average daily dose of 500 µg/day. A very small percentage of individuals taking this dose will present as B_{12} deficient postsurgically. When oral administration fails, then monthly injection of B_{12} is recommended. Some adolescents may prefer the injectable form.

10.7.5 VITAMIN B₁ (THIAMIN)

Thiamin deficiency (beriberi) is rare but has been reported following gastric bypass surgery. There are minimal stores present in the body. Deficiency has been reported as early as 18 days following dietary restriction. Specifically in female adolescents, thiamin deficiency has been reported after gastric bypass surgery presenting 4–6 months postoperatively. It presents as lower extremity weakness and pain, numbness, or tingling.[19] After WLS, thiamin deficiency is most likely to occur in patients who experience persistent vomiting or excessive weight loss postoperatively.

Adolescents who have undergone bariatric surgery should be receiving a minimum of 50 mg of thiamin per day, which can be supplied by including an additional B complex in the vitamin regimen. Most programs recommend supplementation of thiamine during the rapid weight loss phase during the first 6 months postsurgery.

10.7.6 CALCIUM

Calcium deficiency is common and represents a long-term potential risk postsurgically. If calcium levels are low, the bone will release calcium into the blood to normalize serum calcium. Calcium citrate is the recommended form of supplementation, as it does not require stomach acid for absorption. The recommended dosage is 1,200–1,500 mg of calcium citrate per day in three divided doses. The calcium should be taken separate from the iron/prenatal medication. This supports the concept of a medication schedule in order to assure compliance with both the intake and timing of medications/supplementation.

10.8   HYDRATION

After bariatric surgery patients are at risk for dehydration typically due to inadequate intake, vomiting, or diarrhea. Fluid requirements for patients can vary and should be guided by thirst. The recommendation for adolescents is the same as that for the adult patient, a minimum of 48–64 oz of total fluids per day. In order to meet these fluid requirements, the patient is encouraged to carry a water bottle with him or her throughout the day. Students often need to have a written note in order to carry a water bottle with them at school.

10.9   PREGNANCY

Woman having WLS are encouraged to delay pregnancy until after the period of maximum weight loss or 12–18 months. Pregnancy earlier than this time frame requires closer surveillance of maternal weight and nutritional status.[20] Adolescents should receive counseling regarding pregnancy prevention prior to and after WLS. The young woman needs to understand that weight loss will improve fertility, and those that were not consistently using contraception prior to WLS without consequences will now need to be more vigilant for pregnancy prevention. One study found pregnancy rates twice the rate of the general population for adolescents after bariatric surgery.[21] In addition, dietary counseling before, during, and after pregnancy is essential for assessment and prevention of vitamin deficiencies. An evaluation for micronutrient deficiencies should be done at the beginning of pregnancy and in the absence of other deficiencies; monitoring the blood count, iron, ferritin, calcium, and vitamin D levels every trimester should be considered.[20]

10.10 TRANSITION OF CARE

Young adults require a thoughtful transition to an adult care model; this process ideally begins early in the care of the adolescent and family. This can be achieved by allowing the adolescent as he or she becomes developmentally capable to take more responsibility for the management of his or her health at home and in the medical office. This includes having opportunities to speak with the health care team privately to become more comfortable with discussing health concerns and understanding medical instructions. The young adult will need an understanding of the importance of ongoing follow-up with a primary care provider or an adult bariatric team to monitor laboratory values and weight.

10.11 CONCLUSION

The prevalence of adolescent severe obesity is increasing. Nonsurgical treatment is seldom successful, and due to medical comorbidities, surgery is increasingly considered. There are now well-accepted guidelines for use of surgery in adolescents and for the composition of multidisciplinary teams offering surgical care for adolescent severe obesity. In addition to the understanding of general principles of bariatric medicine and surgery, successful bariatric care of adolescents requires an understanding of other unique aspects of adolescents: development psychology, developmental physiology, medicine, dietary/eating behaviors, nutrition, and issues surrounding transition of care for older adolescents. By incorporating expertise in all of these areas, bariatric procedures can be used safely and effectively in this age group.

REFERENCES

1. Ogden, C.L. et al. Prevalence of high body mass index in US children and adolescents, 2007–2008. *JAMA*, 2010; 303(3): 242–49.
2. Skelton, J.A. et al. Prevalence and trends of severe obesity among US children and adolescents. *Acad Pediatr*, 2009; 9(5): 322–29.
3. Parsons, T.J. et al. Childhood predictors of adult obesity: a systematic review. *Int J Obes Relat Metab Disord*, 1999; 23(Suppl 8): S1–107.
4. Sjoberg, R.L., K.W. Nilsson, and J. Leppert. Obesity, shame, and depression in school-aged children: a population-based study. *Pediatrics*, 2005; 116(3): e389–92.
5. Danielsson, P. et al. Response of severely obese children and adolescents to behavioral treatment. *Arch Pediatr Adolesc Med*, 2012; 166(12): 1103–8.
6. Tsai, W.S., T.H. Inge, and R.S. Burd. Bariatric surgery in adolescents: recent national trends in use and in-hospital outcome. *Arch Pediatr Adolesc Med*, 2007; 161(3): 217–21.

7. Kelleher, D.C. et al. Recent national trends in the use of adolescent inpatient bariatric surgery: 2000 through 2009. *JAMA Pediatr*, 2013; 167(2): 126–32.

8. Pratt, J.S. et al. Best practice updates for pediatric/adolescent weight loss surgery. *Obesity (Silver Spring)*, 2009; 17(5): 901–10.

9. Aikenhead, A., T. Lobstein, and C. Knai. Review of current guidelines on adolescent bariatric surgery. *Clinical Obesity*, 2011; 1(1): 3–11.

10. Michalsky, M. et al. Developing criteria for pediatric/adolescent bariatric surgery programs. *Pediatrics*, 2011; 128: S65–70.

11. Michalsky, M. et al. ASMBS pediatric committee best practice guidelines. *Surg Obes Relat Dis*, 2012; 8(1): 1–7.

12. Kelly, A.S. et al. Severe obesity in children and adolescents: identification, associated health risks, and treatment approaches: a scientific statement from the American Heart Association. Submitted to *Circulation*, 2013; 128: 1689–1712.

13. Miller, W.R., and S. Rollnick. Ten things that motivational interviewing is not. *Behav Cogn Psychother*, 2009; 37(2): 129–40.

14. Benotti, P.N. et al. Preoperative weight loss before bariatric surgery. *Arch Surg*, 2009; 144(12): 1150–55.

15. Kruger, A.J. et al. Preparation of a severely obese adolescent for significant and long-term weight loss: an illustrative case. *Pediatr Surg Int* 2013; 29: 835–839.

16. Modi, A.C. et al. Adherence to vitamin supplementation following adolescent bariatric surgery. *Obesity (Silver Spring)*, 2013; 21(3): 190–95.

17. Mechanick, J.I. et al. Clinical practice guidelines for the perioperative nutritional, metabolic, and nonsurgical support of the bariatric surgery patient—2013 update: cosponsored by American Association of Clinical Endocrinologists, The Obesity Society, and American Society for Metabolic and Bariatric Surgery. *Obesity (Silver Spring)*, 2013; 21(Suppl 1): S1–27.

18. Hillman, J.B., R.J. Miller, and T.H. Inge. Menstrual concerns and intrauterine contraception among adolescent bariatric surgery patients. *J Womens Health*, 2011; 20(4): 533–38.

19. Towbin, A. et al. Beriberi after gastric bypass surgery in adolescence. *J Pediatr*, 2004; 145(2): 263–67.

20. American College of Obstetrics and Gynecology Committee on Obstetric Practice. Committee opinion: obesity in pregnancy. *Obstet Gynecol*, 2005; 3(106): 671–75.

21. Roehrig, H.R. et al. Pregnancy after gastric bypass surgery in adolescents. *Obes Surg*, 2007; 17(7): 873–77.

22. Fullmer, M.A. et al. Nutritional strategy for adolescents undergoing bariatric surgery: report of a working group of the Nutrition Committee of NASPGHAN/NACHRI. *J Pediatr Gastroenterol Nutr*, 2012; 54(1): 125–35.

11 Special Populations
Pregnancy and Lactation after Bariatric Surgery

Michelle A. Kominiarek

CONTENTS

11.1 INTRODUCTION

According to the National Health and Nutrition Examination Survey (NHANES) from 2009 to 2010, the prevalence of obesity among women ≥20 years of age was 35.8%.[1] This same survey found that the prevalence of class 2 and 3 obesity was greater in women (18.1% and 8.1%, respectively) compared to men (12.5% vs. 4.4%, respectively).[1] Of further interest, the number of obese women of reproductive age (20–39 years) increased by 64.2% (from 20.7% to 34.0%) between 1988–1994 and 2007–2008, the greatest increase in obesity for women of any age category.[2] In light of this information about obesity prevalence and its sex differences, it is not surprising that more than 80% of bariatric surgery procedures are performed in women who have a mean age of 42 years.[3]

Infertility, one of the common obesity comorbidities, often improves after a bariatric surgery procedure.[4,5] Not only is pregnancy a possibility after a bariatric surgery, but pregnancy is often an intention of women who plan to have bariatric surgery.[6] A woman's preconception weight is important because women with a higher prepregnancy body mass index (BMI) have a greater risk for adverse perinatal outcomes.[7,8] The combination of obesity and pregnancy introduces morbidities in addition to the underlying morbidities associated with obesity alone. These include both maternal (e.g., gestational diabetes, pregnancy-related hypertension, cesareans, and infectious complications from cesareans) and fetal (e.g., birth defects, stillbirth, and abnormal fetal growth) risks. As such, weight loss prior to pregnancy is strongly recommended to reduce complications and improve outcomes.[9]

The evidence to support weight loss prior to pregnancy is derived primarily from studies that evaluate perinatal outcomes in women before and after bariatric surgery or in women with and without bariatric surgery. These studies and systematic reviews suggest that a pregnancy after bariatric surgery is safe and several perinatal outcomes are improved, but a pregnancy occurring after a bariatric surgery procedure creates unique management issues.[3,10,11] These include timing a pregnancy after bariatric surgery, managing a laparoscopic adjustable gastric band (LAGB), altering the screening approach for gestational diabetes, identifying and treating nutritional deficiencies, and managing surgical complications. Unfortunately, many women are still obese when they conceive after having a bariatric surgery procedure.[12–14] Noncompliance to the bariatric surgery postoperative recommendations (e.g., ongoing behavioral modifications, intake of a daily multivitamin, and recommended follow-up visits) also compounds these issues. For example, only 59% of patients after bariatric surgery took the prescribed multivitamin supplements based on surveys performed 1–2 years after the surgery.[15] Given that bariatric procedures can create nutritional deficiencies of micro- and macronutrients, a pregnancy occurring after a bariatric surgery procedure requires particular attention to nutritional deficiencies so that both maternal and offspring health are optimized. The purpose of this chapter is to review the nutritional management of pregnancies that occur after bariatric surgery. This is perhaps the most important element in the prenatal and postpartum care of these women, not only for the optimization of immediate perinatal outcomes such as gestational diabetes or birth defects, but also because intrauterine exposures such as those related to nutrition can influence the risk for chronic disease in the offspring (e.g., obesity, diabetes).[16–20]

11.2 NORMAL PREGNANCY

11.2.1 NUTRITION DURING PREGNANCY

During pregnancy, the traditional teaching is that caloric intake should increase by approximately 300 kcal/day. This is derived from an estimate of 80,000 kcal needed to support a full-term pregnancy and accounts for increased maternal and fetal metabolism as well as fetal and placental growth. Dividing this gross energy cost by the mean pregnancy duration (250 days after the first month) yields the 300 kcal/day estimate for the entire pregnancy.[21,22] However, energy requirements vary significantly depending on a woman's age, BMI, and activity level. Caloric intake should therefore be individualized.

Changes in protein, nitrogen, carbohydrate, and lipid metabolism occur continuously throughout the pregnancy to ensure a supply of nutrients to the developing fetus. Pregnancy is also a period of insulin resistance, which develops progressively during the pregnancy and is attributed to placental hormones such as human placental lactogen (hPL), progesterone, and estrogen. Insulin action is approximately 50% to 60% lower in the third trimester compared to a nonpregnant state.[23]

Protein recommendations during pregnancy are 60 g/day, which is an increase from 46 g/day in a nonpregnant state. This also reflects a change to 1.1 g of protein/kg/day during pregnancy from 0.8 g of protein/kg/day for a nonpregnant state.[22] Table 11.1 shows the recommended daily allowances for vitamins and minerals for pregnant and lactating women and how they differ compared to nonpregnant women.[24] Although approximately 19 million pregnant women worldwide have vitamin A deficiency, severe vitamin A deficiency is rare in the United States.[25] Vitamin A is essential for cell differentiation and proliferation as well as development of the spine, heart, eyes, and ears. Vitamin A is transported rapidly across the placenta to the fetus by retinal-binding protein receptors.[26-29] Offspring of mothers with vitamin A deficiency have a higher mortality rate, which may be associated with decreased immune function.[30] On the other hand, excessive doses of vitamin A can also have a teratogenic effect and have been associated with cranial-facial and cardiac birth defects. The upper limit for vitamin A intake is 3000 µg/day. Vitamin D is not only essential for calcium homeostasis and maternal bone health, but it also plays a role in fetal growth and the regulation of genes responsible for implantation and angiogenesis. In the United States, vitamin D deficiency is common during pregnancy.[31-33] Vitamin D supplementation is advised for women who are strict vegetarians and for those who avoid sunlight or dairy foods. Vitamin B_{12} is required for methylation reactions in several metabolic pathways, especially related to DNA synthesis, and it is also important to maintain normal vitamin B_{12} levels during pregnancy.

Although vitamin and mineral supplementation for women with appropriate dietary intake is not mandatory, most clinicians prescribe a prenatal vitamin because many women do not have an adequate diet, especially during the first trimester, and therefore cannot meet the increased nutritional requirements for pregnancy. Table 11.2 shows the typical composition of a prenatal vitamin. The critical difference compared to other multivitamins is the folic acid dose, which is necessary to support rapid cell growth, cell replications, cell division, and nucleotide synthesis

TABLE 11.1
Recommended Daily Dietary Allowances for Pregnant and Lactating Women

Nutrient	Nonpregnant	Pregnant[a]	Lactation[a]
Vitamin A (µg/day)	700	770	1300
Vitamin D (µg/day)	5	15	15
Vitamin E (mg/day)	15	15	19
Vitamin K (µg/day)	90	90	90
Folate (µg/day)	400	600	500
Niacin (mg/day)	14	18	17
Riboflavin (mg/day)	1.1	1.4	1.6
Thiamin (mg/day)	1.1	1.4	1.4
Vitamin B_6 (mg/day)	1.3	1.9	2
Vitamin B_{12} (µg/day)	2.4	2.6	2.8
Vitamin C (mg/day)	75	85	120
Calcium (mg/day)	1000	1000	1000
Iron (mg/day)	18	27	9
Phosphorus (mg/day)	700	700	700
Selenium (µg/day)	55	60	70
Zinc (mg/day)	8	11	12

Source: Otten, J. J. et al., eds., *Dietary Reference Intakes: The Essential Guide to Nutrient Requirements*, National Academies Press, Washington, DC, 2006.[24] With permission.

[a]   Applies to women >18 years old.

TABLE 11.2
Prenatal Vitamin Composition

Component	Amount	Percent Daily Value for Pregnancy and Lactation
Vitamin A	4000 IU as beta carotene	50%
Vitamin D_3	400 IU	100%
Vitamin E	11 IU	37%
Folic acid	800 µg	100%
Niacin	18 mg	90%
Riboflavin	1.7mg	85%
Thiamin	1.5 mg	88%
Vitamin B_6	2.6 mg	104%
Vitamin B_{12}	4 µg	50%
Vitamin C	100 mg	167%
Calcium	250 mg	19%
Iron	27 mg	150%
Zinc	25 mg	167%

for fetal and placental development. Humans are dependent on dietary sources or supplements to meet the requirements for folate during pregnancy. Women of child-bearing age should take 400 µg/day of folic acid, whereas women should take 600 µg/day during pregnancy.

11.2.2   PHYSIOLOGICAL AND ANATOMICAL CHANGES DURING PREGNANCY

Physiological gastrointestinal changes that occur during pregnancy include decreased stomach tone and motility, decreased gastric acid secretion, delayed gastric empty-ing, increased gastric mucous secretion, and decreased lower esophageal sphincter pressure. In light of these changes, several gastrointestinal complaints worsen during pregnancy. Nausea and vomiting is common during pregnancy and can start as early as 5 weeks.[34] Although it typically resolves by 16–18 weeks, nausea and vomiting can persist until delivery.[34,35] Nearly 90% of women will have some degree of nausea, but severe nausea and vomiting during pregnancy accompanied by weight loss and dehy-dration is less common.[36] The exact etiology for nausea and vomiting in pregnancy is unclear, but it is likely related to increases in human chorionic gonadotropin (hCG), which typically peaks at 12 weeks gestation.[35] Vitamin B_6 supplements (10 to 25 mg three times a day) are one of the most effective treatments for nausea and vomiting during pregnancy.[37,38] Heartburn and indigestion are also common symptoms during pregnancy. These symptoms may worsen during the third trimester as the enlarging uterus compresses adjacent organs. Lastly, 50% of pregnant women experience con-stipation at some point during the pregnancy.

11.2.3   LABORATORY CHANGES DURING PREGNANCY

Several laboratory values are altered as a result of physiological changes during pregnancy. Specific attention is addressed to the values that pertain to nutritional status in pregnancy. Both total red blood cell mass and plasma volume increase early in gestation, but plasma volume increases to a greater extent, resulting in hemodilu-tion and a physiological anemia during pregnancy. As a result, a hemoglobin of <10.5 g/dl and a hematocrit of <32% are used to establish the diagnosis of anemia during the second trimester. A hemoglobin of <11 g/dl is considered anemic for the first or third trimester. Serum total proteins and albumin decrease during pregnancy and are 30% lower than nonpregnant values.[39] Additionally, estrogen increases the hepatic production of certain proteins, and there is greater protein binding of corticoste-roids, sex steroids, thyroid hormones, and vitamin D during pregnancy. An accurate assessment of a disease state in pregnancy usually requires evaluation of the free or unbound forms (e.g., free T4 vs. total T4) in the evaluation of thyroid disorders.

11.2.4   WEIGHT GAIN AND LOSS DURING PREGNANCY

Regardless of a woman's prepregnancy BMI, pregnancy has traditionally been con-sidered a time for weight gain, not weight loss. The obligatory weight gain during pregnancy is approximately 8 kg and takes into account contributions to maternal tissues (e.g., uterus, breast, blood volume), the fetus, and the placenta. A weight gain

TABLE 11.3

Gestational Weight Gain Recommendations

Prepregnancy BMI	Total Weight Gain	Rate of Weight Gain in Second and Third Trimester; Mean (Range)
Underweight	12.5–18 kg	0.51 (0.44–0.58) kg/week
(<18.5 kg/m²)	28–40 lb	1 (1–1.3) lb/week
Normal weight	11.5–16 kg	0.42 (0.35–0.50) kg/week
(18.5–24.9 kg/m²)	25–35 lb	1 (0.8–1) lb/week
Overweight	7–11.5 kg	0.28 (0.23–0.33) kg/week
(25.0–29.9 kg/m²)	15–25 lb	0.6 (0.5–0.7) lb/week
Obese	5–9 kg	0.22 (0.17–0.27) kg/week
(≥30.0 kg/m²)	11–20 lb	0.5 (0.4–0.6) lb/week

Source: Weight Gain during Pregnancy: Reexamining the Guidelines, Institute of Medicine, Washington, DC, 2009.

less than this amount would imply that maternal adipose and protein stores would need to be mobilized to support a developing pregnancy. The literature is sparse regarding metabolic changes of women who lose weight during pregnancy, but it is known that ketonemia, increased urinary nitrogen excretion, and decreased gluconeogenic amino acid production result after a period of fasting during pregnancy.[40] Because of the increase in insulin resistance, pregnancy is often considered a time of "accelerated starvation," with an increased risk for developing ketonuria and ketonemia regardless of a woman's glucose tolerance status.[41] This is critical to consider during pregnancy because there may be significant consequences related to fetal growth and later neurocognitive development in the presence of maternal ketonemia or ketonuria.[42–44]

The recommendations for the total amount of weight gain and rate of weight gain during pregnancy are based on the woman's prepregnancy BMI (Table 11.3).[23] Of note, the guidelines for gestational weight gain published in 2009 by the Institute of Medicine (IOM) differ from the original 1990 recommendations in that women with a prepregnancy BMI of ≥30kg/m² should gain 5–9 kg or 11–20 lb during pregnancy.[23,45] In general, overweight or obese women have lower total gestational weight gains than normal-weight women, yet >40% of all women exceed the gestational weight gain recommendations.[46] The IOM 2009 guidelines also recommend that women begin pregnancy at a healthy weight so that optimal maternal and neonatal outcomes are achieved.[23]

11.3 LACTATION PHYSIOLOGY

Breastfeeding and breast milk are the global standard for infant feeding. Several organizations, including the World Health Organization, the U.S. Surgeon General, the American Academy of Pediatrics, the American College of Obstetricians and Gynecologists, the American Academy of Family Practice, and the Academy of Breastfeeding Medicine, support this statement. Furthermore, the American Academy of Pediatrics recommends breastfeeding at least through the first year of life and exclusive breastfeeding for the first 6 months.[47] Similar to pregnancy, energy and nutritional requirements also differ during lactation and breastfeeding.

In terms of energy requirements, lactating women require approximately 500 additional kcal/day than what is recommended for nonpregnant and nonlactating women.[48] The estimate comes from the mean volume of breast milk produced per day (780 ml, range 450–1200 ml) and the energy content of milk (67 kcal/100 ml).[49] These goals can typically be achieved by consuming increased calories; however, many women do not consume these extra calories, which means that body stores are used to maintain lactation. During pregnancy, most women store an extra 2 to 5 kg (19,000 to 48,000 kcal) in tissue, mainly as fat, in physiologic preparation for lactation. These calories and nutrients are then mobilized to supplement the maternal diet during lactation. If weight loss is occurring, it will usually not influence the quantity or quality of breast milk, but it may increase the risk for maternal deficiencies in magnesium, vitamin B_6, folate, calcium, and zinc.[49,50] As such, a common recommendation is for women to continue to take a prenatal vitamin daily while they are breastfeeding (Tables 11.1 and 11.2). Even if a woman has a limited diet and restricted nutrients, milk quality is usually sufficient for infant feeding and growth. Both fat- and water-soluble vitamins are secreted into breast milk. Fat-soluble vitamins (vitamins A, D, and K) are reduced in breast milk when there is a maternal vitamin deficiency.[51–52] Water-soluble vitamins (vitamins C, B_1, B_6, and B_{12}, folate) are also influenced by maternal diet and are reduced in breast milk when there are deficiencies. Calcium, phosphorus, and magnesium levels in breast milk are independent of maternal serum levels and diet.[53] Maternal stress, anxiety, and smoking can decrease milk production, but the quantitative and caloric value of breast milk does not change with dieting and exercise.[54–61] Moreover, a woman's weight, BMI, body fat percentage, and weight gain during pregnancy do not influence milk production.[62–64]

11.4 OVERVIEW OF PERINATAL OUTCOMES AFTER BARIATRIC SURGERY

There are no prospective randomized trials that study pregnancies of women after bariatric surgery. Instead, the literature is limited to retrospective cohort studies with varying control groups (i.e., a single woman whose pregnancy before bariatric surgery is compared to her pregnancy after bariatric surgery, a comparison of pregnancy outcomes in obese women vs. women after bariatric surgery, etc.), differing outcome measures (i.e., chronic hypertension and preeclampsia combined vs. reported individually), and differing types of surgeries (i.e., restrictive vs. combined restriction-malabsorption). The literature can be summarized by stating that occurrences of gestational diabetes and hypertensive disorders,[3,65–69] as well as macrosomia (defined as a birth weight of >4200 g or >4500 g),[67,70,71] appear to decrease after bariatric surgery. Conversely, other studies have reported no influence on macrosomia[65,66] and increases in small for gestational age (SGA) (a birth weight of <10th% for the gestational age) infants.[71,72] As such, the literature on perinatal outcomes after bariatric surgery needs to be interpreted with caution. Several studies have also shown that gestational weight gain decreases in women after bariatric surgery.[10,51] For example, in a study of 27 matched pregnancies before and after a LAGB in predominantly obese women, the mean gestational weight gain was 14.8 ± 10.1 vs. 6.6 ± 7.9 kg, respectively, $p < 0.001$.[10]

11.4.1 REVIEW OF DIET AND NUTRITIONAL INDICES IN PREGNANCIES AFTER BARIATRIC SURGERY

Since nutritional requirements increase during pregnancy, nutritional deficiencies in the pregnant bariatric surgery patient, who may already have nutritional deficiencies at conception, can be exacerbated during pregnancy. Chapters X in this textbook have discussed some of the most common micro- and macronutrient deficiencies that occur after bariatric surgery—vitamin B_{12}, folate, and iron.[73] Literature supports that these specific vitamins and nutrients are critical to a developing fetus and a breastfed infant (Sections 11.2.1 and 11.3).[74] Two reports that describe nutritional measures (e.g., food diaries, laboratory studies) in pregnancies after bariatric surgery can give some insight into the management of these high-risk pregnancies and are detailed below.

Dietary intake and nutritional assessment was described in a study of 14 women who had a pregnancy up to 5 years after a Roux-en-Y gastric bypass (RYGBP).[75] During these pregnancies, women had nutritional counseling and were recommended to consume 15–25 kcal/kg/day and advised to gain 7–11 kg during the pregnancy. Multivitamins and minerals were prescribed. The mean time from the bariatric surgery until conception was 24.2 months, and the mean BMI was 36 kg/m² in the second trimester. During pregnancy, the mean intakes of protein (71 ± 17 g/day), folic acid (1000 µg/day), and iron (60 mg/day) met the nutritional guidelines, but calcium (250 mg/day) and vitamin B_{12} (12 µg/day) were significantly below what other investigators have recommended during pregnancy.[76,77] Additional analysis compared dietary intake and nutritional laboratory values prior to the bariatric surgery and during the pregnancy (second or third trimester recordings). Women consumed more total calories (2330 ± 515 vs. 1789 ± 659 kcal/day, $p = 0.046$) and a greater proportion of carbohydrates (51.3 ± 13.5% vs. 43.3 ± 11.5%, $p = 0.048$) before the bariatric surgery compared to the second trimester, but the intake of fat and protein did not differ between the two time periods. Lymphocytes, markers of nutrition and immunity, decreased during pregnancy (3.1 ± 1.1 vs. 2.0 ± 0.5/mm³, $p = 0.04$). Although both hemoglobin (13.9 ± 1.6 vs. 11.4 ± 1.5 g/dl, $p = 0.038$) and albumin (4.3 ± 0.3 vs. 4.1 ± 0.4 g/dl, $p = 0.047$) decreased during pregnancy compared to before the bariatric surgery, the mean values were within the standard pregnancy ranges. Iron levels decreased during pregnancy (107 ± 73 vs. 78 ± 50 µg/dl, $p = 0.049$), but neither ferritin nor transferrin differed between the two time periods. Remarkably, glycosylated hemoglobin improved during pregnancy (5.9 ± 1.5 vs. 4.4 ± 0.3%, $p = 0.036$), but mean glucose did not differ (94 ± 25 vs. 80 ± 8 mg/dl, $p = 0.134$). Calcium levels decreased during pregnancy (9.5 ± 0.6 vs. 9.2 ± 0.6 mg/dl, $p = 0.048$), but there was never frank hypocalcemia. Folate levels increased dramatically (2.7 ± 0.3 vs.

10.7 ± 4.3 ng/ml, $p = 0.011$), but vitamin B_{12} did not differ (256 ± 70 vs. 193 ± 102 pg/ml, $p = 0.182$) between the two time periods. These latter three levels were appropriate for second trimester gestations.

In another study, Guelinckx obtained 7-day dietary records from 49 pregnant women during the first and second trimesters with a prior bariatric surgery procedure.[78] The records were analyzed according to the Healthy Eating Index (HEI), which represents the degree to which a diet meets the guidelines of the U.S. Department of Agriculture Food Guide Pyramid.[79,80] The HEI has 10 components (e.g., grains, vegetables, fruits, etc., and diet variety), each receiving a score range of 0–10. For each component, a score of 10 means the consumed servings conformed to the recommendations. A HEI score of <51 (50% of maximum score) indicated an "unhealthy diet," 51–80 indicated the diet "needed improvement," and >80 indicated a "healthy diet." In the first trimester, only 15% had a healthy diet, 82% needed improvement, and 3% had a poor quality diet. The diet quality did not improve from the first to the second trimester. The highest scores (indicating a healthier diet) pertained to cholesterol, meat, and sodium components and diet variety, whereas the lowest scores (indicating a poorer diet) were grains and total fat components, with fruit having the lowest score overall (range 4.4–5.2). The daily composition of macronutrient intake also differed slightly from the recommended values: 35% fat intake (recommended 30–35%), 13% saturated fat intake (recommended upper limit 10%), 15% protein (recommended 9–11%), and 48% carbohydrates (recommended 50%) The dietary fiber intake was the most striking result: 18.5 g/day, which is less than the recommended 30 g/day. A mean calcium intake of 702–833 mg/day clearly did not meet the requirements for pregnant women (1000 mg/day). Only iron met the recommendations (9–11 mg/day compared to recommended 10 mg/day). Further analysis revealed that there were no differences in the total HEI score between women with a restrictive vs. gastric bypass procedure except for the intake of grains (6.0 ± 1.5 vs. 4.5 ± 1.6, $p = 0.01$), which was higher in women who had a restrictive procedure. Of note, only 24% of the women in the study met the 2009 IOM gestational weight gain recommendations.

Both of these studies have limitations, which are primarily due to the small number of pregnancies reported after bariatric surgery. Nonetheless, the findings are significant in that despite continued nutritional advice and monitoring, several nutritional deficiencies were noted in these women. The increased folate levels were likely a reflection of supplementation in preparation for or during a pregnancy. The pregnancies described by Faintuch et al. occurred after a RYGBP, which is more likely to result in malabsorption and nutritional deficiencies than purely restrictive procedures.[75] Because malabsorptive procedures have a higher risk for nutritional deficiencies, closer surveillance in pregnancies that occur after these types of surgeries is appropriate.

11.4.2 ADVERSE PERINATAL OUTCOMES RELATED TO NUTRITIONAL STATUS IN PREGNANCIES AFTER BARIATRIC SURGERY

Several studies suggest that birth defects and infant mortality in pregnancies occurring after bariatric surgery do not differ compared to the general population.[81–83] There are several case reports and case series that describe unexpected infant morbidity and mortality that were potentially related to the maternal nutritional status and specific deficiencies during pregnancies after bariatric surgery. Given the high prevalence of vitamin and nutrient deficiencies reported after gastric bypass-type bariatric surgeries outside of pregnancy (i.e., 53% vitamin A deficiency, 38% folate deficiency, 64% vitamin B_{12} deficiency), it is particularly important to review the potential consequences of these deficiencies during and after a pregnancy.[84–86]

Although the biliopancreatic diversion (BPD) procedure is less commonly performed today, several case reports describe both maternal and neonatal complications from vitamin A deficiency, including maternal night blindness, preterm deliveries, and neonatal micropthalmia.[87,88]

Deficiencies in vitamin K have also been linked to adverse outcomes in infants born to mothers after bariatric surgery. One case report attributed a fetal cerebral hemorrhage to vitamin K deficiency in a mother who experienced complications from a gastric banding procedure and required parenteral feeding for several weeks before delivery.[89] The infant had diffuse subarachnoid and subdural hemorrhages and died on day of life 7. In another case series, severe intracranial neonatal bleeding occurred in three infants born to mothers after bariatric surgery (two after LAGB, one after BPD).[90] Although not substantiated by neonatal laboratory testing, the presumed cause was maternal vitamin K deficiency.

One report describes a woman who delivered a full-term infant weighing 3400 g approximately 6 years after a gastric bypass surgery.[91] At 4 months of age, the exclusively breastfed infant was evaluated for pallor, decreased activity, shaking movements, and poor weight gain. A brain computer tomography (CT) showed cortical and subcortical atrophy, and congenital vitamin B_{12} deficiency was diagnosed. Although the hematological parameters improved after treatment, the infant had significant gross motor and language developmental delay. The woman's vitamin B_{12} level had never been assessed until her infant was evaluated for these issues. Her vitamin B_{12} deficiency (vitamin B_{12} level = 84 pg/ml) was concomitantly diagnosed and treated.[91] Grange et al. also describe a 10-month-old exclusively breastfed infant with failure to thrive, anemia, and neutropenia who was born to a mother 2 years after a gastric bypass procedure. She took a standard prenatal vitamin containing 8 μg of vitamin B_{12}, but her levels were never evaluated during or after the pregnancy. Laboratory studies showed undetectable levels of vitamin B_{12} in the mother and infant. One month later they were both showing an appropriate response to intramuscular vitamin B_{12}. Several other case reports describe vitamin B_{12} deficiencies in infants born to women after a gastric bypass procedure.[92,93,94]

It is well known that adequate maternal folic acid intake can prevent fetal neural tube defects.[95] Neural tube defects, one of the most common birth defects estimated at 0.76 per 1000 births, and concomitant folate deficiency after bariatric surgery have been described in case reports.[96–99] Lastly, another report describes a 4-month-old exclusively breastfed infant with failure to thrive who was born to a woman after gastric bypass surgery. She did not have any dietary restrictions, but she was not compliant with multivitamins, iron supplements, and vitamin B_{12} injections during the pregnancy.[100] As part of the infant's evaluation, an analysis of the breast milk was also performed, which showed that the fat composition was only 39% of the expected value. Formula supplements were recommended and the infant's growth subsequently returned to normal. Although a specific nutrient deficiency was not identified in this particular case, it highlights the potential for breast milk to lack the required composition for adequate infant growth and development.

Although a cause-effect cannot be established from these case reports and case series alone, important relationships between maternal nutrition status and off-spring risks have been discovered. The larger cohort studies often lack information on these specific outcomes. Of greater interest, LAGBs are less frequently associated with nutrient or vitamin deficiencies, but the vitamin K deficiencies described above should alert the clinician to monitor these levels in women who might be experiencing complications related to the bariatric surgery. The potential for serious consequences in the offspring also highlights the need for nutritional evaluation and treatment during both pregnancy and breastfeeding.

11.5 NUTRITIONAL MANAGEMENT IN PREGNANCIES AFTER BARIATRIC SURGERY

11.5.1 DIAGNOSIS OF NUTRITIONAL DEFICIENCIES DURING PREGNANCY

Screening for nutritional deficiencies after bariatric surgery primarily applies to malabsorptive-type procedures such as the RYGBP and BPD.[101] However, micronutrient deficiencies can occur just as commonly after restrictive-type procedures, so one recommendation is to screen all postoperative patients for nutritional deficiencies.[102] Since pregnancy in general is a time to recognize and treat nutritional issues, it is reasonable to screen for nutritional deficiencies in all pregnancies that occur after bariatric surgery, regardless of the procedure type. Guidelines are limited with respect to screening in pregnancy, but recommendations are adapted from those designed for nonpregnant patients and include testing once a trimester or every 3 months if the levels are normal (Table 11.4).[101,103] Testing should start early, i.e., at the first prenatal visit. Abnormal levels or persistent deficiencies despite supplementation require more frequent testing and management in consultation with the bariatric surgery team. In general, bariatric surgery patients do require lifelong follow-up of hematological and iron parameters because iron deficiency anemia can be a long-term complication, occurring in 6% to 50% of patients after RYGBP.[104–107] In pregnancy, iron deficiency anemia can be diagnosed in the usual manner with a low mean corpuscular volume, and abnormal iron studies (e.g., low serum iron, high total iron-binding capacity, and a low serum ferritin), keeping in mind the physiologic anemia that occurs during pregnancy (Section 11.2.3).

11.5.2 RECOMMENDATIONS FOR DIET AND NUTRITIONAL SUPPLEMENTS

Because the evidence for nutritional management of pregnancies after bariatric surgery is lacking, these guidelines also mirror what is recommended in nonpregnant populations with adjustments for pregnancy.[51,78,101,108] The American Dietetic Association recommends a total caloric intake of 2200–2900 kcal/day during pregnancy, but the advice for pregnant bariatric patients is unknown. As such, the energy intake should be individualized with modifications for the woman's prepregnancy

TABLE 11.4

Diagnostic Testing Along with Prophylaxis and Treatment of Micro- and Macronutrient Deficiencies in Pregnancies after Bariatric Surgery

Component	Diagnostic Testing	Prophylaxis	Treatment if Deficient
Protein	Serum albumin and prealbumin	60 g protein/day	Protein supplements
Vitamin A	Vitamin A	4000 IU/day in prenatal vitamin	Vitamin A not to exceed 3000 µg/day
Vitamin D	Serum 25-hydroxy vitamin D	400–800 IU/day in prenatal vitamin	Oral calcitriol (vitamin D) 1000 IU/day
Vitamin K	Serum vitamin K₁, if clinically indicated	Not routinely given	Vitamin K 1 mg/day Consult with hematologist
Folic acid	Complete blood count, red blood cell folate	600–800 µg/day in prenatal vitamin	Folic acid 1000 µg/day
Vitamin B$_{12}$	Complete blood cell count, vitamin B$_{12}$	4 µg/day in prenatal vitamin	Oral vitamin B$_{12}$ 350 µg/day or intramuscular 1000 µg/month Consult with hematologist
Calcium	Total and ionized calcium	250 mg/day in prenatal vitamin	Calcium citrate 1000 mg/day with vitamin D
Iron	Complete blood count, iron, ferritin, total iron-binding capacity	30 mg/day in prenatal vitamin	Ferrous sulfate 325 mg two or three times/day with vitamin C

Source: *Guidelines for Perinatal Care*, 7th ed., American Academy of Pediatrics and the American College of Obstetricians and Gynecologists, Washington, DC, 2012; Mechanick, J. I. et al., *Obesity (Silver Spring)*, 17(Suppl 1), S1–S70, v, PMID19319140, 2009.

BMI and physical activity level. Regardless, weight loss during pregnancy has never been recommended.

The recommendation for protein intake (60 g/day) does not change based on the bariatric surgery status. In general, a daily long-term multivitamin supplement for all bariatric surgery patients has been recommended. During pregnancy, this should be replaced with a prenatal vitamin, which contains most of the required vitamins and nutrients (Table 11.2).

Additional modifications for a pregnancy after bariatric surgery are found in Table 11.4.

In pregnancy, vitamin A supplementation should not exceed 3000 µg/day. Other multivitamin supplements may contain excessive vitamin A doses and should not be continued during pregnancy. Although some studies recommend two multivitamins daily during pregnancy, this should not be the case because excessive doses of vitamin A can be teratogenic.[109,110] Treatment of vitamin D deficiency entails 1000–5000 mg/day of vitamin D₃ depending on the level of deficiency. Similar to recommendations outside of pregnancy, calcium should be taken with meals and calcium citrate preparations are preferred in bariatric surgery patients because they are better absorbed when gastric acid production is diminished.[111,112] The usual calcium requirements for pregnancy are 1000 mg/day, and this dose is also appropriate for pregnancies after bariatric surgery. Treatment and follow-up testing for iron deficiency anemia is recommended as in any other pregnant patient. Only ferrous iron formulations should be prescribed (e.g., ferrous sulfate 325 mg and ferrous fumarate 200 mg, both of which provide 65 mg of elemental iron per tablet). Iron should be taken on an empty stomach and not in close proximity to teas and calcium. Concomitant vitamin C ingestion may help increase iron absorption and ultimately improve hematological parameters.[113]

11.6   OTHER UNIQUE ASPECTS TO CONSIDER IN THE NUTRITIONAL MANAGEMENT OF PREGNANCIES AFTER BARIATRIC SURGERY

Timing a pregnancy after a bariatric surgery is a topic of considerable debate. The rapid weight loss that occurs immediately after bariatric surgery could theoretically increase the risk for malnourishment during pregnancy, potentially leading to low birth weight or malformations. Because the period of rapid weight loss lasts approximately 12–18 months, most experts recommend waiting at least 12–18 months prior to conception,[101,103,114] yet no untoward effects on pregnancies that occurred prior to this period have been reported.[12,109,115]

Another unique aspect in the management of pregnancies after bariatric surgery pertains to the management of the adjustable band. There are several options in terms of completely removing, maintaining, or actively adjusting the fluid in the band during pregnancy.[10,14,66–68,116] A common approach is to deflate the band entirely upon the diagnosis of pregnancy to maximize nutrition and minimize nausea and vomiting. In one study, 17% of 83 women had the band deflated during pregnancy because they were not meeting nutritional requirements or were having frequent vomiting,[10] though many asymptomatic women requested to loosen the band due to fear of inadequate nutrition. In another study, all women had the band deflated due to nausea and vomiting.[14] Citing excessive gestational weight gain in women with a band deflation, another study concluded that the LAGB is generally well tolerated during pregnancy and should only be deflated in symptomatic women.[117]

One recommended practice during pregnancy is to screen for gestational diabetes, usually between 24 and 28 weeks gestation. This is typically done with a 50 g glucose load. Because the consumption of simple carbohydrates can precipitate dumping syndrome (i.e., abdominal pain, cramping, nausea, diarrhea, flushing, tachycardia, and even syncope) in patients who have had a RYGBP, this test should be avoided during pregnancy. An alternative method to screen for gestational diabetes is home glucose monitoring with fasting and postprandial values during 1 week in the 24- to 28-week period.

Pregnancy is a transitional period or a naturally occurring "teachable moment."[118,119] Women are frequently motivated to change their health behaviors to have a healthy pregnancy. This unparalleled and nearly universal desire for a healthy pregnancy makes it an ideal time for health behavior interventions. Similar to the preoperative and immediate postoperative care of nonpregnant bariatric surgery patients, continued nutritional counseling and promotion of healthy behaviors from the clinical team has the potential to help pregnant women improve their perinatal outcomes by maintaining healthy diets and exercise practices during and beyond the pregnancy. A multidisciplinary team approach consisting of the obstetrician-gynecologist in addition to the surgeons, endocrinologists, obesity medicine specialists, psychologists, dieticians, and behavioral therapists should continue to manage weight-related issues during the pregnancy. Motivational interviewing has been shown to be an effective tool in behavioral change-related smoking cessation, psychological diseases, and weight-related issues.[120] This approach may continue to benefit the pregnant bariatric surgery patient because disordered eating patterns, mood disorders, and coping issues are also common during pregnancy.

11.7   BREASTFEEDING

Women who have had bariatric surgery are also advised to follow the WHO recommendation of breastfeeding for 6 months. There are no contraindications to breastfeeding based on the bariatric surgery status alone. Laboratory evaluation, as described in Table 11.4 for the pregnancy, also needs to be done for breastfeeding women. One team of investigators evaluates these parameters every 3 months in breastfeeding women.[121] The infant's care provider also should be aware of the mother's bariatric surgery status as well as any of her specific dietary restrictions or nutrient deficiencies. For women who have a LAGB, there is also a recommendation to keep the band deflated until breastfeeding has been successfully initiated and infant growth is established.[13] It is assumed that the nutritional content of breast milk produced by lactating women after bariatric surgery is similar to that of other women, but few studies have evaluated this. Infants who are predominantly breastfed may have a reduced risk of early childhood obesity.[122–124] As such, there may be additional long-term benefits for women who have had bariatric surgery to breastfeed their infants.

11.8   CONCLUSION

Pregnancy after bariatric surgery appears to be safe, but nutritional needs are at the forefront in the evaluation and management of these pregnancies. Future research should address long-term maternal and offspring outcomes in terms of weight loss goals, nutritional status, and development of chronic diseases. Because this is a unique population in which appropriate nutrition is critical for the health of future generations, further strides in determining the best nutritional management, including the evaluation of deficiencies and supplementation, are needed from evidence-based medicine.

ACKNOWLEDGMENT

This work was supported by Grant K12HD055892 from the NICHD and NIH Office of Research on Women's Health (ORWH).

REFERENCES

1. K. M. Flegal, M. D. Carroll, B. K. Kit, and C. L. Ogden. Prevalence of obesity and trends in the distribution of body mass index among US adults, 1999–2010. *JAMA* 2012; 307: 491–97. PMID22253363.

2. M. Shields, M. D. Carroll, and C. L. Ogden. Adult obesity prevalence in Canada and the United States. NCHS data brief no. 56, Hyattsville, MD: National Center for Health Statistics, 2011. *Adv Nutr* 2011; 2: 368–69. PMCID3125686, PMID22332078.

3. M. Maggard, Z. Li, I. Yermilov, M. Maglione, M. Suttorp, J. Carter, C. Tringale, L. Hilton, S. Chen, and P. Shekelle. Bariatric surgery in women of reproductive age: special concerns for pregnancy. Evidence Report/Technology Assessment 169. Prepared by the Southern California Evidence-Based Practice Center under Contract 290-02-003). Rockville, MD: Agency for Healthcare Research and Quality. November 2008.

4. M. E. Paulen, L. B. Zapata, C. Cansino, K. M. Curtis, and D. J. Jamieson. Contraceptive use among women with a history of bariatric surgery: a systematic review. *Contraception* 2010; 82: 86–94. PMIDISI:000279445300010.

5. M. Teitelman, C. A. Grotegut, N. N. Williams, and J. D. Lewis. The impact of bariatric surgery on menstrual patterns. *Obes Surg* 2006; 16: 1457–63. PMID17132411.

6. G. G. Gosman, W. C. King, B. Schrope, K. J. Steffen, G. W. Strain, A. P. Courcoulas, D. R. Flum, J. R. Pender, and H. N. Simhan. Reproductive health of women electing bariatric surgery. *Fertil Steril* 2010; 94: 1426–31. PMCID2888936, PMID19815190.

7. M. S. Hauger, L. Gibbons, T. Vik, and J. M. Belizan. Prepregnancy weight status and the risk of adverse pregnancy outcome. *Acta Obstet Gynecol Scand* 2008; 87: 953–59. PMID18720038.

8. S. Cnattingius, R. Bergstrom, L. Lipworth, and M. S. Kramer. Prepregnancy weight and the risk of adverse pregnancy outcomes. *N Engl J Med* 1998; 338: 147–52. PMID9428815.

9. Obesity in pregnancy. Committee Opinion No. 549. American College of Obstetricians and Gynecologists. *Obstet Gynecol* 2012; 12(1): 213–217.

10. A. Lapolla, M. Marangon, M. G. Dalfra, G. Segato, M. De Luca, D. Fedele, F. Favretti, G. Enzi, and L. Busetto. Pregnancy outcome in morbidly obese women before and after laparoscopic gastric banding. *Obes Surg* 2010; 20: 1251–57. PMID20524157.

11. D. Bar-Zohar, F. Azem, J. Klausner, and S. Abu-Abeid. Pregnancy after laparoscopic adjustable gastric banding: perinatal outcome is favorable also for women with relatively high gestational weight gain. *Surg Endosc* 2006; 20: 1580–83. PMID16902748.

12. J. R. Wax, A. Cartin, R. Wolff, S. Lepich, M. G. Pinette, and J. Blackstone. Pregnancy following gastric bypass surgery for morbid obesity: maternal and neonatal outcomes. *Obes Surg* 2008; 18: 540–44. PMID18317852.

13. J. B. Dixon, M. E. Dixon, and P. E. O'Brien. Pregnancy after Lap-Band surgery: management of the band to achieve healthy weight outcomes. *Obes Surg* 2001; 11: 59–65. PMID11361170.

14. H. G. Weiss, H. Nehoda, B. Labeck, K. Hourmont, C. Marth, and F. Aigner. Pregnancies after adjustable gastric banding. *Obes Surg* 2001; 11: 303–6. PMID11433905.

15. J. B. Dixon. Elevated homocysteine with weight loss. *Obes Surg* 2001; 11: 537–38. PMID11594089.

16. J. Smith, K. Cianflone, S. Biron, F. S. Hould, S. Lebel, S. Marceau, O. Lescelleur, L. Biertho, S. Simard, J. G. Kral, and P. Marceau. Effects of maternal surgical weight loss in mothers on intergenerational transmission of obesity. *J Clin Endocrinol Metab* 2009; 94: 4275–83. PMID19820018.

17. P. M. Catalano. Obesity and pregnancy—the propagation of a viscous cycle? *J Clin Endocrinol Metab* 2003; 88: 3505–6. PMID12915626.

18. D. J. Barker, C. Osmond, J. Golding, D. Kuh, and M. E. Wadsworth. Growth in utero, blood pressure in childhood and adult life, and mortality from cardiovascular disease. *BMJ* 1989; 298: 564–67. PMCID1835925. PMID2495113.

19. D. J. Barker. In utero programming of cardiovascular disease. *Theriogenology* 2000; 53: 555–74. PMID10735050.

20. E. Oken and M. W. Gillman. Fetal origins of obesity. *Obes Res* 2003; 11: 496–506. PMID12690076.

21. E. Forsum and M. Lof. Energy metabolism during human pregnancy. *Annu Rev Nutr* 2007; 27: 277–92. PMID17465854.

22. P. R. Trumbo, A. A. Yates, and M. Poos. *Food and Nutrition Board, Institute of Medicine: Dietary Reference Intakes for energy, carbohydrate, fiber, fat, fatty acids, cholesterol, protein, and amino acids.* Washington, DC: National Academies Press; 2002. http://www.nal.usda.gov/fnc/PRI/DRI_Energy/energy_full_report.pdf

23. *Weight gain during pregnancy: reexamining the guidelines.* Washington, DC: Institute of Medicine; 2009.

24. J. J. Otten, J. P. Hellwig, and L. D. Meyers, eds. *Dietary Reference Intakes. The essential guide to nutrient requirements.* Washington, DC: National Academies Press; 2006.

25. WHO (World Health Organization). Guideline: Vitamin A supplementation in infant and children 6–59 months of age. Geneva: World Health Organization. 2011.

26. G. M. Morriss-Kay and N. Sokolova. Embryonic development and pattern formation. *FASEB J* 1996; 10: 961–68. PMID8801178.

27. P. Chambon. The retinoid signaling pathway: molecular and genetic analyses. *Semin Cell Biol* 1994; 5: 115–25. PMID8068884.

28. V. Sapin, M. C. Alexandre, S. Chaib, J. A. Bournazeau, P. Sauvant, P. Borel, B. Jacquetin, P. Grolier, D. Lemery, B. Dastugue, and V. Azais-Braesco. Effect of vitamin A status at the end of term pregnancy on the saturation of retinol binding protein with retinol. *Am J Clin Nutr* 2000; 71: 537–43. PMID10648269.

29. M. Sundaram, A. Sivaprasadarao, M. M. DeSousa, and J. B. Findlay. The transfer of retinol from serum retinol-binding protein to cellular retinol-binding protein is mediated by a membrane receptor. *J Biol Chem* 1998; 273: 3336–42. PMID9452451.

30. J. H. Humphrey, K. P. West Jr., and A. Sommer. Vitamin A deficiency and attributable mortality among under-5-year-olds. *Bull World Health Org* 1992; 70: 225–32. PMID1600583.

31. J. M. Lee, J. R. Smith, B. L. Philipp, T. C. Chen, J. Mathieu, and M. F. Holick. Vitamin D deficiency in a healthy group of mothers and newborn infants. *Clin Pediatr (Phila)* 2007; 46: 42–44. PMID17164508.

32. A. C. Looker, C. M. Pfeiffer, D. A. Lacher, R. L. Schleicher, M. F. Picciano, and E. A. Yetley. Serum 25-hydroxyvitamin D status of the US population: 1988–1994 compared with 2000–2004. *Am J Clin Nutr* 2008; 88: 1519–27. PMCID2745830. PMID19064511.

33. L. M. Bodnar and H. N. Simhan. Vitamin D may be a link to black-white disparities in adverse birth outcomes. *Obstet Gynecol Surv* 2010; 65: 273–84. PMCID3222336, PMID20403218.

34. C. Holmgren, K. M. Aagaard-Tillery, R. M. Silver, T. F. Porter, and M. Varner. Hyperemesis in pregnancy: an evaluation of treatment strategies with maternal and neonatal outcomes. *Am J Obstet Gynecol* 2008; 198: 56.e1–4. PMID18166306.

35. M. S. Fejzo, S. A. Ingles, M. Wilson, W. Wang, K. MacGibbon, R. Romero, and T. M. Goodwin. High prevalence of severe nausea and vomiting of pregnancy and hyperemesis gravidarum among relatives of affected individuals. *Eur J Obstet Gynecol Reprod Biol* 2008; 141: 13–17. PMCID2660884, PMID18752885.

36. L. Dodds, D. B. Fell, K. S. Joseph, V. M. Allen, and B. Butler. Outcomes of pregnancies complicated by hyperemesis gravidarum. *Obstet Gynecol* 2006; 107: 285–92. PMID16449113.

37. D. Jewell and G. Young. Interventions for nausea and vomiting in early pregnancy. *Cochrane Database Syst Rev* 2003: CD000145. PMID14583914.

38. P. Chittumma, K. Kaewkiattikun, and B. Wiriyasiriwach. Comparison of the effectiveness of ginger and vitamin B_6 for treatment of nausea and vomiting in early pregnancy: a randomized double-blind controlled trial. *J Med Assoc Thai* 2007; 90: 15–20. PMID17621727.

39. C. G. Hytten F. *Clinical physiology in obstetrics.* Oxford: Blackwell Scientific Publications; 1991.

40. P. Felig. Maternal and fetal fuel homeostasis in human pregnancy. *Am J Clin Nutr* 1973; 26: 998–1005. PMID4600999.

41. N. Freinkel. Banting lecture 1980. Of pregnancy and progeny. *Diabetes* 1980; 29: 1023–35. PMID7002669.

42. J. A. Stehbens, G. L. Baker, and M. Kitchell. Outcome at ages 1, 3, and 5 years of children born to diabetic women. *Am J Obstet Gynecol* 1977; 127: 408–13. PMID835641.

43. T. Rizzo, B. E. Metzger, W. J. Burns, and K. Burns. Correlations between antepartum maternal metabolism and child intelligence. *N Engl J Med* 1991; 325: 911–16. PMID1881416.

44. B. L. Silverman, T. Rizzo, O. C. Green, N. H. Cho, R. J. Winter, E. S. Ogata, G. E. Richards, and B. E. Metzger. Long-term prospective evaluation of offspring of diabetic mothers. *Diabetes* 1991; 40(Suppl 2): 121–25. PMID1748240.

45. *Nutrition during pregnancy.* Washington, DC: Institute of Medicine; 1990.

46. S. Y. Chu, W. M. Callaghan, C. L. Bish, and D. D'Angelo. Gestational weight gain by body mass index among US women delivering live births, 2004–2005: fueling future obesity. *Am J Obstet Gynecol* 2009; 200: 271.e1–7. PMID19136091.

47. American Academy of Pediatrics policy statement breastfeeding and the use of human milk. *Pediatrics* 2013; 129: e827–841.

48. *Guidelines for perinatal care.* 7th ed. Washington, DC: American Academy of Pediatrics and the American College of Obstetricians and Gynecologists; 2012.

49. *Nutrition during lactation.* Washington, DC: Institute of Medicine, National Academy Press; 1991.

50. L. M. Gartner and F. R. Greer. Prevention of rickets and vitamin D deficiency: new guidelines for vitamin D intake. *Pediatrics* 2003; 111: 908–10. PMID12671133.

51. N. F. Butte and D. H. Calloway. Evaluation of lactational performance of Navajo women. *Am J Clin Nutr* 1981; 34: 2210–15. PMID7293949.

52. B. Hollis, P. W. Lambert, and R. L. Horst. Factors affecting the antirachitic sterol content of native milk. 1983; 157.

53. A. Prentice. Calcium supplementation during breast-feeding. *N Engl J Med* 1997; 337: 558–59. PMID9262501.

54. R. J. Schanler and N. M. Hurst. Human milk for the hospitalized preterm infant. *Semin Perinatol* 1994; 18: 476–84. PMID7701350.

55. J. M. Hopkinson, R. J. Schanler, J. K. Fraley, and C. Garza. Milk production by mothers of premature infants: influence of cigarette smoking. *Pediatrics* 1992; 90: 934–38. PMID1437437.

56. F. Vio, G. Salazar, and C. Infante. Smoking during pregnancy and lactation and its effects on breast-milk volume. *Am J Clin Nutr* 1991; 54: 1011–16. PMID1957815.

57. A. N. Andersen, C. Lund-Andersen, J. F. Larsen, N. J. Christensen, J. J. Legros, F. Louis, H. Angelo, and J. Molin. Suppressed prolactin but normal neurophysin levels in cigarette smoking breast-feeding women. *Clin Endocrinol (Oxf)* 1982; 17: 363–68. PMID7139967.

58. K. G. Dewey. Effects of maternal caloric restriction and exercise during lactation. *J Nutr* 1998; 128: 386S–89S. PMID9478032.

59. K. G. Dewey, C. A. Lovelady, L. A. Nommsen-Rivers, M. A. McCrory, and B. Lonnerdal. A randomized study of the effects of aerobic exercise by lactating women on breast-milk volume and composition. *N Engl J Med* 1994; 330: 449–53. PMID8289849.

60. L. B. Dusdieker, D. L. Hemingway, and P. J. Stumbo. Is milk production impaired by dieting during lactation? *Am J Clin Nutr* 1994; 59: 833–40. PMID8147327.
61. M. A. McCrory, L. A. Nommsen-Rivers, P. A. Mole, B. Lonnerdal, and K. G. Dewey. Randomized trial of the short-term effects of dieting compared with dieting plus aerobic exercise on lactation performance. *Am J Clin Nutr* 1999; 69: 959–67. PMID10232637.
62. K. G. Dewey, M. J. Heinig, L. A. Nommsen, and B. Lonnerdal. Maternal versus infant factors related to breast milk intake and residual milk volume: the DARLING study. *Pediatrics* 1991; 87: 829–37. PMID2034486.
63. N. F. Butte, C. Garza, J. E. Stuff, E. O. Smith, and B. L. Nichols. Effect of maternal diet and body composition on lactational performance. *Am J Clin Nutr* 1984; 39: 296–306. PMID6695830.
64. K. F. Michaelsen. Nutrition and growth during infancy. The Copenhagen Cohort Study. *Acta Paediatr Suppl* 1997; 420: 1–36. PMID9185902.
65. A. J. Skull, G. H. Slater, J. E. Duncombe, and G. A. Fielding. Laparoscopic adjustable banding in pregnancy: safety, patient tolerance and effect on obesity-related pregnancy outcomes. *Obes Surg* 2004; 14: 230–35. PMID15018752.
66. J. B. Dixon, M. E. Dixon, and P. E. O'Brien. Birth outcomes in obese women after laparoscopic adjustable gastric banding. *Obstet Gynecol* 2005; 106: 965–72. PMID16260513.
67. G. Ducarme, A. Revaux, A. Rodrigues, F. Aissaoui, I. Pharisien, and M. Uzan. Obstetric outcome following laparoscopic adjustable gastric banding. *Int J Gynaecol Obstet* 2007; 98: 244–47. PMID17433814.
68. A. Karmon and E. Sheiner. Timing of gestation after bariatric surgery: should women delay pregnancy for at least 1 postoperative year? *Am J Perinatol* 2008; 25: 331–33. PMID18493884.
69. M. M. Kjaer, J. Lauenborg, B. M. Breum, and L. Nilas. The risk of adverse pregnancy outcome after bariatric surgery: a nationwide register-based matched cohort study. *Am J Obstet Gynecol* 2013. PMID23467053.
70. P. Marceau, D. Kaufman, S. Biron, F. S. Hould, S. Lebel, S. Marceau, and J. G. Kral. Outcome of pregnancies after biliopancreatic diversion. *Obes Surg* 2004; 14: 318–24. PMID15072650.
71. V. Belogolovkin, H. M. Salihu, H. Weldeselasse, B. J. Biroscak, E. M. August, A. K. Mbah, and A. P. Alio. Impact of prior bariatric surgery on maternal and fetal outcomes among obese and non-obese mothers. *Arch Gynecol Obstet* 2012; 285: 1211–18. PMID22057892.
72. P. Santulli, L. Mandelbrot, E. Facchiano, C. Dussaux, P. F. Ceccaldi, S. Ledoux, and S. Msika. Obstetrical and neonatal outcomes of pregnancies following gastric bypass surgery: a retrospective cohort study in a French referral centre. *Obes Surg* 2010; 20: 1501–8. PMID20803358.
73. P. Shankar, M. Boylan, and K. Sriram. Micronutrient deficiencies after bariatric surgery. *Nutrition* 2010; 26: 1031–37. PMID20363593.
74. L. Hark, P. M. Catalano. Nutritional management during pregnancy. In: S.G. Gabbe, J.R. Niebyl, J.L. Simpson et al., eds. *Obstetrics: Normal and Problem Pregnancies*. 6th ed. Philadelphia, PA: Saunders Elsevier; 2012, Chapter 7.
75. J. Faintuch, M. C. Dias, E. de Souza Fazio, F. C. de Oliveira, R. M. Nomura, M. Zugaib, and I. Cecconello. Pregnancy nutritional indices and birth weight after Roux-en-Y gastric bypass. *Obes Surg* 2009; 19: 583–89. PMID18953618.
76. J. H. Beard, R. L. Bell, and A. J. Duffy. Reproductive considerations and pregnancy after bariatric surgery: current evidence and recommendations. *Obes Surg* 2008; 18: 1023–27. PMID18392904.
77. J. I. Mechanick, R. F. Kushner, H. J. Sugerman, J. M. Gonzalez-Campoy, M. L. Collazo-Clavell, A. F. Spitz, C. M. Apovian, E. H. Livingston, R. Brolin, D. B. Sarwer, W. A. Anderson, J. Dixon, and S. Guven. American Association of Clinical Endocrinologists, The Obesity Society, and American Society for Metabolic and Bariatric Surgery medical

guidelines for clinical practice for the perioperative nutritional, metabolic, and nonsurgical support of the bariatric surgery patient. *Obesity (Silver Spring)* 2009; 17(Suppl 1): S1–70, v. PMID19319140.

78. I. Guelinckx, R. Devlieger, P. Donceel, S. Bel, S. Pauwels, A. Bogaerts, I. Thijs, K. Schurmans, P. Deschilder, and G. Vansant. Lifestyle after bariatric surgery: a multicenter, prospective cohort study in pregnant women. *Obes Surg* 2012; 22: 1456–64. PMID22644802.

79. E. T. Kennedy, J. Ohls, S. Carlson, and K. Fleming. The Healthy Eating Index: design and applications. *J Am Diet Assoc* 1995; 95: 1103–8. PMID7560680.

80. C. S. Hann, C. L. Rock, I. King, and A. Drewnowski. Validation of the Healthy Eating Index with use of plasma biomarkers in a clinical sample of women. *Am J Clin Nutr* 2001; 74: 479–86. PMID11566646.

81. E. Sheiner, A. Levy, D. Silverberg, T. S. Menes, I. Levy, M. Katz, and M. Mazor. Pregnancy after bariatric surgery is not associated with adverse perinatal outcome. *Am J Obstet Gynecol* 2004; 190: 1335–40. PMID15167839.

82. A. Y. Weintraub, A. Levy, I. Levi, M. Mazor, A. Wiznitzer, and E. Sheiner. Effect of bariatric surgery on pregnancy outcome. *Int J Gynaecol Obstet* 2008; 103: 246–51. PMID18768177.

83. L. B. Knudsen and B. Kallen. Gastric bypass, pregnancy, and neural tube defects. *Lancet* 1986; 2: 227. PMID2873476.

84. B. M. Rhode, P. Arseneau, B. A. Cooper, M. Katz, B. M. Gilfix, and L. D. MacLean. Vitamin B_{12} deficiency after gastric surgery for obesity. *Am J Clin Nutr* 1996; 63: 103–9. PMID8604656.

85. S. Pereira, C. Saboya, G. Chaves, and A. Ramalho. Class III obesity and its relationship with the nutritional status of vitamin A in pre- and postoperative gastric bypass. *Obes Surg* 2009; 19: 738–44. PMID18392900.

86. R. E. Brolin, J. H. Gorman, R. C. Gorman, A. J. Petschenik, L. J. Bradley, H. A. Kenler, and R. P. Cody. Are vitamin B_{12} and folate deficiency clinically important after Roux-en-Y gastric bypass? *J Gastrointest Surg* 1998; 2: 436–42. PMID9843603.

87. S. Huerta, L. M. Rogers, Z. Li, D. Heber, C. Liu, and E. H. Livingston. Vitamin A deficiency in a newborn resulting from maternal hypovitaminosis A after biliopancreatic diversion for the treatment of morbid obesity. *Am J Clin Nutr* 2002; 76: 426–29. PMID12145017.

88. K. J. Smets, T. Barlow, and P. Vanhaesebrouck. Maternal vitamin A deficiency and neonatal microphthalmia: complications of biliopancreatic diversion? *Eur J Pediatr* 2006; 165: 502–4. PMID16718478.

89. T. Van Mieghem, D. Van Schoubroeck, M. Depiere, A. Debeer, and M. Hanssens. Fetal cerebral hemorrhage caused by vitamin K deficiency after complicated bariatric surgery. *Obstet Gynecol* 2008; 112: 434–36. PMID18669754.

90. A. Eerdekens, A. Debeer, G. Van Hoey, C. De Borger, V. Sachar, I. Guelinckx, R. Devlieger, M. Hanssens, and C. Vanhole. Maternal bariatric surgery: adverse outcomes in neonates. *Eur J Pediatr* 2010; 169: 191–96. PMID19562372.

91. M. Y. Celiker and A. Chawla. Congenital B_{12} deficiency following maternal gastric bypass. *J Perinatol* 2009; 29: 640–42. PMID19710657.

92. C. D. Campbell, J. Ganesh, and C. Ficicioglu. Two newborns with nutritional vitamin B_{12} deficiency: challenges in newborn screening for vitamin B_{12} deficiency. *Haematologica* 2005; 90: ECR45. PMID16464760.

93. D. K. Grange and J. L. Finlay. Nutritional vitamin B_{12} deficiency in a breastfed infant following maternal gastric bypass. *Ped Hematol Onc* 1994; 11: 311–8.

94. T. D. Wardinsky, R. G. Montes, R. L. Friederich, R. B. Broadhurst, V. Sinnhuber, and D. Bartholomew. Vitamin B_{12} deficiency associated with low breast-milk vitamin B_{12} concentration in an infant following maternal gastric bypass surgery. *Arch Pediatr Adolesc Med* 1995; 149: 1281–84. PMID7581767.

95. MRC Vitamin Study Research Group. Prevention of neural tube defects: results of the Medical Research Council Vitamin Study. *Lancet* 1991; 338: 131–37. PMID1677062.

96. D. Friedman, S. Cuneo, M. Valenzano, G. M. Marinari, G. F. Adami, E. Gianetta, E. Traverso, and N. Scopinaro. Pregnancies in an 18-year follow-up after biliopancreatic diversion. *Obes Surg* 1995; 5: 308–13. PMID10733817.

97. J. A. Moliterno, M. L. DiLuna, S. Sood, K. E. Roberts, and C. C. Duncan. Gastric bypass: a risk factor for neural tube defects? Case report. *J Neurosurg Pediatr* 2008; 1: 406–9. PMID18447680.

98. J. E. Haddow, L. E. Hill, E. M. Kloza, and D. Thanhauser. Neural tube defects after gastric bypass. *Lancet* 1986; 1: 1330. PMID2872457.

99. Folic acid for the prevention of neural tube defects: U.S. Preventive Services Task Force recommendation statement. *Ann Intern Med* 2009; 150: 626–31. PMID19414842.

100. W. S. Martens 2nd, L. F. Martin, and C. M. Berlin Jr. Failure of a nursing infant to thrive after the mother's gastric bypass for morbid obesity. *Pediatrics* 1990; 86: 777–78. PMID2235232.

101. J. I. Mechanick, A. Youdim, D. B. Jones, W. T. Garvey, D. L. Hurley, M. M. McMahon, L. J. Heinberg, R. Kushner, T. D. Adams, S. Shikora, J. B. Dixon, and S. Brethauer. Clinical practice guidelines for the perioperative nutritional, metabolic, and nonsurgical support of the bariatric surgery patient—2013 update: cosponsored by American Association of Clinical Endocrinologists, The Obesity Society, and American Society for Metabolic and Bariatric Surgery. *Obesity (Silver Spring)* 2013; 21(Suppl 1): S1–27. PMID23529939.

102. K. A. Gudzune, M. M. Huizinga, H. Y. Chang, V. Asamoah, M. Gadgil, and J. M. Clark. Screening and diagnosis of micronutrient deficiencies before and after bariatric surgery. *Obes Surg* 2013. PMID23515975.

103. Bariatric surgery and pregnancy. Practice Bulletin 105. American College of Obstetricians and Gynecologists. *Obstet Gynecol* 2009; 113(6): 1405–1413.

104. S. R. Simon, R. Zemel, S. Betancourt, and B. L. Zidar. Hematologic complications of gastric bypass for morbid obesity. *South Med J* 1989; 82: 1108–10. PMID2772679.

105. D. Heber, F. L. Greenway, L. M. Kaplan, E. Livingston, J. Salvador, and C. Still. Endocrine and nutritional management of the post-bariatric surgery patient: an Endocrine Society clinical practice guideline. *J Clin Endocrinol Metab* 2010; 95: 4823–43. PMID21051578.

106. R. Alvarez-Cordero and E. Aragon-Viruette. Post-operative complications in a series of gastric bypass patients. *Obes Surg* 1992; 2: 87–89. PMID10765170.

107. J. D. Halverson. Micronutrient deficiencies after gastric bypass for morbid obesity. *Am Surg* 1986; 52: 594–98. PMID3777703.

108. S. A. Shikora, J. J. Kim, and M. E. Tarnoff. Nutrition and gastrointestinal complications of bariatric surgery. *Nutr Clin Pract* 2007; 22: 29–40. PMID17242452.

109. T. Dao, J. Kuhn, D. Ehmer, T. Fisher, and T. McCarty. Pregnancy outcomes after gastric-bypass surgery. *Am J Surg* 2006; 192: 762–66. PMID17161090.

110. A. C. Wittgrove, L. Jester, P. Wittgrove, and G. W. Clark. Pregnancy following gastric bypass for morbid obesity. *Obes Surg* 1998; 8: 461–64; discussion 465–66. PMID9731683.

111. L. R. Goode, R. E. Brolin, H. A. Chowdhury, and S. A. Shapses. Bone and gastric bypass surgery: effects of dietary calcium and vitamin D. *Obes Res* 2004; 12: 40–47. PMID14742841.

112. R. D. Bloomberg, A. Fleishman, J. E. Nalle, D. M. Herron, and S. Kini. Nutritional deficiencies following bariatric surgery: what have we learned? *Obes Surg* 2005; 15: 145–54. PMID15802055.

113. B. M. Rhode, C. Shustik, N. V. Christou, and L. D. MacLean. Iron absorption and therapy after gastric bypass. *Obes Surg* 1999; 9: 17–21. PMID10065575.

114. R. Magdaleno Jr., B. G. Pereira, E. A. Chaim, and E. R. Turato. Pregnancy after bariatric surgery: a current view of maternal, obstetrical and perinatal challenges. *Arch Gynecol Obstet* 2012; 285: 559–66. PMID22205187.

115. E. Sheiner, A. Edri, E. Balaban, I. Levi, and B. Aricha-Tamir. Pregnancy outcome of patients who conceive during or after the first year following bariatric surgery. *Am J Obstet Gynecol* 2011; 204: 50 e1–6. PMID20887972.

116. L. F. Martin, K. M. Finigan, and T. E. Nolan. Pregnancy after adjustable gastric banding. *Obstet Gynecol* 2000; 95: 927–30. PMID10831994.

117. Y. Jasaitis, F. Sergent, V. Bridoux, M. Paquet, L. Marpeau, and P. Teniere. [Management of pregnancies after adjustable gastric banding]. *J Gynecol Obstet Biol Reprod (Paris)* 2007; 36: 764–69. PMID17512137.

118. S. Phelan. Pregnancy: a "teachable moment" for weight control and obesity prevention. *Am J Obstet Gynecol* 2010; 202: 135 e1–8. PMCID2815033. PMID19683692.

119. M. Kominiarek. Discussing the risks of obesity in pregnancy with your patients: recommendations for the obstetrician-gynecologist. *Female Patient* 2008; 33: 1–5.

120. Motivational interviewing: a tool for behavior change. Committee Opinion 423. American College of Obstetricians and Gynecologists. *Obstet Gynecol* 2009; 113(1): 243–246.

121. K. J. Kaska L, Abacjew-Chmylko A, et al. Nutrition and pregnancy after bariatric surgery. *ISRN Obesity* 2013; 2013: 6.

122. S. Arenz, R. Rückerl, B. Koletzko, and R. von Kries. Breast-feeding and childhood obesity—a systematic review. *Int J Obes Relat Metab Disord* 2004; 28(10): 1247–56.

123. C. G. Owen, R. M. Martin, P. H. Whincup, G. D. Smith, and D. G. Cook. Effect of infant feeding on the risk of obesity across the life course: a quantitative review of published evidence. *Pediatrics* 2005; 115(5): 1367–77.

124. S. Ip, M. Chung, G. Raman et al. Breastfeeding and maternal and infant health outcomes in developed countries. *Evid Rep Technol Assess* (Full Rep) 2007; (153): 1–186.

12 Psychological Issues and Eating Behavior before and after Bariatric Surgery

David B. Sarwer and Rebecca J. Dilks

CONTENTS

12.1   INTRODUCTION

This chapter will review the psychosocial and behavioral issues commonly seen in persons who undergo bariatric surgery. The chapter begins with a discussion of psychological characteristics and eating behaviors of candidates for surgery. The chapter then will highlight the typically positive changes in these domains that are seen after surgery. The chapter concludes with an overview of the psychological and behavioral issues that may present themselves postoperatively and, as a result, threaten the long-term success of bariatric surgery.

12.2   PSYCHOSOCIAL STATUS OF BARIATRIC SURGERY CANDIDATES

The vast majority of bariatric surgery programs and third-party payers in the United States require that candidates for bariatric surgery undergo a behavioral health evaluation prior to surgery. In general, the evaluation serves two purposes. First, it can identify potential contraindications to surgery, such as substance abuse, poorly controlled depression, or other major psychiatric illness. The evaluation also can help identify potential postoperative challenges and facilitate behavioral changes that can enhance long-term weight management.[1]

There are a number of published recommendations regarding the structure and content of these evaluations.[2–5] Almost all rely on clinical interviews with patients; approximately two-thirds also include questionnaires to further assess psychiatric symptoms or objective tests of personality or psychopathology. More comprehensive evaluations assess the patients' knowledge of bariatric surgery, weight and dieting history, eating and activity habits, as well as both potential obstacles and resources that may influence postoperative outcomes.

Between 20 and 70% of persons with extreme obesity (BMI > 40 kg/m^2) who pursue bariatric surgery are thought to suffer from a psychiatric illness. For example, among 288 bariatric surgery candidates who were assessed by the Structured Clinical Interview based on DSM-IV (SCID), 38% received a current axis I diagnosis and 66% were given a lifetime diagnosis.[6] The most common diagnoses are mood disorders, eating disorders, anxiety disorders, and substance abuse.

12.2.1   MOOD DISORDERS

Several studies have suggested a relationship between excess body weight and depression.[7–8] More specifically, persons with extreme obesity are almost five times more likely to have experienced an episode of major depression in the past year compared to average weight individuals.[7] The relationship between obesity and depression appears to be stronger for women than men.[9] Among candidates for bariatric surgery, 38% of patients meet diagnostic criteria for a mood disorder at the time of surgery and 50% report a lifetime history of a mood disorder diagnosis.[6]

12.2.2 Eating Disorders

Disordered eating is common among candidates for bariatric surgery and likely contributed to the development of extreme obesity. The most common eating disorder among bariatric surgery patients is binge eating disorder (BED), which is characterized by the consumption of a large amount of food in a brief period of time (less than 2 h), during which the individual experiences a loss of control.[10] The most recent, methodologically rigorous studies have indicated that the disorder occurs in 5–15% of patients who present for surgery.[11,12] Approximately 2% of candidates for surgery have bulimia nervosa, where the binge eating is accompanied by self-induced vomiting or other compensatory behaviors, such as inappropriate laxative use or excessive exercise.

12.2.3 Anxiety

Anxiety disorders also are common among bariatric surgery candidates. In the study by Kalarchian and colleagues, almost 24% of surgery candidates were found to have an anxiety disorder. The most common was social anxiety disorder, found in 9% of patients.[6] Despite the rate of anxiety disorders in candidates for surgery, there is no evidence suggesting that they contraindicate surgery. However, intuitive thought and clinical experience suggest that uncontrolled anxiety may negatively impact surgical decision making, postoperative recovery, and the patient's ability to adhere to the postoperative diet.

12.2.4 Substance Abuse

Candidates for bariatric surgery report higher rates of substance abuse than estimates from the general population. Approximately 10% of candidates report a history of drug use or alcoholism. Active use or abuse of illegal drugs or alcohol is widely considered a contraindication to surgery, in part as there is concern that substance abuse problems may reappear postoperatively, as discussed below.[13]

12.2.5 Ongoing Mental Health Treatment

Current or past mental health treatment, including both psychotherapy and the use of psychiatric medications, can be seen as a marker of psychopathology. Studies have found that between 16 and 40% of patients report ongoing mental health treatment at the time of bariatric surgery.[12,14–16] Up to 50% have reported a history of psychiatric treatment, most commonly use of antidepressant medications.[12] Unfortunately, little is known about how these medications interact with the different surgical procedures.[17] Potentially dramatic changes in absorption of medications may occur due to a reduction in gastrointestinal surface area and other changes, and rapid changes in body weight and fat mass may also affect the efficacy and tolerability of antidepressant medications.[18]

12.3 OTHER RELEVANT PSYCHOSOCIAL AND BEHAVIORAL CONSIDERATIONS IN CANDIDATES FOR BARIATRIC SURGERY

12.3.1 MOTIVATIONS AND EXPECTATIONS

Given the comorbid medical problems associated with extreme obesity, improvement in overall health and longevity is likely the primary motivation for bariatric surgery for most people. Candidates for surgery should be internally motivated—seeking surgery for improvements in their health and well-being. Those who are externally motivated—interested in surgery for some secondary gain such as saving a troubled marriage—are not believed to be good candidates for surgery.

Persons with extreme obesity often have unrealistic expectations regarding the amount of weight they will lose with bariatric surgery. These unrealistic expectations were once thought to put individuals at risk for weight regain; recent evidence suggests that they may be unrelated to postoperative weight loss.[19] Nevertheless, individuals interested in bariatric surgery are encouraged to listen carefully to their surgeon regarding the amount of weight loss and improvements in their health that they can realistically expect after surgery.

12.3.2 BODY IMAGE, SELF-ESTEEM, AND QUALITY OF LIFE

Many people who present for surgery do so with the hope that the weight loss will improve their health, but also their physical appearance and body image. Individuals who are overweight or obese report greater body image dissatisfaction than average weight individuals, and those who lose weight, whether by behavioral modification, weight loss medications, or surgery, report improvements in their body image.[20]

Body image is an important aspect of self-esteem and quality of life for many individuals. Extreme obesity can dramatically impact self-esteem, such that it is difficult for persons to recognize and appreciate their other talents and abilities because of their struggles with their weight. Numerous studies have shown a relationship between excess body weight and impairments in both health and weight-related quality of life.[21–25] These impairments likely motivate many individuals to seek bariatric surgery. At the same time, obesity (and extreme obesity in particular) is associated with stigmatization if not outright discrimination in a number of settings, including educational, employment, and even health care.[26]

12.3.3 INTERPERSONAL AND ROMANTIC RELATIONSHIPS

Individuals may have expectations about the impact of bariatric surgery on their interpersonal relationships. Many people may intuitively think that as they lose weight, their social or romantic relationships will improve. This does occur for many individuals. However, for some, the experience of a major weight loss becomes an unsettling experience. Some individuals may experience unwanted attention related to their weight loss and physical appearance that may make them uncomfortable. For these reasons, men and women interested in bariatric surgery should consider the potential impact of their weight loss on their interpersonal and romantic relationships.[27]

12.3.4   FAMILY SUPPORT

The decision to undergo bariatric surgery can impact family relationships. During the preoperative mental health evaluation, patients are asked about living arrangements, their satisfaction with their spouse (partner) and other intimate relationships, and whether family members and friends support the decision to undertake surgery. Patients should identify relatives and friends who can assist in their care, both in the initial days after surgery and with the lifelong dietary and behavioral changes required of surgery. In rare cases, family members may be opposed to surgery or may try to sabotage the dietary and behavioral changes required of surgery.

12.3.5   WEIGHT AND DIETING HISTORY

The bariatric surgery candidate's weight and dieting history is typically reviewed by a registered dietitian prior to surgery. Many mental health professionals also review this information during the mental health evaluation, with the goal of identifying positive behaviors as well as maladaptive ones that may impact long-term postoperative outcomes.[1] Persons with extreme obesity typically have an earlier age of onset of obesity and stronger family history of the disorder than do persons with less severe obesity.[28] Such characteristics may well be associated with a greater genetic predisposition to obesity. Most candidates for bariatric surgery have had multiple attempts at a range of more conservative weight loss treatments.[29] A small minority of patients, however, have not participated in any organized weight loss programs prior to surgery. As a result, they do not have the fount of dietary knowledge seen in other patients and likely necessary for long-term success with bariatric surgery. With these patients, it is often useful to recommend some preoperative dietary counseling as well as attendance in preoperative support groups to help provide additional education.

12.3.6   EATING BEHAVIOR AND PHYSICAL ACTIVITY

Many mental health professionals also assess current eating behavior and physical activity levels. The purpose of this is to identify changes in eating and activity habits that will be required after surgery. Physical activity is briefly assessed to determine the patient's pattern of lifestyle and programmed activity and any physical conditions that limit mobility. Most bariatric surgery candidates report very low levels of activity[30]; strategies to enhance physical activity after bariatric surgery are among the great unmet needs in the field at the present time.

12.3.6.1   Timing for Surgery

The mental health professional, along with other members of the bariatric team, also assesses the timing of surgery in relation to other life events. Patients should undergo surgery at times that are relatively free of major life stressors, such as starting a new job, changing homes, or ending a romantic relationship. Ideally, the patient should have 3–4 weeks of time to undergo the operation, recover from it physically, and begin to adopt new lifestyle habits, the most important of which is adhering to the postoperative diet.

12.4   OUTCOMES FROM THE PREOPERATIVE MENTAL HEALTH EVALUATION

Several studies have found that approximately 70% of patients are uncondition-ally recommended for surgery by the mental health professional who evaluates them.[12,14,31–33] Other patients are recommended to undergo additional treatment (men-tal health or dietary) and are asked to return for further evaluation, typically in about 3 months. Most patients who follow these treatment recommendations ultimately undergo surgery. A patient's inability to follow these recommendations is likely a poor prognostic sign regarding the ability to make the lifestyle changes required by bariatric surgery. Nevertheless, the potential benefits of recommending a delay in surgery need to be balanced with two other issues. First, there is the risk that patients will not return for surgery and receive the care they likely need. Second, even a suboptimal outcome following bariatric surgery (e.g., a 20% weight loss rather than 35% weight loss following a RYGB procedure), and the health benefits that may be associated with it, may be far superior to what could be achieved with a nonsurgical weight loss treatment.

Many professionals who work in the area of bariatric surgery likely have wondered about the relationship between preoperative psychological status and postoperative outcomes. Several reviews over the past decade suggested that the early evidence was inconclusive.[2,34–37] Some studies identified a relationship between preopera-tive mental health issues and postoperative outcomes; others did not. Unfortunately, many of these studies suffered from a range of methodological problems that make it difficult to draw definitive conclusions from this literature.

A number of more recent studies that have used more rigorous psychometric meth-odologies seem to suggest a relationship between preoperative psychopathology and suboptimal postoperative outcomes. For example, patients with a lifetime diagnosis of any axis I clinical disorder, particularly mood or anxiety disorders, experienced smaller weight losses 6 months after RYGB than those who never had an axis I dis-order.[38] Bariatric surgery patients with two or more psychiatric diagnoses were found to be significantly more likely to experience weight loss cessation or weight regain after 1 year than those with zero or one diagnosis.[39] Several studies, but not all, also have suggested that the presence of binge eating is associated with either suboptimal weight losses or premature weight regain.[40–44] Thus, while the relationship between preoperative psychopathology and postoperative outcomes awaits further investiga-tion, the presence of significant, uncontrolled psychopathology—active substance abuse, psychosis, bulimia nervosa, severe depression—contraindicates surgery.[13] Given the evidence above, those patients with a history of psychiatric illness would likely benefit from close follow-up from the bariatric team after surgery.

12.5   POSTOPERATIVE PSYCHOSOCIAL AND EATING OUTCOMES

Bariatric surgery is, for most individuals, associated with significant improvements in psychosocial status. Most psychosocial characteristics—including symptoms of depression and anxiety, health-related quality of life, self-esteem, and body image—improve dramatically in the first year after surgery.[2,3,34,36,45–47] Many of these benefits appear to endure through the first four postoperative years. Longer-term psychosocial outcomes have not been well studied.

The impact of bariatric surgery on formal psychopathology, such as depression, is unclear. Psychosocial distress that is secondary to obesity—such as significant body image dissatisfaction or distress about weight-related limitations on functioning—may facilitate weight loss following surgery. In contrast, the presence of significant psychopathology that is independent of the degree of obesity—such as a long-standing history of major depression—may inhibit patients' ability to make the necessary dietary and behavioral changes to have the most successful postoperative outcome possible.[36]

Just as some patients experience medical complications, some also will experience poor behavioral or psychological outcomes. Some of the most commonly seen untoward outcomes are discussed below.

12.6   DEPRESSION AND SUICIDE

As noted above, studies have identified a relationship between depression and obesity. A number of studies also have found a higher than expected rate of suicide after bariatric surgery. For example, Adams and colleagues examined mortality and causes of death over a mean of 7 years in 7925 postoperative bariatric surgery patients and 7925 nonpatient controls who were matched for age, gender, and body mass index (BMI). All-cause mortality was significantly reduced in surgery patients compared to controls.[48] However, nearly twice as many surgery patients ($n = 43$) as controls ($n = 24$) died by suicide. Given the overall psychosocial benefits seen with bariatric surgery, these results are both surprising and concerning. These findings underscore the importance of the preoperative mental health evaluation as well as the need to ensure that patients with a psychiatric history receive appropriate mental health care after surgery.

12.7   SUBSTANCE ABUSE

A small number of studies have suggested that there is an increased risk of substance abuse—both alcohol and other drugs—following bariatric surgery.[49–51] For example, a large prospective study by King and colleagues found an increased rate of alcohol use disorders in patients who have undergone Roux-en-Y gastric bypass in the second postoperative year, compared to the year prior to surgery or in the first postoperative year.[52] The increased risk of alcohol use disorders was associated with male sex, younger age, and other lifestyle variables, such as smoking, regular alcohol consumption, and lack of social support.[52]

These findings hint at the potential for addiction transfer in persons who undergo bariatric surgery. *Addiction transfer* is a mass media-created term that refers to the idea that patients who undergo bariatric surgery may develop addictions to substances, gambling, sex, etc., to replace their preoperative "addiction" to food. Addiction transfer is not an accepted clinical or scientific term. The term and construct have several shortcomings, as detailed by Sogg.[53] Chief among these is that the view of food as an addictive substance, or eating as an addictive behavior, is not supported by scientific consensus. Additionally, there is little support for the notion that a treated symptom (e.g., compulsive eating) will resurface in a different form (e.g., compulsive drinking or shopping) unless the psychological basis for the original problem is resolved.

12.8   WEIGHT REGAIN/DIETARY NONADHERENCE

Between 20 and 30% of persons who undergo bariatric surgery fail to reach the typical postoperative weight loss or begin to regain weight within the first few postoperative years.[48,54] Suboptimal results are typically attributed to poor adherence to the postoperative diet or a return of maladaptive eating behaviors, rather than to surgical factors.[55] A number of studies have found that adherence to the postoperative diet is poor. Caloric intake often increases significantly during the postoperative period, which likely contributes to the weight regain.[56,57]

Adherence to the dietary and behavioral changes necessary for success after bariatric surgery likely requires ongoing care. Clinical reports have suggested that postoperative follow-up with the bariatric surgery program is frequently suboptimal and can negatively impact weight loss, in some cases within the first postoperative year.[55,58]

12.9   BODY IMAGE DISSATISFACTION

The massive weight loss seen with bariatric surgery is associated with significant improvements in body image.[20] Unfortunately, some patients who lose large amounts of weight report residual body image dissatisfaction associated with loose, sagging skin of the breasts, abdomen, thighs, and arms. This dissatisfaction likely motivates some individuals to seek plastic surgery to address these concerns.

According to the American Society of Plastic Surgeons, in 2013 approximately 50,000 patients underwent body contouring procedures after weight loss. The most common procedure was abdominoplasty, which is designed to eliminate the excessive skin around the abdomen and lower torso, which was performed on approximately 18,000 people. Breast lift (mastopexy) is also common and was performed on approximately 16,000 women.[59] There is a rapidly growing body of knowledge related to the surgical aspects of these procedures. Far less, however, is known about the psychological aspects of these procedures.

12.10   SEXUAL ABUSE, ROMANTIC RELATIONSHIPS, AND SEXUAL FUNCTIONING

There appears to be a modest association between sexual abuse and obesity.[60] Studies have suggested that between 16 and 32% of bariatric surgery candidates reported a history of sexual abuse, which is higher than most estimates from the general population.[61,62] Interestingly, several studies have suggested that a history of previous sexual abuse is unrelated to weight loss following bariatric surgery.[27] Nevertheless, patients with a history of sexual abuse often struggle with a range of psychological issues, including body image, sexual, and romantic relationship issues, following bariatric surgery. Some may experience distress that leads them to sabotage their weight loss efforts. These individuals would likely benefit from mental health treatment.

12.11   SUMMARY

Individuals who suffer from extreme obesity often do so with a wide range of unique behavioral and psychosocial issues. These issues represent a threat to the long-term success of bariatric surgery, in terms of both the size and durability of the weight loss and the adaptation of the postoperative lifestyle changes required of surgery. As a result, the preoperative mental health evaluation is widely considered to be a critical element of the preoperative evaluation of persons with extreme obesity interested in bariatric surgery. Encouragingly, persons who undergo bariatric surgery often experience significant improvements in a wide range of psychosocial and behavioral domains after surgery. At the same time, a sizable minority of patients experience psychosocial distress after surgery. This distress can threaten the long-term sustainability of the weight losses and health improvements seen in bariatric surgery. Interventions to address these issues are greatly needed to ensure the long-term success of bariatric surgery for patients as well as contribute to the further development of the medical specialty as a whole.

REFERENCES

1. Wadden T.A., Sarwer D.B. 2006. Behavioral assessment of candidates for bariatric surgery: a patient oriented approach. *Surgery for Obesity and Related Diseases* 2(2):171–79.
2. Sarwer D.B., Wadden T.A., Fabricatore A.N. 2005. Psychosocial and behavioral aspects of bariatric surgery. *Obesity Research* 14: 479–88.
3. Mitchell J.E., de Zwaan M. 2005. *Bariatric surgery: a guide for mental health professionals.* New York: Routledge.
4. Sogg S., Mori D.L. 2004. The Boston interview for gastric bypass: determining the psychological suitability of surgical candidates. *Obesity Surgery* 14(3):370–80.
5. Heinberg L.J., Ashton K., Windover A. 2010. Moving beyond dichotomous psychological evaluation: the Cleveland Clinic Behavioral Rating System for weight loss surgery. *Surgery for Obesity and Related Diseases* 6(2):185–90.
6. Kalarchian M.A., Marcus M.D., Levine M.D., Courcoulas A.P., Pilkonis P.A., Ringham R.M., et al. 2007. Psychiatric disorders among bariatric surgery candidates: relationship to obesity and functional health status. *American Journal of Psychiatry* 164:328–34.
7. Onyike C.U., Crum R.M., Lee H.B., Lyketsos C.G., Eaton W.W. 2003. Is obesity associated with major depression? Results from the Third National Health and Nutrition Examination Survey. *American Journal of Epidemiology* 158(12):1139–47.
8. Petry N.M., Barry D., Pietrzak R.H., Wagner J.A. 2008. Overweight and obesity are associated with psychiatric disorders: results from the National Epidemiologic Survey on Alcohol and Related Conditions. *Psychosomatic Medicine* 70(3):288–97.

9. Carpenter K.M., Hasin D.S., Allison D.B., Faith M.S. 2000. Relationships between obesity and DSM-IV major depressive disorder, suicide ideation, and suicide attempts: results from a general population study. *American Journal of Public Health* 90:251–57.

10. American Psychiatric Association. 2013. *Diagnostic and statistical manual of mental disorders.* 5th edition. Washington, DC: APA Press.

11. Allison K.C., Wadden T.A., Sarwer D.B., Fabricatore A.N., Crerand C.E., et al. 2006. Night eating syndrome and binge eating disorder among persons seeking bariatric surgery: prevalence and related features. *Surgery for Obesity and Related Diseases* 2(2):153–58.

12. Sarwer D.B., Cohn N.I., Gibbons L.M., Magee L., Crerand C.E., Raper S.E., et al. 2004. Psychiatric diagnoses and psychiatric treatment among bariatric surgery candidates. *Obesity Surgery* 14(9):1148–56.

13. Mechanick J.I., Youdim A., Jones D.B., Garvey W.T., Hurley D.L., McMahon M.M., et al. 2013. Clinical practice guidelines for the perioperative nutritional, metabolic, and nonsurgical support of the bariatric surgery patient—2013 update: cosponsored by American Association of Clinical Endocrinologists, The Obesity Society, and American Society for Metabolic and Bariatric Surgery. *Obesity (Silver Spring)* 21(Suppl 1):S1–27.

14. Friedman K.E., Applegate K.L., Grant J. 2007. Who is adherent with preoperative psychological treatment recommendations among weight loss surgery candidates? *Surgery for Obesity and Related Diseases* 3:376–82.

15. Larsen J.K., Greenen R., van Ramshorst B., Brand N., de Wit P., Stroebe W., et al. 2003. Psychosocial functioning before and after laparoscopic adjustable gastric banding: a cross-sectional study. *Obesity Surgery* 13(4):629–36.

16. Clark M.M., Balsiger B.M., Sletten C.D., Dahlman K.L., Ames G., Williams D.E., et al. 2003. Psychosocial factors and 2-year outcome following bariatric surgery for weight loss. *Obesity Surgery* 13(5):739–45.

17. Sarwer D.B., Faulconbridge L.F., Steffen K.J., Roerig J.L., Mitchell J.E. 2010. Managing patients after surgery: changes in drug prescription, body weight can affect psychotropic prescribing. *Current Psychiatry* 10(1):3–9.

18. Seaman J.S., Bowers S.P., Dixon P., Schindler L. 2005. Dissolution of common psychiatric medications in a Roux-en-Y gastric bypass model. *Psychosomatics* 46(3):250–53.

19. Casazza K., Fontaine K.R., Astrup A., Birch L.L., Brown A.W., Bohan Brown M.M., et al. 2013 Myths, presumptions, and facts about obesity. *New England Journal of Medicine* 368(5):446–54.

20. Sarwer D.B., Dilks R.J., Spitzer J.C. 2011. Weight loss and changes in body image. In Cash T.F., Smolak L., eds., *Body image: a handbook of science, practice and prevention* (pp. 369–377). New York: Guilford Press.

21. Schok M., Greenen R., van Antwerpen T., de Wit P., Brand N., van Ramshorst B. 2000. Quality of life after laparoscopic adjustable gastric banding for severe obesity: postoperative and retrospective preoperative evaluations. *Obesity Surgery* 10:502f–8f.

22. Kolotkin R.L., Crosby R.D., Pendleton R., Strong M., Gress R.E., Adams T. 2003. Health-related quality of life in patients seeking gastric bypass surgery vs nontreatment-seeking controls. *Obesity Surgery* 13(3):371–77.

23. Kolotkin R.L., Crosby R.D., Gress R.E., Hunt S.C., Engel S.G., Adams T.D. 2008. Health and health related quality of life: differences between men and women who seek gastric bypass surgery. *Surgery for Obesity and Related Diseases* 4:651–58.

24. Fontaine K.R., Cheskin L.J., Barofsky I. 1996. Health-related quality of life in obese persons seeking treatment. *Journal of Family Practice* 43:265 -70.

25. Heo M., Allison D.B., Faith M.S., Zhu S., Fontaine K.R. 2003. Obesity and quality of life: mediating effects of pain and comorbidities. *Obesity Research* 11:209–16.

26. Depierre J.A., Puhl R.M. 2012. Experiences of weight stigmatization: a review of self-report assessment measures. *Obesity Facts* 5(6):897–918.

27. Sarwer D.B., Lavery M., Spitzer J.C. 2012. A review of the relationships between extreme obesity, quality of life, and sexual function. *Obesity Surgery* 22(4):668–76.
28. Crerand C.E., Wadden T.A., Sarwer D.B., Fabricatore A.N., Kuehnel R.H., Gibbons L.M., et al. 2006. A comparison of weight histories in women with class III vs. class I-II obesity. *Surgery for Obesity and Related Diseases* 2(2):165–70.
29. Gibbons L.M., Sarwer D.B., Crerand C.E., Fabricatore A.N., Kuehnel R.H., Lipschutz P.E., et al. 2006. Previous weight loss experiences of bariatric surgery candidates: how much have patients dieted prior to surgery? *Obesity* 14(S3):70S–76S.
30. Bond D.S., Jakicic J.M., Vithiananthan S., Thomas J.G., Leahey T.M., Sax H.C., et al. 2010. Objective quantification of physical activity in bariatric surgery candidates and normal-weight controls. *Surgery for Obesity and Related Diseases* 6(1):72–78.
31. Fabricatore A.N., Crerand C.E., Wadden T.A., Sarwer D.B., Krasucki J.L. 2006. How do mental health professionals evaluate candidates for bariatric surgery? Survey results. *Obesity Surgery* 16:567–73.
32. Pawlow L.A., O'Neil P.M., White M.A., Byrne T.K. 2005. Findings and outcomes of psychological evaluations of gastric bypass applicants. *Surgery for Obesity and Related Diseases* 1:523–27.
33. Zimmerman M., Francione-Witt C., Chelminski I., Young D., Boerescu D., Attiullah N., et al. 2007. Presurgical psychiatric evaluations of candidates for bariatric surgery. Part 1. Reliability and reasons for and frequency of exclusion. *Journal of Clinical Psychiatry* 68:1557–62.
34. Bocchieri L.E., Meana M., Fisher B.L. 2002. A review of psychosocial outcomes of surgery for morbid obesity. *Journal of Psychosomatic Research* 52:155–65.
35. Greenberg I., Perna F., Kaplan M., Sullivan M.A. 2005. Behavioral and psychological factors in the assessment and treatment of obesity surgery patients. *Obesity Research* 13(2):244–49.
36. Herpertz S., Kielmann R., Wolfe A.M., Hebebrand J., Senf W. 2004. Do psychosocial variables predict weight loss or mental health after obesity surgery? A systematic review. *Obesity Research* 12:1554–69.
37. van Hout G.C., Verschure S.K., van Heck G.L. 2005. Psychosocial predictors of success following bariatric surgery. *Obesity Research* 15:552–60.
38. Kalarchian M.A., Marcus M.D., Levine M.D., Soulakova J.N., Courcoulas A.P., Wisinski M.S. 2008. Relationship of psychiatric disorders to 6-month outcomes after gastric bypass. *Surgery for Obesity and Related Diseases* 4:544–49.
39. Rutledge T., Groesz L.M., Savu M. 2011. Psychiatric factors and weight loss patterns following gastric bypass surgery in a veteran population. *Obesity Surgery* 21(1):29–35.
40. Kinzl J.F., Schrattenecker M., Traweger C., Mattesich M., Fiala M., Biebl W. 2006. Psychosocial predictors of weight loss after bariatric surgery. *Obesity Surgery* 16:1609–14.
41. Alger-Mayer S., Rosati C., Polimeni J.M., Malone M. 2009. Preoperative binge eating statis and gastric bypass surgery: a long-term outcome study. *Obesity Surgery* 19:139–45.
42. White M.A., Kalarchian M.A., Masheb R.M., Marcus M.D., Grilo C.M. 2010. Loss of control over eating predicts outcome in bariatric surgery patients: a prospective 24-month follow-up study. *Journal of Clinical Psychiatry* 71:175–84.
43. de Zwaan M., Hilbert A., Swan-Kremeier L., Simonich H., Lancaster K., Howell L.M., et al. 2010. Comprehensive interview assessment of eating behavior 18–35 months after gastric bypass surgery for morbid obesity. *Surgery for Obesity and Related Diseases* 6:79–87.
44. Livhits M., Mercado C., Yermilov I., Parikh J.A., Dutson E., Mehran A., et al. 2012. Preoperative predictors of weight loss following bariatric surgery: systematic review. *Obesity Surgery* 22:70–89.

45. Herpertz S., Kielmann R., Wolf A.M., Langkafel M., Senf W., Hebebrand J. 2003. Does obesity surgery improve psychosocial functioning? A systematic review. *International Journal of Obesity and Related Metabolic Disorders* 27:1300–14.
46. van Hout G.C., Leibbrandt A.J., Jakimowicz J.J., Smulders J.F., Schoon E.J. 2003. Bariatric surgery and bariatric psychology: general overview and the Dutch approach. *Obesity Surgery* 13(6):926–31.
47. van Hout G.C., Boekestein P., Fortuin, F A., Pelle A.J., van Heck G.L. 2006. Psychosocial functioning following bariatric surgery. *Obesity Surgery* 16:787–94.
48. Adams T., Gress R., Smith S., Halverson R.C., Simper S.C., Rosamond W.D., et al. 2007. Long-term mortality following gastric bypass surgery. *New England Journal of Medicine* 357:753–61.
49. Mitchell J.E., Lancaster K.L., Burgard M.A., Howell L.M., Krahn D.D,. Crosby R.D., et al. 2001. Long-term follow-up of patients' status after gastric bypass. *Obesity Surgery* 11:464–78.
50. Suzuki J., Haimovici F., Chang G. 2012. Alcohol use disorders after bariatric surgery. *Obesity Surgery* 22(2):201–7.
51. Ertelt T.W., Mitchell J.E., Lancaster K., Crosby R.D., Steffen K.J., Marino J.M. 2008. Alcohol abuse and dependence before and after bariatric surgery: a review of the literature and report of a new data set. *Surgery for Obesity and Related Diseases* 4(5):647–50.
52. King W.C., Chen J.Y., Mitchell J.E., Kalarchian M.A., Steffen K.J., Engel S.G., et al. 2012. Prevalence of alcohol use disorders before and after bariatric surgery. *Journal of the American Medical Association* 307(23):2516–25.
53. Sogg S. 2007. Alcohol misuse after bariatric surgery: epiphenomenon or "Oprah" phenomenon? *Surgery for Obesity and Related Diseases* 3:366–68.
54. Sjöström L., Lindroos A.K., Peltonen M., Torgerson J., Bouchard C., Carlsson B., et al. 2004. Swedish Obese Subjects study scientific group. Lifestyle, diabetes, and cardiovascular risk factors 10 years after bariatric surgery. *New England Journal of Medicine* 351(26):2683–93.
55. Sarwer D.B., Dilks R.J., West-Smith L. 2011. Dietary intake and eating behavior after bariatric surgery: threats to weight loss maintenance and strategies for success. *Surgery for Obesity and Related Diseases* 7(5):644–51.
56. Faria S.L., de Oliveira Kelly E., Faria O.P., Ito M.K. 2008. Snack-eating patients experience lesser weight loss after Roux-en-Y gastric bypass surgery. *Obesity Surgery* 19:1293–96.
57. Sarwer D.B., Wadden T.A., Moore R.H., Baker A.W., Gibbons L.M., Raper S.E., et al. 2008. Preoperative eating behavior, postoperative dietary adherence and weight loss following gastric bypass surgery. *Surgery for Obesity Related Diseases* 5:640–46.
58. Madan A.K., Tichansky D.S. 2005. Patients postoperatively forget aspects of preoperative patient education. *Obesity Surgery* 15:1066–106.
59. American Society of Plastic Surgeons. 2014. *Report of the 2013 National Clearinghouse of Plastic Surgery statistics.* Arlington Heights, IL.
60. Gustafson T.B., Sarwer D.B. 2004. Childhood sexual abuse and obesity. *Obesity Review* 5:129–35.
61. Grilo C.M., Masheb R.M., Brody M., Toth C., Burke-Martindale C.H., Rothschild B.S. 2005. Childhood maltreatment in extremely obese male and female bariatric surgery candidates. *Obesity Research* 13:123–30.
62. Gustafson T.B., Gibbons L.M., Sarwer D.B., Crerand C.E., Fabricatore A.N., Wadden T.A., et al. 2006. History of sexual abuse among bariatric surgery candidates. *Surgery for Obesity and Related Diseases* 2:369–74.

13 Nutrition and Body Contouring Procedures

Siamak Agha-Mohammadi

CONTENTS

13.1 SUMMARY

With advances in post-bariatric plastic surgery, more and more patients are requesting body contouring surgery to reshape their body, especially after extensive weight loss. These patients may need multiple surgical procedures to correct forearms, breasts, torso, back, and thigh laxity, with extensive incisions and undermining. However, often, optimal healing in this patient population is hampered by existing nutritional deficiencies that directly impact their wound healing process and immune response competency. Many of these deficiencies are well established and may have detrimental effects on the healing, even at subclinical levels. It is essential that health care providers who treat post-bariatric patients are aware of these nutritional deficiencies, which can be prevented by adhering to eating guidelines and supplemental prescriptions.

13.2   INTRODUCTION

According to the latest data from the World Health Organization, 1.5 billion adults over 20 years of age are overweight, including 200 million men and 300 million women who are clinically obese.[1] Overweight and obesity prevalence have increased steadily among all U.S. population groups over the past 30 years.[2,3] If these trends continue, 86.3% of adults will be overweight or obese, and 51.1% obese by 2030.[4]

Of all the available methods, weight loss or bariatric surgery has been shown to be an effective approach to the treatment of obesity by providing sustained weight loss, resolution of obesity-related comorbidities,[5,6] improved quality of life[7] and psychological conditions,[8,9] and reductions in disease risk factors[10] and mortality.[11] Thus, the number of weight loss surgeries has risen each year by a factor of 5 from 1996 to 2003.[12] The bariatric techniques employed can be divided into three categories. Restrictive procedures reduce the size of the stomach so that satiety is reached with small food portions. Malabsorptive procedures change the anatomy of the stomach and intestines to reduce absorptive capacity. Combination procedures utilize aspects of both restrictive and malabsorptive procedures.[13] In the United States, the two most commonly performed bariatric surgeries are laparoscopic adjustable gastric banding (LAGB) and Roux-en-Y gastric bypass (RYGBP). LAGB is a restrictive procedure, in which a small gastric pouch is created, resulting in early and prolonged satiety. Since the normal absorptive surface is preserved, specific nutrient deficiencies are rare. The RYGBP procedure involves both restrictive and malabsorptive components. The stomach size is decreased to about 30 ml proximal gastric pouch with a 75 to 150 cm Roux limb connected as an enteroenterostomy to the jejunum, 30 to 50 cm from the ligament of Trietz.[14] This combined restrictive-malabsorptive procedure results in greater risk nutrient deficiency postoperatively.

Less popular procedures such as biliopancreatic diversion (BPD) and BPD with duodenal switch (BPD-DS) result in more severe malabsorption and carry a higher risk of nutritional deficiencies.[14] The sleeve gastrectomy is growing in popularity as a primary procedure; however, there are not yet sufficient data to implicate nutritional deficiencies.

Depending on the procedure employed, patients typically lose about 25 to 40% of their initial weight at 12 to 18 months, and maintain the majority of the lost weight for many years to come.[15] The success of gastric bypass surgeries has led to an increasing population of post-bariatric patients with sagging skin who need body contouring surgery for both aesthetic and functional goals. According to the American Society of Plastic Surgeons, more than 45,000 body contouring procedures were performed on weight loss patients in 2012.[16]

A disturbing feature of these complex body contouring operations is the high rate of complications reported in post-bariatric patients. Multiple studies have shown complication rates of 20 to 75% in post-bariatric body contouring patients.[17–21] Specifically, wound-related complications occur more frequently in this patient population. Recently, Greco et al. reported a 41% rate of wound-related complications in weight loss patients relative to 22% of non-bariatric patients. Furthermore, compared to non-weight loss patients, post-bariatric patients had an increase in all categories of wound complications: healing disturbance 11%, wound infection 12%, hematoma 6%, and seroma 14%.[21] On the other hand, Kitzinger et al. reported 60%

rate of wound dehiscence, 34% seroma, 8% infection, and 8% hematoma in their lower-body lift patients.[22] A number of factors may be responsible for this higher rate of complication in post-bariatric patients. These include the following:

1. Post-bariatric patients often require multiple procedures that are often combined in two or more stages. With more extensive operations and longer incisions, typically a larger surface area of tissue is removed. Neaman and Hansen have shown increased complications when a larger volume of tissue is removed during body contouring surgery.[23]
2. Body mass indices (BMIs) of over 25 have been shown to be correlated with a three times increase in postoperative complications.[24]
3. Both max BMI and change in BMI have been shown to be strong predictors of postoperative complications.[25]
4. The majority of bariatric patients in the United States have a malabsorptive procedure and may be macronutrient and micronutrient deficient.[26] Many of these deficient nutrients are essential for efficient wound healing.

The aim of this chapter is to highlight the nutritional deficiencies of the weight loss surgery patients as they may relate to their subsequent planned plastic surgery procedures.

13.3   BODY CONTOURING AND PLASTIC SURGERY AFTER MASSIVE WEIGHT LOSS

The success of bariatric surgery has generated a large population of post-bariatric patients who desire plastic surgery for aesthetic or functional concerns. With the increasing demand and cases, we have gained a greater understanding of the dysmorphic anatomical changes of the massive weight loss patient. The nature of the anatomical changes that a patient may experience is determined by the patient's gender, age, prebariatric weight, actual weight loss, and genetic predisposition. The typical weight loss patient experiences significant changes in the form, shape, and contour of his or her face, arms, axilla, upper chest, breasts, back, buttocks, abdomen, thighs, and even calves. Many of these changes follow a predictable course. The aim of body contouring surgery is correction of the lost shape and form. These often require multiple procedures, such as a brachioplasty, upper-body lift, breast reshaping and lift, lower-body lift, and thigh reduction and lift (Figure 13.1).

13.4   NUTRITIONAL RISKS OF THE POST-BARIATRIC PATIENT

There are six primary causes of nutritional deficiency in a bariatric patient:

1. It is now well established that many overweight and obese children and adults suffer from micronutrient deficiencies. These include deficiency of vitamin A, vitamin C, vitamin D, thiamine, folate, vitamin B_{12}, iron, zinc, selenium, and ferritin (Table 13.1).[27] The higher prevalence of nutrient deficiency in overweight, obese, and morbidly obese patients, compared to

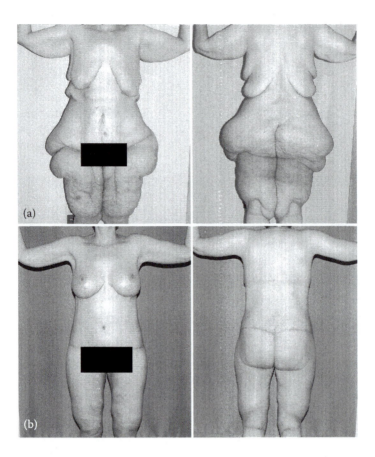

FIGURE 13.1 Fifty-year-old female who had a biliary diversion procedure and lost over 260 lb of weight. The patient presented for plastic surgery after weight loss at a weight of 230 lb. The patient underwent multiple surgeries, including a lower-body lift, vertical thigh plasty, thigh lift, upper-body lift, buttock augmentation with autologous tissue, breast augmentation and lift, and liposuction. Postoperative pictures were taken at 3 months after her last surgical stage.

normal weight patients, may be due to the poor nutritional value of their diets. Obese and morbidly obese patients, based on their economic status, may consume diets of lower quality that may not meet their entire nutritional needs. Moreover, the absorption, distribution, metabolism, and excretion of these micronutrients in overweight and obese individuals might be altered.[28]

2. All forms of weight loss surgery restrict caloric intake, and thereby restrict nutrient intake. The energy and protein intake for the first postoperative month is oftentimes suboptimal, but steadily increases throughout the first postop year. At 1 year, the average energy intake is approximately 1,000 kcal/day, and protein intake averages 60 to 80 g/day.[29] Dias et al. have shown that the daily energy intakes at 3, 6, 9, and 12 months were 529,

TABLE 13.1

Abnormal and Deficient Nutritional Levels in Preoperative Obese and Postoperative Bariatric Patients

Nutrient	Obese Patients Deficiency (%)	Post-Bariatric Patients Deficiency (%)
Protein	N/A	0–25%
Vitamin B$_{12}$	5%	0–37%
Folate	2%	9–35%
		11%
Thiamine	15.5–29%	18.3% (1 year postop)[a]
		11.2% (2 years postop)[a]
Vitamin A	7%	11% (1 year postop)[a]
		8.3% (2 years postop)[a]
		61–69%[b]
Vitamin B$_2$		13.6% (1 year postop)[a]
		7.1% (2 years postop)[a]
Vitamin B$_6$		17.6% (1 year postop)[a]
		14.2% (2 years postop)[a]
Vitamin E		22%[a]
Vitamin K		68%[b]
Vitamin C		34.6% (1 year postop)[a]
		35.4% (2 years postop)[a]
25(OH)D	40%	19%
Iron	14%	0–100%
Ferritin	6%	16%
Zinc	28%	36%
Selenium	58%	3%

[a] RYGBP patients.
[b] BPD and BPD-DS.

710, 833, and 866 kcal/day, respectively. Protein intake was increased in the same proportion at 6, 9, and 12 months as well.[30]

3. Intolerance of certain food after surgery, such as meat and dairy intolerance, or carbohydrate restriction.

4. Deficiency from malabsorption and maldigestion. Procedures that have a malabsorptive component such as RYGBP and the bileopancreatic diversion with duodenal switch may produce more extensive nutritional problems since surgical changes in digestive physiology interfere with normal nutrient digestion and absorption. Even purely restrictive procedures such as LAGB and sleeve gastrectomy increase the risk for nutrient deficiency. Nutritional deficiencies reported in LAGB include deficiencies of folate, vitamin B$_{12}$, thiamine, iron, and bone loss (Table 13.2).[31]

TABLE 13.2
Nutritional Deficiencies Associated with Bariatric Surgery

Deficiency	VBG	RYGBP	BDP
Severe malnutrition	Rare	Less common	Common
Fat malabsorption	None	Less common	Common
Vitamin B$_{12}$	None	Common	Common
Folate	None	Less common	Common
Thiamine	Rare	Common	Common
Vitamins A, K, E	None	Less common	Common
Iron	Rare	Common	Common
Zinc	Rare	Common	Common
Calcium	Rare	Less common	Common

5. Patients' compliance makes a significant contribution to postoperative nutritional status in bariatric surgery patients. Despite emphasis and recommendations, only 60% of patients take their multivitamins after RYGBP,[32] and intake of most vitamins and minerals is below 50% of the recommended daily average.[33]

Thus, it is not surprising many macronutrient and micronutrient deficiencies have been noted with the various weight loss surgeries.[34,35] The following sections will concentrate on those deficiencies that are implicated in wound healing.

13.5   NUTRITIONAL DEFICIENCY OF THE BARIATRIC PATIENT

13.5.1   MACRONUTRIENT DEFICIENCIES

13.5.1.1   Fat Deficiency

Fat malabsorption reduces calorie intake and, in part, may facilitate weight loss in bariatric patients. Fat malabsorption, evidenced by steatorrhea, is not seen with LAGB or sleeve gastrectomy, and is rare in RYGBP, but not uncommon with BPD.

Although, the role of fat in wound healing is not completely understood, fat malabsorption may impact wound healing both directly and indirectly. Indirectly, as a source of calories other than glucose and protein, fat malabsorption may theoretically expedite protein catabolism in the stressed or wounded state. Directly, lipids are responsible for the primary structure of all cell membranes, and deficiencies of essential fatty acids impair wound healing in both humans and animals.[36]

13.5.1.2   Protein Deficiency

Red meat, dairy, and other high-quality protein sources are often poorly tolerated in the immediate postoperative period after bariatric surgery. If the patient does not consume enough alternative protein sources, protein deficiency can develop for months after surgery (Table 13.1). All stages of wound healing require protein. Protein is necessary for the synthesis of enzymes involved in wound healing, proliferation of cells and collagen, and formation of connective tissue. Protein depletion results in decreased skin and fascial wound breaking strength, impaired fibroblast proliferation, angiogenesis, collagen production, and increased wound infection rates. Furthermore, protein deficiency is closely associated with immunosuppression, decreased T-cell function, phagocytic activity, complement and antibody levels, and ultimately diminished immune response against infection.[35]

Protein deficiency is clearly associated with amino acid deficiency. Arginine and glutamine are two amino acids that have been extensively studied for their role in wound healing. Arginine is a semiessential amino acid that acts as a substrate for protein synthesis, collagen deposition, and cellular growth. At times of stress or injury, arginine synthesis is insufficient to meet the demands of increased protein turnover. At pharmacological levels (17 to 24.8 g of free arginine per day), arginine enhances wound tensile strength in acute wounds by increasing the amount of hydroxyproline and total protein deposition at the wound site. Furthermore, arginine has been shown to increase nitric oxide production and enhance immune function. Nitric oxide is a powerful vasodilator, an autocrine stimulator of fibroblast contractile and collagen synthesis, and a mediator of macrophage-induced bacterial killing. Another role of arginine in wound healing relates to stimulation of the T-cell, which is essential for normal wound healing.[35]

Another amino acid of importance is glutamine. Glutamine plays a significant role in wound healing as a major respiratory fuel source in gluconeogenesis, and serves as a nitrogen donor for the synthesis of amino acids and a precursor for the synthesis of nucleotides in proliferating cells. Glutamine is also involved in immune function via lymphocyte proliferation, and is important in stimulating the inflammatory response during the inflammatory phase of wound healing. Glutamine levels fall rapidly after an injury, and supplementation has been shown to improve nitrogen balance and enhance immune function after major surgery, trauma, and sepsis.[35]

Other amino acids may influence wound healing. Methionine stimulates fibroblast proliferation and collagen synthesis. Cysteine functions as a cofactor for enzyme processes in the formation of collagen. Lysine and proline are other amino acids that contribute to wound healing as precursors of collagen.

The Recommended Dietary Allowance (RDA) for protein in healthy adults is 0.8 g/kg body weight. In the context of weight loss surgery patients, previous studies have indicated a minimum of 60 to 70 g of protein per day is needed to avert any protein deficiency. However, for the purpose of surgical wounds, 1.25 to 2.1 ± 0.9 g protein/kg is needed for optimal healing (Table 13.3).[35]

13.5.2 MICRONUTRIENT DEFICIENCIES

The reduction in the small intestine's absorptive capacity can lead to specific vitamins, minerals, trace metals, and electrolytes deficiencies after malabsorptive procedures (Table 13.1).

TABLE 13.3

Pharmacological Doses of Vitamins and Minerals Recommended for Optimal Healing

Ingredient	Dose per Day
Protein	120–150 g
Folate	400 µg
Vitamin B$_{12}$	500–600 µg
Vitamin C	2 g
Vitamin A	25,000 IU
Vitamin B$_2$	6–30 mg
Iron	100–200 mg
Zinc	40 mg
Selenium	100 µg

13.5.2.1 Vitamin Deficiency

Most vitamins are coenzymes or cofactors involved in the metabolism of carbohydrate, fat, and protein. Others function in oxidation-reduction reactions, as antioxidants or as hormones. Since the small intestine remains intact in restrictive procedures, micronutrient deficiencies are rare among commonly noted malabsorptive procedures.

13.5.2.1.1 Vitamin B$_{12}$ and Folate

Vitamin B$_{12}$ (cobalamin) deficiency and folate deficiency are fairly prevalent after bariatric operations as early as 6 months after surgery. The risk for vitamin B$_{12}$ and folate deficiencies is highest in RYGBP patients, although other malabsorptive procedures can also increase the risk.

Folate is a generic term for the water-soluble B-complex vitamin that exists in many different forms. It is an essential cofactor in metabolic pathways, especially amino acid conversion and DNA synthesis, and is necessary for erythrocyte formation and growth. Vitamin B$_{12}$ also plays an important role in DNA synthesis and neurologic function.[35]

Most RYGBP patients with Vitamin B$_{12}$ or folate deficiency are asymptomatic or suffer from subclinical disease. Over time, a deficiency in either vitamin B$_{12}$ or folate can lead to macrocytic anemia, a condition characterized by the production of fewer, but larger, red blood cells and a decreased ability to carry oxygen. Those with severe deficiency present with megaloblastosis. Megaloblastosis is a generalized disorder since it also affects nonhematopoietic cells, such as gastrointestinal and uterine cervical mucosal cells, which have megaloblastic features. A common basis for megaloblastosis is impaired DNA and protein synthesis. Thus, deficiencies of these vitamins can potentially contribute to poor cellular proliferation and repair in the post-bariatric patient. Furthermore, the associated megaloblastic anemia will adversely affect circulation in the healing tissues. Given the fact that body contouring patients can lose a significant amount of blood during multiple procedures, it is essential that erythropoesis is not hampered by inadequate vitamin B$_{12}$/folate reserves.[35]

The majority of RYGBP patients cannot maintain normal vitamin B$_{12}$ levels with an oral diet alone, and will require supplementation. Supplementation for postsurgical patients ranges from 500 to 600 μg/day in an oral form, or 100 μg monthly via intramuscular injection. Folate deficiency can be prevented by ingestion of 400 μg of folate per day after RYGBP surgery (Table 13.3).[35]

13.5.2.1.2 Vitamin C

Vitamin C (ascorbic acid) deficiency has been recently reported in RYGBP patients up to 24 months after the surgery. Vitamin C is required for wound healing by increasing collagen synthesis and angiogenesis, and fibroblast proliferation. It also enhances neutrophil function and complement activity. While deficiency is asymptomatic in post-bariatric patients, vitamin C levels decrease with stress and injury since humans lack long-term storage. This observation is obviously of concern in post-bariatric patients seeking body contouring surgery. Vitamin C deficiency is associated with capillaries leakage due to decreased collagen production and susceptibility to wound infections.[35]

Vitamin C supplementation would be of benefit in post-bariatric patients who are about to undergo body contouring procedures. For optimal healing, supplementation of 1,000 to 2,000 mg/day orally has been suggested in major burn victims (Table 13.3).[35]

13.5.2.1.3 Vitamin B$_1$ (Thiamine)

Although thiamine stores can usually last 3 to 6 weeks, deficiency can set in after an unbalanced intake of carbohydrate in post-bariatric patients. Thus, a continuous supply of thiamine is necessary on a regular basis in gastric bypass patients. In uncomplicated post-bariatric patients, thiamine deficiency is likely to be subclinical, as clinical manifestations (weakness, peripheral neuropathy, etc.) are very rare.[51] Thiamine plays an essential role in the metabolism of carbohydrates and branched-chain amino acids and thus may be involved in the healing process.

13.5.2.1.4 Vitamin B$_2$ (Riboflavin) Deficiency

Riboflavin is not stored in ample amounts, and thus a constant supply is needed. In RYGBP patients, deficiency of this vitamin is usually part of a multiple-nutrient deficiency (Table 13.1). Riboflavin is important for energy production, enzyme function, and normal fatty acid and amino acid synthesis and is necessary for the reproduction of glutathione, a free radical scavenger. A deficiency should be treated by 6 to 30 mg of riboflavin daily (Table 13.3).[35]

13.5.2.1.5 Vitamin B$_6$ (Pyridoxine)

Vitamin B$_6$ deficiency has been reported in RYGBP patients up to 24 months after surgery. Vitamin B$_6$ is an essential cofactor in DNA synthesis and various transamination, decarboxylation, and synthesis pathways involving carbohydrate, sphingolipid, sulfur-containing amino acids, heme, and neurotransmitter metabolism. Although the role of vitamin B$_6$ in wound healing is not clearly defined, supplementation is advisable in deficient patients. Recommendation for treatment of deficiency is variable and depends on the clinical presentation.[35]

13.5.2.1.6   Vitamin A

Vitamin A deficiency is noted in both RYGBP and BPD patients (Table 13.1). Vitamin A is necessary for night vision and also influences the healing process. While the clinical consequences of vitamin A deficiency are few, continued deficiency will adversely impact the healing process of the post-bariatric body contouring patient. Vitamin A plays an important role in wound healing during the inflammatory phase through enhanced lysosomal membrane lability. It enhances wound healing by stimulating epithelization and increasing collagen deposition by fibroblasts. Furthermore, vitamin A is an essential factor in the healing patient since it functions as an immunostimulant by increasing the number of monocytes and macrophages in the wound and by stabilizing the intracellular lysosomes of the white blood cells.[35]

To enhance wound healing, documented recommendations include a vitamin A supplementation at 10,000 to 50,000 IU/day orally or 10,000 IU intramuscularly for 10 days (Table 13.3).[35]

13.5.2.1.7   Vitamin K

Vitamin K is a group of structurally similar, fat-soluble vitamins that the human body needs for posttranslational modification of certain proteins required for blood coagulation, and in metabolic pathways in bone and other tissue. Although deficiency of vitamin K is noted in BPD and BPD-DS procedures (Table 13.1), its implications in post-bariatric patients are unknown.[35] Certainly in terms of clinical manifestation, no incidence of increased bleeding has been reported in body contouring patients.

13.5.2.1.8   Vitamin E

Vitamin E, or tocopherol, refers to a group of eight fat-soluble compounds that act as an antioxidant. Vitamin E deficiency is clinically uncommon in most post-bariatric patients who receive supplementation. Vitamin E has many biological functions, the antioxidant function being the most important or best known. The function of this vitamin group in wound healing is largely unknown, but excess supplementation can inhibit collagen synthesis, and decreases the tensile strength of wounds.[35]

13.5.2.2   Mineral Deficiencies

13.5.2.2.1   Iron

There is a significant risk of persistent iron deficiency with all types of bariatric surgery (Table 13.1). Iron deficiency is associated with both restrictive and malabsorptive procedures. In terms of optimal wound healing, iron plays an important role in oxygen transport and collagen production. Iron is required for the hydroxylation of specific prolyl and lysyl residues in collagen, and severe iron deficiency can impair collagen production. Iron deficiency presents with microcytic anemia, generalized fatigue, and weakness. This can be further compounded by the blood loss of multiple body contouring procedures. Also, anemia-related fatigue and weakness can exacerbate immobilization of the postoperative patient, which can increase the risk of coagulopathy. Treatment is usually accomplished with single daily doses of 100 to 200 mg of elemental iron per day (Table 13.3).[35]

13.5.2.2.2 Zinc

Zinc deficiency is noted in a significant percentage of post-bariatric patients (Table 13.1). Zinc is an essential trace mineral that is required for cellular growth and replication. Zinc is needed in multiple aspects of wound healing. It is important in DNA synthesis, protein synthesis, synthesis of structural proteins such as collagen, function of several hundred zinc metalloproteinases and zinc finger proteins, and normal insulin-like growth factor (IGF-1) production. Therefore, zinc deficiency can result in decreased fibroblast proliferation and collagen synthesis, leading to decreased wound strength and delayed epithelization.[35]

Zinc also plays an important role in both cellular and humoral immune functions. Zinc plays a vital role in leukocyte function and cell-mediated immunity. Zinc deficiency may result in an increased susceptibility to wound infection and delayed healing. The recommendation for zinc supplementation to enhance wound healing is up to 40 mg (176 mg zinc sulfate) for 10 days (Table 13.3).[35]

13.5.2.2.3 Selenium

Few studies have been published regarding selenium deficiency after bariatric surgery. Although no clinical consequences of selenium deficiency are noted, this trace element is important for thyroid function, muscle metabolism, and immune function (Table 13.3).[35]

13.6 DISCUSSIONS

Today, with the success of bariatric surgery, there is an increasing population of post-bariatric patients who need body contouring procedures to relieve the excess skin and hanging tissues that result in rash, infection, ulceration, inflammation, and skin disorders, not to mention hygiene problems and inability to engage in regular daily activities. Often these patients will present with extreme anatomical changes of their tissues and require multiple procedures to regain their contour. Patients may require multiple surgical procedures, which is often termed a total body lift. These procedures are often planned in two to more stages with a 3-month gap in between each. A common and disappointing feature of these extensive and often complex body contouring surgeries is their high rate of wound healing complication rates: 20 to 75%.[17–21] This is common denominator in the complications related to the nutritional deficiencies of obese and postoperative bariatric patients.[34]

Several studies have highlighted the suboptimal nutritional status of the morbidly obese patients, referred to as high-energy malnutrition. Preoperative deficiencies have been noted for vitamin A, vitamin B_{12}, zinc, selenium, folate, iron, ferritin, thiamine, and 25-OH vitamin D in morbidly obese patients.[37] Following bariatric surgery, many of these nutritional deficiencies can become more profound and chronic. Many post-bariatric patients are deficient in protein, vitamin A, vitamin B_{12}, vitamin D_{25}, zinc, iron, ferritin, selenium, and folate at 1 year post-bariatric surgery (Table 13.1). In studies of post-bariatric patients who were within 1 month of planned plastic surgery, 33% of patients had vitamin A deficiency, 9.5% vitamin B_{12} deficiency, 16.3% iron deficiency, 28.6% transferrin deficiency, and 38% a prealbumin of less than 20 mg/dl.[27]

Surgeons are at the crossroads of wound making and wound healing. Common predicaments of all healing wounds are perfusion, nutritional competency, optimal immune response, and hemostatic physiological environment. The physiological environment of the wound is influenced by such factors as inflammation and temperature. Whereas perfusion is much dependent on healthy living and the surgical technique, both nutritional status and competency of the immune response are integrally dependent on adequate nutritional intake.

With ample scientific data on importance of nutrition in the healing process and defense mechanisms, many surgical disciplines have evaluated the impact of nutrition on perioperative outcome of their surgical patients. Many publications have confirmed a significant reduction in postoperative infectious complications, length of hospital stay, and morbidity and mortality rates in subjects receiving nutritional supplementation in their perioperative period. The greatest improvement was observed in patients receiving specialized nutritional support preoperatively.[27] Between 2004 and 2005, under the auspices of the European Society for Clinical Nutrition and Metabolism (ESPEN), a steering committee of 88 experts in clinical nutrition from 20 countries developed guidelines on enteral nutrition that included enhanced recovery of surgical patients. Enhanced recovery of patients after surgery emphasizes the importance of avoidance of long periods of preoperative fasting, reestablishment of oral feeding as early as possible after surgery, integration of nutritional support into the overall operative management, metabolic control of blood glucose, and reduction of factors that exacerbate stress-related catabolism or impair gastrointestinal function. More recently, The Obesity Society published guidelines for bariatric patients as well.[38] Adequate protein, arginine, glutamine, vitamin A, vitamin B_{12}, vitamin C, folate, thiamine, iron, zinc, and selenium have been deemed essential in many studies for the healing of wounds and optimization of the immune system. Nutritional supplementation containing protein, free amino acids, arginine, glutamine, and dietary nucleotides, as well as vitamins A, C, B_6, and B_{12}, folate, thiamine, iron, zinc, and selenium, clearly reduced postoperative complication rates in obese and post-bariatric patients to those of the normal weight non-bariatric control group.[27]

13.7 CONCLUSION

While many obese and post-bariatric patients have clear nutritional deficiencies, many more patients will have low subclinical levels of these nutrients. At times of surgery or stress, subclinical nutritional deficiency can rapidly become clinical when demand for calorie, protein, amino acids, vitamins, and minerals increase proportionally to the injury and level of stress. With this in mind, supplementation of these elements is appealing in all body contouring patients.

REFERENCES

1. World Health Organization. WHO: obesity and overweight. Available at http://www. who.int/mediacentre/factsheets/fs311/en/index.html (accessed October 2, 2012).
2. Wang, Y., and Beydoun, M.A. 2007. The obesity epidemic in the United States—gender, age, socioeconomic, racial/ethnic, and geographic characteristics: a systematic review and meta-regression analysis. *Epidemiol Rev* 29:6–28.
3. Ogden, C.L., Carroll, M.D., Curtin, L.R. et al. 2006. Prevalence of overweight and obesity in the United States, 1999–2004. *JAMA* 295:1549–55.
4. Wang, Y., Beydoun, M.A., Liang, L., Caballero, B., and Kumanyika, S.K. 2008. Will all Americans become overweight or obese? Estimating the progression and cost of the US obesity epidemic. *Obesity (Silver Spring)* 16(10):2323–30.
5. Fisher, B.L., and Schauer, P. 2002. Medical and surgical options in the treatment of severe obesity. *Am J Surg* 184(6B):9S.
6. Santry, H.P., Gillen D.L., and Lauderdale, D.S. 2005. Trends in bariatric surgical procedures. *JAMA* 294(15):1909.
7. Dixon, J.B., Dixon, M.E., and O'Brien, P.E. 2001. Quality of life after Lap-Band placement: influence of time, weight loss, and comorbidities. *Obes Res* 9:713–21.
8. Mamplekou, E., Komesidou, V., Bissias, C. et al. 2005. Psychological condition and quality of life in patients with morbid obesity before and after surgical weight loss. *Obes Surg* 15:1177–84.
9. Dixon, J.B., Dixon, M.E., and O'Brien, P.E. 2002. Body image: appearance orientation and evaluation in the severely obese. Changes with weight loss. *Obes Surg* 12:65–71.
10. Sjostrom, L., Lindroos, A.K., Peltonen, M. et al. 2004. Lifestyle, diabetes, and cardiovascular risk factors 10 years after bariatric surgery. *N Engl J Med* 351:2683–93.
11. Adams, T.D., Gress, R.E., Smith, S.C. et al. 2007. Long-term mortality after gastric bypass surgery. *N Engl J Med* 357:753–61.
12. Steinbrook, R. 2004. Surgery for severe obesity. *N Engl J Med* 350(11):1075–79.
13. Matarasso, A., Roslin, M.S., and Kurian, M. 2007. Bariatric surgery: an overview of obesity surgery. *Plast Reconstr Surg* 119(4):1357.
14. National Institutes of Health. 1991. Gastrointestinal surgery for severe obesity: National Institutes of Health Consensus Development Conference Panel. *Ann Intern Med* 115:956–61.
15. Fobi, M.A., Lee, H., Holness, R., and Cabinda, D. 1998. Gastric bypass operation for obesity. *World J Surg* 22(9):925–35.
16. American Society of Plastic Surgeons. 2013. Massive weight loss patients create mass appeal for body contouring procedures (press release). http:www.plasticsurgery.org.
17. Araco, A., Gravante, G., Araco, F. et al. 2006. Body contouring after weight loss: the plastic-bariatric surgery symbiosis. *Aesthetic Plast Surg* 30:374–76.
18. Shermak, M.A., Chang, D., Magnuson, T.H. et al. 2006. An outcomes analysis of patients undergoing body contouring surgery after massive weight loss. *Plast Reconstr Surg* 118:1026–31.
19. Fraccalvieri, M., Datta, G. et al. 2007. Abdominoplasty after weight loss in morbidly obese patients: a 4-year clinical experience. *Obes Surg* 17(10):1319–24.
20. Hurwitz, D.J., Agha-Mohammadi, S., Ota, K., Unadkat, J. 2008. A review of total body lift surgery. *Aesthet Surg J* 28(3):294–303.
21. Greco, J.A., Castaldo, E.T., Nanney, L.B. et al. 2008. The effect of weight loss surgery and body mass index on wound complications after abdominal contouring operations. *Ann Plast Surg* 61(3):235–42.
22. Kitzinger, H.B., Cakl, T., Wenger, R., Hacker, S., Aszmann, O.C., and Karle, B. 2013. Prospective study on complications following a lower body lift after massive weight loss. *J Plast Reconstr Aesthet Surg* 66(2):231–38.

23. Neaman, K.C., and Hansen, J.E. 2007. Analysis of complications from abdominoplasty: a review of 206 cases at a university hospital. *Ann Plast Surg* 58(3):292–98.

24. Arthurs, Z.M., Cuadrado, D., Sohn, V. et al. 2007. Post-bariatric panniculectomy: pre-panniculectomy body mass index impacts the complication profile. *Am J Surg* 193(5):567–70.

25. Nemerofsky, R.B., Oliak, D.A., and Capella, J.F. 2006. Body lift: an account of 200 consecutive cases in the massive weight loss patient. *Plast Reconstr Surg* 117(2):414–30.

26. Kaidar-Person, O., Person, B., Szomstein, S., and Rosenthal, R.J. 2008. Nutritional deficiencies in morbidly obese patients: a new form of malnutritions? Part B. Minerals. *Obes Surg* 18(8):1028–34.

27. Agha-Mohammadi, S., and Hurwitz, D.J. Enhanced recovery after body-contouring surgery: reducing surgical complication rates by optimizing nutrition. *Aesthetic Plast Surg* 34(5):617–25.

28. Kaidar-Person, O., Person, B., Szomstein, S., and Rosenthal, R.J. 2008. Nutritional deficiencies in morbidly obese patients: a new form of malnutrition? Part B. Minerals. *Obes Surg* 18(8):1028–34.

29. Coughlin, K., Bell, R.M., Bivins, B.A., Wrobel, S., and Griffen, W.O. 1983. Preoperative and postoperative assessment of nutrient intakes in patients who have undergone gastric bypass surgery. *Arch Surg* 118(7):813–16.

30. Dias, M.C., Ribeiro, A.G., Scabim, V.M. et al. 2006. Dietary intake of female bariatric patients after anti-obesity gastroplasty. *Clinics* 61:93.

31. Marcason, W. 2004. What are the dietary guidelines following bariatric surgery? *J Am Diet Assoc* 104(3):487.

32. Bloomberg, R.D., Fleishman, A., Nalle, J.E., Herron, D.M., and Kini, S. 2005. Nutritional deficiencies following bariatric surgery: what have we learned? *Obes Surg* 15:145.

33. Trostler, N., Mann, A., Zilberbush, N. et al. 1995. Nutrient intake following vertical banded gastroplasty or gastric bypass. *Obes Surg* 5(4):403.

34. Agha-Mohammadi, S., and Hurwitz, D.J. 2008. Nutritional deficiency of post-bariatric surgery body contouring patients: what every plastic surgeon should know. *Plast Reconstr Surg* 122(2):604–13.

35. Agha-Mohammadi, S., and Hurwitz, D.J. 2008. Potential impacts of nutritional deficiency of postbariatric patientson body contouring surgery. *Plast Reconstr Surg* 122(6):1901–14.

36. Flancbaum, L., Belsley, S., Drake, V., Colarusso, T., and Tayler, E. 2006. Preoperative nutritional status of patients undergoing Roux-en-Y gastric bypass for morbid obesity. *J Gastrointest Surg* 10(7):1033–37.

37. Madan, A.K., Orth, W.S., Tichansky, D.S., and Ternovits, C.A. 2006. Vitamin and trace mineral levels after laparoscopic gastric bypass. *Obes Surg* 16(5):603–6.

38. Heber, D., Greenway, F.L., Kaplan, L.M., Livingston, E., Salvador, J., Still, C. 2010. Endocrine and nutritional management of the post-bariatric surgery patient: an Endocrine Society Clinical Practice Guideline. *J Clin Endocrinol Metab* 95(11): 4823–43.

14 Obesity in Critical Illness
Implications for Nutrition Therapy

Stephen A. McClave, Thomas H. Frazier,
Samir D. Vermani, and Ryan T. Hurt

CONTENTS

14.1 INTRODUCTION

A paucity of information exists from societal guidelines to direct the nutritional management of the critically ill obese bariatric patient. Such an absence of guidelines in the middle of an epidemic of obesity implies that obese patients are treated no differently in the intensive care unit (ICU) than their lean counterparts. A single management strategy that has emerged from the literature is the provision of high-protein hypocaloric feeding (misconstrued as permissive underfeeding), which is based on mostly retrospective studies and a few small randomized trials.

No information or guidance is provided on many topics related to the obese critically ill patient, such as the optimal formula, appropriate ratio of nonprotein calories to nitrogen, use of pharmaconutrition, appropriate monitors and measures to determine tolerance, and what changes occur in body composition in response to high-protein hypocaloric feeding.

14.2   HAS OBESITY REACHED THE ICU?

Data from the Centers for Disease Control and Prevention (CDC) indicate that with the current epidemic of obesity, 67% of the U.S. population is overweight or obese.[1] A third of U.S. adults are obese, and 17% of U.S. children are obese.[2] It is not surprising that similar numbers are seen in the ICU, with 33% of ICU patients having a body mass index (BMI) of >30, and 7% of ICU patients having severe obesity with a BMI of >40.[2] By the year 2030, the CDC predicts that 50% of the U.S. population will be obese, with a BMI of >30. Of greater concern is the disproportionate increase in severe obesity (with the greatest increase in those patients with a BMI of >50),[3] a change that is also associated with an increase in chronic disease and comorbid conditions.[4–6]

14.3   PREDISPOSITION TO INFLAMMATION

A variety of mechanisms predispose the obese subject to inflammation, creating in effect a low-grade systemic inflammatory response syndrome (SIRS). Such a baseline response sets the obese subject up for the classic one-hit, two-hit immunologic model. The first hit represents the low-grade SIRS response. When the patient sustains the second hit (such as pneumonia, trauma, burns, myocardial infarction, or any event that brings him or her into the ICU), the baseline SIRS leads to a maladaptive immune response.[12]

Alterations in the gut microbiota in the obese bariatric patient are characterized by an increase in the Firmicutes:Bacteroidetes ratio. This alteration in the intestinal milieu is associated with increased gut permeability, increased generation of lipopolysaccharide endotoxin and inflammation, and reduced insulin sensitivity. In lean subjects, dramatic changes occur in the intestinal biome within 6 h of severe injury, with an up to 90% reduction of commensal organisms and an emergence of virulent pathogenic organisms. How critical illness affects the Firmicutes:Bacteroidetes ratio in the obese subject is not clear. In the absence of critical illness, a high-fat Western diet increases the Firmicutes:Bacteroidetes ratio and promotes weight gain. Provision of prebiotics or probiotics seems to have the reverse phenomenon and contributes to weight loss. With increasing use of probiotics in the ICU to prevent ventilator-associated pneumonia, acquisition of *Clostridium difficile* pseudomembranous colitis, and antibiotic-related diarrhea, it is not clear whether the obese critically ill patient would benefit more or less than his or her lean counterparts.[7]

Alteration in the hunger satiety signals in the obese subject likewise promotes inflammation. As visceral adiposity and BMI go up, insulin levels are higher, but receptor abnormalities are greater, predisposing to insulin resistance and hyperglycemia. Leptin levels are increased, with greater increases in BMI as well. Surprisingly, leptin has a proinflammatory effect on macrophages, stimulating inducible nitric oxide synthase, raising the level of reactive oxygen species. Leptin also stimulates the release of tumor necrosis factor (TNF) and interleukin-1 (IL-1), both proinflammatory cytokines from macrophages. Resistin levels are also higher with increasing adiposity, again having a direct effect on production of TNF and IL-1, with a proinflammatory response. The degree to which bariatric surgery reverses these phenomena is not clear.[8]

14.4 CONTRIBUTION OF COMORBIDITIES TO CRITICAL ILLNESS

Many of the over 60 comorbidities associated with obesity predispose the obese ICU patient to organ dysfunction, infection, and total complications.[9] Metabolic consequences of diabetes and insulin resistance increase risk for nosocomial infection in the ICU. Underlying nonalcoholic fatty liver disease and nonalcoholic steatohepatitis create a baseline of hepatic dysfunction, which may worsen with critical illness.[10] Increased abdominal pressure with increasing BMI causes exacerbation of gastroesophageal reflux and risk of aspiration.[11,12] The heavy chest wall in obesity creates restrictive lung disease, such that obese ICU patients cannot take advantage of the strategy of low-title-volume mechanical ventilation. Underlying sleep apnea and obstructive airway problems lead to impaired ventilation and disordered gas exchange.[10] The baseline abnormalities in inflammation that predispose the patient to arthritis and autoimmune disorders may contribute to exaggerated immune responses to critical illness.[13] Lipotoxicity with fat deposition in the heart may contribute to cardiomyopathy and increased risk for congestive heart failure.[10] Fat deposition in the skeletal muscle further promotes insulin resistance. The hyperglycemia that results contributes to glycosylation of muscle, which may affect ambulation, motor function, and the rapidity of return to baseline after discharge from the ICU. Worsening control of hypertension as adiposity increases may further contribute to congestive heart failure. For those patients with severe obesity and a BMI of >40, the risk of venous thrombosis and thromboembolism increases dramatically.[10,11]

Postoperative bariatric surgery admissions to the ICU are common, as both planned and unplanned admissions. Planned postoperative ICU admissions are often the result of obesity-related comorbidities, such as obstructive sleep apnea requiring ICU management. Complications from bariatric surgery lead to ICU unplanned admission as well. Complications from bariatric surgery leading to such admissions include anastomotic leak, internal hernia, small bowel obstruction, wound infection, pulmonary embolism, and rhabdomyolysis.

14.5 EFFECT ON PATIENT MANAGEMENT ISSUES

Hospitals are ill-equipped to manage the critically ill obese patient. Positioning and transport of the obese patient requires lift teams and specific bariatric equipment, such as increased weight-bearing beds, wheelchairs, and gurneys. Hospital personnel are at increased risk for work-related injuries in the management of such patients. Problems occur with technical monitoring. Use of echocardiogram to monitor volume status may be rendered less accurate because of increased chest wall thickness. Obtaining vascular access in the patient with a thick neck may be difficult, as can be tracheal intubation and airway maintenance.[9,14] Little guidance is provided for altering doses of the common medications used in the ICU, despite information that pharmacokinetics is grossly altered by increasing BMI and obese habitus.

14.6   HOW DOES OBESITY AFFECT MORTALITY IN THE ICU?

One of the leading controversies in critical care is whether obesity protects or increases risk for the patient with regard to mortality. Whether comparing trauma or postop patients in the surgical ICU with those patients in a medical ICU, obesity clearly appears to increase morbidity in all obese patients compared to lean counterparts. Infection, hospital and ICU length of stay, multiple organ failure, and duration on mechanical ventilation are all increased in the obese patient compared to lean counterparts (both surgical and medical critically ill patients).[2.11] A key difference, however, appears to be present with respect to mortality. Obesity is associated with a sevenfold increase in mortality in the surgical ICU for the trauma patient. However, in the medical ICU, obese subjects appear to have reduced mortality compared to lean counterparts.[15] The literature clearly contains conflicting reports with regard to this effect of obesity on mortality. A mortality benefit from obesity is more likely to be seen in a medical ICU patient, in observational studies, or when the controls have a low BMI below 20. Obesity is more likely to be seen as increasing risk for mortality in a trauma surgical ICU patient, in a patient with H1N1 viral infection, in prospective randomized control trials (or meta-analyses of those trials), or when the controls have a normal weight with BMI above 20.[16] The morbidity can be artificially inflated for the obese ICU patient. Compared to lean controls, obese patients are more likely to have a longer ICU length of stay because of management issues. Such patients cannot be managed easily on the floor and, as a result, are admitted earlier to the ICU and remain longer.[2] APACHE II scores may be artificially inflated with obesity, as obesity-related diseases contribute to this score. In a recent study by Moock et al., obese subjects in an ICU had a higher mean APACHE II score of 16 (versus 12 in lean controls, $p < 0.05$). Length of stay in the ICU was also significantly longer for the obese subject at 3.6 days (versus 2.7 days in lean controls, $p = 0.029$). However, there were no significant differences between the two groups in mortality, duration of mechanical ventilation, or nosocomial infection. In fact, there was a tendency toward a higher frequency of identifiable disease in lean subjects in the ICU than with those patients who were obese.[17] A possible explanation for this phenomenon is that obese subjects in the medical ICU tend to be younger, have less disease severity, and have an early admission to the ICU with a late discharge. In contrast, obese subjects in a surgical ICU are more likely to have uniform injury from trauma, burns, or an epidemic infection from the H1N1 virus.

One explanation for the discrepancy in the effect of obesity on mortality may be that the curve for mortality versus increasing BMI is U-shaped. Clearly for patients with BMI below 20, mortality is increased compared to normal weight controls. Patients with BMIs above 40 are also at higher mortality than lean controls.[9.18] The nadir of the curve in the range of BMI from 25 to 40 would imply that obesity is actually a benefit to the critically ill patient, reducing mortality. This may be misleading, as BMI in this weight range may not be the best predictor of risk.[19] Higher risk for the critically ill patient in these lower overweight, class I, and class II obesity may be better identified by presence or absence of the metabolic syndrome. Increased waist circumference with associated comorbidities of diabetes, cardiovascular disease, renal disease, and hepatic steatosis contributes to the systemic inflammatory response and may be associated with increased mortality compared to patients of similar BMI without the metabolic syndrome. In one study with ICU patients with similar BMIs, the difference between the absence and presence of central adiposity was an increase in mortality from 25 to 44%.[20] In summary, whether or not obesity is a risk factor for morbidity and mortality in the ICU remains a source of debate. Obesity appears to clearly drive excess morbidity in the ICU for all classes of obesity, regardless of the insult. Obesity also appears to contribute to excess mortality at the higher range of BMI of >40. Obesity may still contribute to excess mortality at lower BMI classes (in the range 30–40), but the increased risk may be better identified by increased waist circumference, presence of metabolic syndrome, and associated comorbidities (than BMI alone).

14.7 PRINCIPLES OF CRITICAL CARE NUTRITION IN THE OBESE ICU PATIENT

The basic principles of critical care nutrition should be applied to the obese critically ill patient. The need for and the benefit gained from early enteral nutrition are no different than those of their lean counterparts.[11,21] The effect of critical illness on the structure and function of the gastrointestinal tract should be no different in the obese versus a lean subject, with increases in gut permeability, reduction in gut and mucosal-associated lymphoid tissue, a diminution of commensal bacteria, and an increase in the gut-lung axis of inflammation with release of cytokines from the serosal side of the epithelial cell.[12]

Misconceptions associated with obesity should be avoided. The perception that obese subjects in the ICU have increased nutrient reserves does not justify prolonged periods of starvation.[11] Critically ill obese subjects may suffer from increased futile fuel cycling. While these patients may have greater fat mass, there may, paradoxically, be reduced availability of fuels to the cell. It is not clear whether obesity in the critically ill patient, with the insulin resistance and increased mobilization and utilization of fatty acids, predisposes to losses of lean body mass compared to similarly critically ill lean subjects.[10,17] Any delays in initiating tube feeding will reduce the value and impact of enteral nutrition for the obese subject.[13]

The critically ill patient at highest risk in the ICU due to obesity-related conditions may be the one identified by a BMI of >40, evidence of hyperglycemia, thrombosis, increased C-reactive protein (CRP) levels, and central adiposity (for classes I and II). Initial assessment of the critically ill obese patient should include anthropometric measures (actual body weight, usual body weight, ideal body weight, height, BMI, and weight circumference) and markers of the metabolic syndrome (triglyceride, constituitive high density lipoprotein [HDLc], and glucose).[11,12] Obese ICU patients should be carefully assessed for preexisting or evolving comorbidities. Specifically, obstructive sleep apnea and restrictive lung disease, non-alcoholic steatohepatitis [NASH]/non-alcoholic fatty liver [NAFL]/cirrhosis, diabetes, cardiomyopathy, hypertension, hyperlipidemia, and evidence of thromboembolic disease should be sought and ruled out as the patient is admitted to the ICU.

14.8   ICU CARE OF THE BARIATRIC PATIENT

For the obese patient admitted to the ICU with a history of bariatric surgery, the rapidity and degree of weight loss postop should be addressed and micronutrient deficiencies, which would compound critical illness, should be looked for.[22] After bariatric surgery approximately a third of patients will develop macronutrient and micronutrient deficiencies. These issues are more common after procedures such as the biliopancreatic diversion and the very long-limb Roux-en-Y gastric bypass. However, they may also be seen following other bariatric interventions in patients with dysfunctional eating habits or protracted vomiting. Protein–energy malnutrition, protein malnutrition, fat malabsorption, and micronutrient deficiencies should be considered upon admission to the ICU. In patients with suspected macronutrient deficiency, refeeding syndrome precautions should be undertaken.

Thiamine should be administered prior to initiation of dextrose-containing IV fluids, to avoid precipitation of acute deficiency and Wernicke's encephalopathy.[23] Potential deficiencies of iron, folate, B_{12}, copper, thiamine, and vitamin D should be addressed and treated if present. It is important to understand that neurologic abnormalities, encephalopathy, nausea, vomiting, and congestive heart failure may herald micronutrient deficiencies in these patients with history of a bariatric procedure.[21,24,25] Delivery of enteral nutrition in patients who have undergone restrictive bariatric surgery can be challenging. Short-term placement of nasogastric tubes in post-bariatric patients can be safely accomplished. If there are difficulties with bedside placement of an enteral access device, endoscopically assisted nasoenteric tubes can be placed. If long-term delivery of EN is needed, then radiologic or surgical placement of a gastrostomy tube into the gastric remnant may be required.

14.9   IS THE TIME OF CRITICAL ILLNESS APPROPRIATE TO PUT A PATIENT ON A STRATEGY OF PERMISSIVE UNDERFEEDING TO PROMOTE WEIGHT LOSS?

Every aspect of obesity interferes with patient care in the ICU.[10,13] Because the patients cannot be turned easily, they are at increased risk for pressure sores, atelectasis, and pneumonia. Difficulties in mechanical ventilation increase the chances for apnea, restrictive lung disease, and prolonged mechanical ventilation.[10,11,13] Difficulty with diagnostic tests relates to problems with transport, and the fact that these patients may not fit in a computed tomography (CT) scanner or magnetic resonance imaging (MRI). The poor ability to ambulate obese subjects increases risk for deep venous thrombosis.[10] For these reasons, a nutritional strategy that promotes weight loss while lessening depletion of lean body mass is appropriate.

Caloric requirements should be determined by indirect calorimetry (IC) when possible.[13] Simplistic weight-based equations are appropriate if IC is not available. For a BMI of 30–50, 11–14 kcal/kg/day actual body weight (ABW) should be used to estimate caloric requirements. For patients with a BMI of >50, however, 22–25 kcal/kg of ideal body weight (IBW)/day should be used instead to avoid overestimating requirements. Nutritionists have shown that for patients with class I and class II obesity, 2.0 g/kg IBW/day is appropriate to determine protein requirements. For patients with class III obesity, however, 2.5 g/kg IBW/day or more may be needed.[26] Nitrogen balance should be followed based on a 24 h urine urea nitrogen to confirm the appropriateness of the protein provision based on these equations.[27]

High-protein hypocaloric feeding should be provided to the obese ICU patient regardless of the route of nutritional therapy (enteral or parenteral).[25,26,28,29] High-protein hypocaloric feeding is not the same as permissive underfeeding, as this strategy attempts to meet protein requirements in order to maximize protein synthesis to match degradation. The strategy suggests providing 60 to 70% of caloric requirements as determined by the previous methods.[9,25,28]

The enteral route is preferred over the parenteral route.[11,20] The importance of early enteral feeding is to maintain gut integrity, avoid increases in permeability, attenuate oxidative stress, and modulate systemic immune responses. A greater benefit from enteral nutrition is seen with greater disease severity.[12] Effective, moderate glucose control is important, keeping the serum glucose between 110 and 150 g/dl.[17] An enteral formulation should be used with as low a nonprotein calorie-to-nitrogen ratio as possible (preferably less than 40 to 50:1, and should be no more than 0.75/kcal/ml). It is important to ensure that obligatory glucose requirements are met, providing a minimum of 100 g glucose/day (but may require up to 150 g/day for wound healing).[27] Unfortunately, many of the current formulations on the market are impractical for these requirements.

A number of pharmaconutrition agents should be considered for provision to the critically ill obese patient, either in a commercial formula or as a supplement. Recent evidence suggests that L-arginine may be essential during sepsis in the ICU. Obese subjects have an alteration in the baseline ratio of arginine to asymmetric dimethyl arginine (ADMA), a ratio that may worsen with critical illness. Arginine is important for wound healing, stimulating immunity, promoting vasodilation and white blood cell function, and acting as a secretagogue stimulating insulin release. ADMA, in contrast, causes hypertension, endothelial damage leading to cardiovascular disease, vasoconstriction, and reduced perfusion of organs. Critical illness causes a decrease in the ratio of arginine to ADMA, as the ADMA levels rise. ADMA increases as a result of catabolism of muscle and reduced clearance by the kidney. The rise in the ADMA level is associated with organ failure and mortality. Providing exogenous arginine is the only treatment strategy that reverses this ratio and promotes vasodilation and perfusion.[12,30]

Provision of omega-3 fish oil has the effect of decreasing macrophage migration, removing fat from the liver, decreasing arachidonic acid generation and the SIRS response, elevating adiponectin levels, and increasing splanchnic blood flow.[12,31,32] Magnesium levels may be depleted in obesity because of reduced dietary provision and increased renal losses. Hypomagnesemia contributes to increased generation of TNF, intracellular calcium, and insulin receptor abnormalities leading to insulin resistance. Hypomagnesemia directly contributes to the metabolic syndrome.[12,33]

Additional factors that theoretically would benefit the obese critically ill patient include zinc, curcumin, leucine, whey, betaine, SAM-e, L-carnitine, and alpha lipoic acid.[12] Unfortunately, none of these agents has been tested in the critical care setting, and thus their addition to nutritional therapy for the obese critically ill patient cannot be recommended at this time.

14.10   FUTURE DIRECTION

Because all of these recommendations are based on a paucity of data, virtually every question generated in this chapter requires further research. An important area of future study should focus on finding a valid biomarker for the high-risk obese ICU patient. The strategy of high-protein hypocaloric feeding needs to be studied in a formal interventional manner, to confirm whether a benefit on patient outcome exists compared to standard feeding, which meets protein and caloric requirements. Research into the optimum content and dose of pharmaconutrients added to an enteral formulation to create an obesity-specific product is important. With the higher ratio of Firmicutes:Bacteroidetes in the gut microbiota of the obese subject, there is likelihood for worsening permeability in the intestinal barrier function contributing to SIRS and the release of inflammatory cytokines. For these reasons, use of probiotics in the obese critically ill patient should be carefully evaluated. It is clear that obesity and its comorbidities exacerbate the complexity of care in the ICU, and little evidence from the literature currently exists to support these strategies of nutrition therapy.

REFERENCES

1. Wang Y, Beydoun MA. The obesity epidemic in the United States—gender, age, socio-economic, racial/ethnic, and geographic characteristics: a systematic review and meta-regression analysis. *Epidemiol Rev* 2007;29:6.
2. Hogue CW Jr, Stearns JD, Colantuoni E, Robinson KA, Stierer T, Mitter N, Pronovost PJ, Needham DM. The impact of obesity on outcomes after critical illness: a meta-analysis. *Intensive Care Med* 2009;35(7):1152–70.
3. Peeters A, Barendregt JJ, Willekens F, Mackenbach JP, Al Mamun A, Bonneux L, for the Netherlands Epidemiology and Demography Compression of Morbidity Research Group (NEDCOM). Obesity in adulthood and its consequences for life expectancy: a life-table analysis. *Ann Intern Med* 2003;138(1):24–32.
4. Field AE, et al. Impact of overweight on the risk of developing common chronic diseases during a 10-year period. *Arch Intern Med* 2001;161(13):1581–86.
5. Gregg EW, et al. Secular trends in cardiovascular disease risk factors according to body mass index in US adults. *JAMA* 2005;293(15):1868–74.
6. Renehan, AG, et al. Body-mass index and incidence of cancer: a systematic review and meta-analysis of prospective observational studies. *Lancet* 2008;371(9612):569–78.
7. DiBaise JK, Zhang H, Crowell MD, Krajmalnik-Brown R, Decker GA, Rittmann BE. Gut microbiota and its possible relationship with obesity. *Mayo Clin Proc* 2008;83(4):460–69.
8. Hurt RT, Frazier TH, Matheson PJ, Cave MC, Garrison RN, McClain CJ, McClave SA. Obesity and inflammation: should the principles of immunonutrition be applied to this disease process? *Curr Gastroenterol Rep* 2007;9(4):305–6.
9. Brodsky JB, Lemmens HJ, Brock-Utne JG, Vierra M, Saidman LJ. Morbid obesity and tracheal intubation. *Anesth Analg* 2002;94(3):732–36.
10. McClave SA, Martindale RG, Vanek VW, McCarthy M, Roberts P, Taylor B, Ochoa JB, Napolitano L, Cresci G. Guidelines for the provision and assessment of nutrition support therapy in the adult critically ill patient: Society of Critical Care Medicine (SCCM) and the American Society for Parenteral and Enteral Nutrition (ASPEN). *JPEN* 2009;33:277–316.

11. Honiden S, McArdle JR. Obesity in the intensive care unit. *Clin Chest Med* 2009;30(3):581–99.
12. Dickerson RN. Hypocaloric feeding of obese patients in the intensive care unit. *Curr Opin Clin Nutr Metab Care* 2005;8(2):189–96.
13. Cave MC, Hurt RT, Frazier TH, Matheson PJ, Garrison RN, McClain CJ, McClave SA. Obesity, inflammation, and the potential application of pharmaconutrition. *Nutr Clin Pract* 2008;23(1):16–34.
14. Joffe A, Wood K. Obesity in critical care. *Curr Opin Anaesthesiol* 2007;20(2):113–18.
15. Sakr Y, Madl C, Filipescu D, Moreno R, Groeneveld J, Artigas A, Reinhart K, Vincent JL. Obesity is associated with increased morbidity but not mortality in critically ill patients. *Int Care Med* 2008;34:1999–2009.
16. Peake SL, Moran JL, Ghelani DR, Lloyd AJ, Walker MJ. The effect of obesity on 12-month survival following admission to intensive care: a prospective study. *Crit Care Med* 2006;34(12):2929–39.
17. Moock M, Mataloun SE, Pandol M et al. Impact of obesity on critical care treatment in adult patients. *Rev Bras Ter Intensiva* 2010;22(2):133–37.
18. Port AM, Apovian C. Metabolic support of the obese intensive care unit patient: a current perspective. *Curr Opin Clin Nutrit Metab Care* 2010;13:184–91.
19. Sharma AM, Kushner RF. A proposed clinical staging system for obesity. *Int J Obesity* 2009. doi:10.1038/ijo.2009.2.
20. Paolini JB, Mancini J, Genestal M, et al. Predictive value of abdominal obesity vs. body mass index for determining risk of intensive care unit mortality. *Crit Care Med* 2010;38(5):1308–14.
21. Elamin EM. Nutritional care of the obese intensive care unit patient. *Curr Opin Crit Care* 2005;11(4):300–3.
22. Schweiger C, Weiss R, Berry E, et al. Nutritional deficiencies in bariatric surgery candidates. *Obes Surg* 2010;20(2):193–97.
23. Al-Fahad T, Ismael A, Soliman MO, et al. Very early onset of Wernicke's encephalopathy after gastric bypass. *Obes Surg* 2006;16:671–72.
24. Kazemi A, Frazier T, Cave M. Micronutrient-related neurologic complications following bariatric surgery. *Curr Gastroenterol Rep* 2010;12(4):288–95.
25. Juhasz-Pocsine K, Rudnicki SA, Archer RL, et al. Neurologic complications of gastric bypass surgery for morbid obesity. *Neurology* 2007;68:1843–50.
26. Choban PS, Dickerson RN. Morbid obesity and nutrition support: is bigger different? *Nutr Clin Pract* 2005;20(4):480–87.
27. Dickerson RN, Tidwell AC, Minard G, Groce MA, Brown RO. Predicting total urinary nitrogen excretion from urine urea nitrogen excretion in multiple trauma patients receiving specialized nutritional support. *Nutrition* 2005;21:332–38.
28. Dickerson RN. Hypocaloric feeding of obese patients in the intensive care unit. *Curr Opin Clin Nutr Metab Care* 2005;8(2):189–96.
29. Reeds DN. Nutrition support in the obese, diabetic patient: the role of hypocaloric feeding. *Curr Opin Gastroent* 2009;25:151–54.
30. Boger RH. The pharmacodynamics of L-arginine. *J Nutr* 2007;137(6 Suppl 2):1650S–55S.
31. Li H, Ruan XZ, Powis SH, et al. EPA and DHA reduce LPS-induced inflammation responses in HK-2 cells: evidence for a PPAR-gamma-dependent mechanism. *Kidney Int* 2005;67(3):867–74.
32. Lo CJ, Chiu KC, Fu M, Lo R, Helton S. Fish oil decreases macrophage tumor necrosis factor gene transcription by altering the NF kappa B activity. *J Surg Res* 1999;82(2):216–21.
33. Barbagallo M, Dominguez LJ. Magnesium metabolism in type 2 diabetes mellitus, metabolic syndrome and insulin resistance. *Arch Biochem Biophys* 2007;458(1):40–47.

15 Nutrition and Weight Regain in the Bariatric Surgical Patient

Kirsten Webb Sorensen, Holly Herrington, and Robert F. Kushner

CONTENTS

Bariatric surgery is an effective treatment for severe obesity. The amount of weight loss and the resolution of comorbid conditions associated with surgical weight loss surpass those of nonsurgical approaches to obesity, leading to an increasing number of bariatric procedures. Approximately 220,000 bariatric surgeries were performed in 2009, a 10-fold increase from 1990.[1] Suboptimal weight loss and weight regain are becoming more of a clinical concern as the number of bariatric procedures continues to rise. This chapter will review the current information regarding weight gain following bariatric surgery and the factors associated with weight regain, and will present a proposed evaluation and treatment strategy.

15.1   OCCURRENCE OF WEIGHT REGAIN IN THE BARIATRIC SURGICAL POPULATION

It is well established that the vast majority of bariatric surgery patients experience significant weight loss and improvement or resolution of type 2 diabetes and cardiovascular risk factors.[2] The amount of weight loss differs between surgical interventions, with biliopancreatic diversion with duodenal switch (BPD/DS) and Roux-en-Y gastric bypass (RYGB) typically producing greater and more rapid average weight loss than the sleeve gastrectomy and adjustable gastric band (AGB). However, the incidence of weight regain following these procedures is not well defined, as definitions used to classify weight loss outcomes have not been standardized. Whereas some studies report outcomes as percent excess weight lost (%EWL), other authors use change in body mass index (BMI) units (kg/m^2) or loss of total body weight measured in kilograms or percentage. Body weights are also often self-reported instead of measured. Additionally, selection bias may occur since follow-up and reporting of patient outcomes is often incomplete. Realizing these limitations, cross-sectional data estimate that significant weight regain occurs in 20–35% of patients, depending upon the procedure performed and duration of time following surgery.[3–6] This number is likely to be an underrepresentation of actual incidence rates.

In addition to uncertain rates of weight regain, it is also unclear how much weight (actual or percent) is regained among post-bariatric surgical patients. The Swedish Obese Subjects (SOS) study, the largest nonrandomized intervention trial comparing weight loss outcomes in a group of over 4000 surgical and nonsurgical subjects, has previously reported 10-year data.[7] Surgically treated subjects underwent fixed or variable banding, vertical banded gastroplasty (VBG) (a procedure that is no longer performed), or RYGB. Total body weight change was maximal after 1 year in the three surgical subgroups (RYGB, $-38 \pm 7\%$; VBG, $-26 \pm 10\%$; and banding, $-21 \pm 10\%$). Weight regain was reported by the second year of follow-up. For the RYGB and banding subgroups, 10-year weight change was $-25 \pm 11\%$ and $-13.2 \pm 13\%$, respectively. Thus, at 10 years, subjects who underwent RYGB experienced a mean weight regain of 12% total body weight, and those who underwent fixed or variable banding regained 8% total body weight. This translates into regaining 34% (for RYGB) and 38% (for banding) of the maximal lost weight at 1 year. Categorical weight regain was not reported.

15.2   DETERMINANTS OF WEIGHT REGAIN

Poor adherence to postoperative recommendations or a return to unhealthy eating habits can contribute to postsurgical weight regain. In addition, a number of patient factors, including a higher presurgical BMI,[8] diabetes,[9] male gender,[9] and older age,[10] also appear to be predictors of poorer weight losses. However, weight regain after bariatric surgery often has a multifactorial cause that is due to a combination of anatomical, behavioral, and psychological factors (Table 15.1).

TABLE 15.1

Etiological Factors for Weight Regain Following Bariatric Surgery

- Anatomical
    - LAGB malfunction or mismanagement
    - RYGB (pouch enlargement, gastrojejunal anastomosis dilation, gastrogastric fistula)
- Physiological
    - Hormonal adaptation
    - Pregnancy
    - Menopause
    - Weight gaining medications
    - Smoking cessation
    - Endocrine disorder
    - Psychological disorder
- Behavioral
    - Dietary: Maladaptive eating patterns, reduced vigilance
    - Physical activity

15.2.1 BRIEF OVERVIEW OF SURGERY FAILURE

Each type of bariatric procedure has its own potential mechanism of surgical failure that can lead to weight gain. In restrictive procedures such as AGB, weight loss is based on the reduction of gastric volume due to the gastric band. Any dilation of the band or insufficient tightening may result in a feeling of decreased restriction, leading to the ability to eat more compared to the initial months after surgery. This is supported by observations that suggest that restrictive procedures fail if the pouch and stoma are too large. In patients who have undergone RYGB, weight regain may occur as a result of a gastrogastric fistula or enlargement of the gastric pouch or stoma outlet. Patients who experience these complications are generally appropriate candidates for a surgical revision procedure. A retrospective review from a bariatric center of excellence identified patients who underwent laparoscopic revisional surgery between 2001 and 2008. Of 384 secondary bariatric operations, 151 reoperative procedures were performed for complications such as pouch enlargements, strictures, and gastrogastric fistulas, with the major morbidity (13.2%) related to leaks.[11] Similarly, another retrospective analysis identifies the major reasons for requiring surgical revision as weight regain (40.3%), type-specific issues (27.8%), dysphagia/reflux (25%), and gastrogastric fistula (6.9%).[12]

15.2.2 BIOLOGICAL ISSUES

The surgical reorganization of gut anatomy causes changes in gut hormones. These changes are often implicated as a mechanism for the benefits of bariatric surgeries, weight loss, and the remission of many obesity-related comorbidities. Ghrelin, peptide YY (PYY), and glucagon-like peptide-1 (GLP-1) are three of the gut hormones that play a paramount role in appetite regulation. Multiple studies have shown that ghrelin levels are reduced following RYGB, though other clinical studies are conflicting.[13] The discrepancy in these findings may be due to the complexity of the ghrelin system or to the poor sensitivity of the techniques used to assess ghrelin levels.[13] PYY is an anorexigenic signal, secreted after food intake, shown to be effective in suppressing appetite. GLP-1 is released into the circulation postmeal to stimulate insulin secretion, inhibit glucagon release, and delay gastric emptying. Both anorexigenic hormones have been shown to increase after RYGB and LSG.

The hormonal causes of weight regain after surgically induced weight loss are not fully understood. Theoretically, it can be thought that there is a disturbance in the metabolic milieu that causes an imbalance in the mechanisms that regulate appetite and metabolic rate, leading to weight regain. Surgically induced alterations in ghrelin, leptin, and incretin hormone levels may diminish over time. Rodent studies have demonstrated that postsurgical weight regain is associated with failure to sustain elevated plasma PYY concentrations. Use of animal models for bariatric surgery should provide further insight into the mechanisms involving the hormonal causes of postsurgical weight regain.

15.2.3 BEHAVIORAL ISSUES

In addition to potential mechanical or medical concerns, suboptimal weight loss or weight regain is often attributed to maladaptive behavioral changes. Eating behaviors that may pose a threat to successful maintenance of weight loss following bariatric surgery include dietary nonadherence, decrease in frequency of dumping syndrome, resolution of food intolerances, maladaptive and disordered eating behaviors, return to preoperative eating or lifestyle patterns that contributed to development of obesity, lack of physical activity, and lack of follow-up care with medical providers.[14] Strategies to improve dietary intake and eating behaviors following weight regain are similar to the nonsurgical obesity treatments for weight loss.[15]

15.2.3.1 Lack of Adherence to the Postsurgical Dietary Recommendations

Lack of adherence to the postsurgical dietary recommendations is likely a key factor in weight regain. Although there are specific nutritional guidelines following bariatric surgery, these guidelines are not taught to patients in a standardized manner, and bariatric programs differ in their degree of follow-up to enforce dietary adherence.[16] It has been suggested that adherence to the recommended postsurgical guidelines is poor, and calorie intake increases significantly during the postoperative period.[17] In 2008, Sarwer et al. conducted a prospective investigation of 200 Roux-en-Y gastric bypass surgery patients to examine eating behaviors both before and after surgery. Patients completed a series of questionnaires both preoperatively and at weeks 20, 40, 66, and 92 weeks postoperatively. The study targeted percentage of weight loss, macronutrient intake, dietary adherence, and eating behavior. Researchers found that baseline cognitive restraint and self-reported adherence to diet at postoperative week 20 were associated with higher percentage of weight loss. Patients reporting high dietary adherence lost 4.5% more weight at postoperative week 90 than those patients that reported low dietary adherence. Caloric intake across the subjects changed significantly as well ($p = .005$). At baseline, average calorie intake was 2390.9 ± 99 kcal/day. At postoperative survey weeks 20, 40, 66, and 90, calories increased to 1172.9 ± 46.5, 1189.5 ± 54.2, 1273.4 ± 56.3, and 1358.1 ± 60.5, respectively. By week 92, all participants had regained some weight, but the group that reported high dietary adherence lost significantly more weight (16.2%) than those patients reporting low dietary adherence (11.7%) ($p = .02$).[17]

In 2008, the Swedish Obese Subjects study compared weight loss, lifestyle, and obesity risk factors of over 4000 subjects who had undergone weight loss surgery. Surgical patients consumed approximately 2900 calories/day prior to receiving surgery. This caloric intake decreased to only 1500 calories/day 6 months after surgery but had increased up to 2000 calories/day 10 years following when patients had regained approximately 10% of their weight loss. This increase in calorie intake is a likely contributor to weight regain.[7]

Patients with disordered eating prior to surgery may be at particular risk for postoperative weight regain. Three factors that relate to the regulation of food intake include cognitive restraint, disinhibition, and hunger. These three factors are measured in the Eating Inventory, or the Three-Factor Questionnaire, widely used in the obesity and eating disorders field of practice and research. Cognitive restraint refers to an individual's ability to intentionally limit food intake in an attempt to lose weight or avoid weight gain. Disinhibition refers to the tendency to lose control over food intake. This is often described by patients as feeling "out of control" with their food intake and is commonly present in binge eating. Lastly, hunger is used to describe the physical and psychological feelings related to the desire to eat.[15] In the study described previously by Sarwer et al.,[17] patients who underwent RYGB surgery reported increased levels of disinhibition and hunger prior to receiving surgery. After surgery, patients reported decreases in disinhibition and hunger accompanied by increases in restraint. The authors hypothesized that the ability to restrain food intake prior to surgery may predict the ability to adhere to a strict postoperative diet. Conversely, patients who fail to develop or experience any restraint in their diet, especially when faced with social or environmental pressures to overeat, and those patients who continue to struggle to control their food intake prior to surgery, may be at a greater risk for weight regain.[17]

15.2.3.2   Resolution of Nausea, Vomiting, Dumping Syndrome, or Plugging

Resolution of nausea, vomiting, dumping syndrome, or "plugging" may also contribute to additional calorie intake over time. Dumping syndrome, which most commonly occurs in patients who have undergone RYGB, can result from ingesting high-sugar or high-fat-containing foods. This results in the patient experiencing nausea, flushing, diarrhea, and vomiting. Plugging, which can occur after a patient receives any bariatric surgery, has been described as the experience of ingested food becoming stuck or lodged within the gastric pouch, resulting in pressure or pain in the chest or abdominal area.[15] This can occur when a patient eats too quickly, consumes foods such as bread, pasta, or dry foods, or as a result of stricture. Both dumping syndrome and plugging can often dissuade patients to stray from the dietary recommendations and promote more strict dietary compliance in the early stages following surgery. However, as time progresses, these symptoms lessen. In most cases, symptoms of dumping syndrome resolve between 18 and 24 months.[18] The disappearance of dumping symptoms and signs may lead the patient to consume high-sugar/high-fat foods, resulting in greater calorie consumption.

15.2.3.3 Development of Substance Abuse

Another behavioral issue that may lead to weight regain is development of substance abuse. Some patients who have undergone weight loss surgery have exhibited an increase in alcohol consumption postoperatively, potentially to compensate for a marked decrease in food intake. This is based on the symptom substitution theory where, upon successful elimination of a particular symptom like excessive eating, a substitute symptom will appear if the underlying cause goes untreated.[19] Another term for this theory is *addiction transfer*, where food may be replaced by an alternate substance as a coping mechanism. Conason et al.[19] investigated the association between substance abuse and weight loss surgery among 155 subjects who underwent laparoscopic RYGB surgery ($n = 100$) or LAGB ($n = 55$). Participants completed the Impulsive Behaviors Questionnaire to assess eating behaviors and substance use preoperatively and 1, 3, 6, 12, and 24 months following surgery. Subjects reported changes in the frequency of substance use (including drug use, alcohol use, and cigarette smoking) 24 months after surgery. In the overall sample population, the frequency of reported alcohol use changed significantly over time. At baseline, 61.3% of patients reported using alcohol. The prevalence rate decreased to 20.2% at 1 month but increased thereafter back up to 63.2% by 24 months.

In the Longitudinal Assessment of Bariatric Surgery observational study, 1945 patients who underwent a RYGB or LAGB procedure completed the Alcohol Use Disorders Identification Test (AUDIT) instrument prior to and 1 and 2 years after surgery.[20] Alcohol use disorder (AUD), defined as a total AUDIT score of at least 8 out of 40, or positive for symptoms of alcohol dependence or alcohol-related harm, increased from 7.6% at the preoperative assessment to 9.6% after the second postoperative year. Male sex and younger age were identified as predictive factors, and AUD was associated with worse postoperative mental health and postoperative treatment for psychiatric or emotional problems.

Patients who undergo RYGB may experience the effects of alcohol more acutely due to the digestive alterations that promote rapid absorption of alcohol into the bloodstream. Weight gain may occur with increased alcohol intake due to the dense calorie composition of alcoholic beverages.[21]

15.2.3.4 Limitation in Physical Activity Following Weight Loss Surgery

A limitation in physical activity following weight loss surgery may also be a predictor for weight regain. Physical activity is often difficult for patients with severe obesity due to osteoarthritis, asthma, joint pain, and stiffness.[22] Many patients may have also suffered emotional discomfort from being embarrassed by working out at health clubs, or experienced frustration at lack of weight loss despite continuous activity prior to bariatric surgery. In contrast, physical activity following bariatric surgery has been associated with a greater estimated weight loss, increased resting energy expenditure, and is a predictive factor in weight maintenance.[23] Bond et al.[24] report that physically active patients lose more weight than those who are sedentary 24 months after surgery. Researchers examined self-reported physical activity participation in relation to excess weight loss and BMI reduction among gastric bypass surgery patients. Researchers hypothesized that physical activity contributes to both greater excess weight loss and a greater reduction in BMI at 2 years postsurgery. Gastric bypass patients who reported physical activity had greater percent excess weight loss and a greater decrease in BMI than gastric bypass patients who reported no physical activity. Additionally, physical activity had a favorable effect on %EWL and BMI among gastric bypass patients at 2 years postsurgery, thus supporting the recommendation of habitual physical activity in a comprehensive gastric bypass postsurgical weight maintenance program.[24] The American College of Sports Medicine (ACSM) and the joint guidelines from the Association of Clinical Endocrinologists (AACE), The Obesity Society (TOS), and American Society for Metabolic and Bariatric Surgery (ASMBS) recommend moderate aerobic physical activity for a minimum of 150 min/week and a goal of 300 min/week, including strength training two to three times per week.[23,25]

15.3 APPROACH TO THE PATIENT WHO PRESENTS WITH WEIGHT REGAIN

15.3.1 MEDICAL

The potential causative factors of weight regain in a postsurgical patient are numerous and varied. Natural life changes such as pregnancy and menopause, use of certain medications or specific medical diseases, and smoking cessation are well known to be associated with weight gain. Therefore, a thorough history and medical examination are required to identify and manage the issues related to weight regain.

Weight gain associated with pregnancy is dependent upon many determinants, including physiological, psychological, and behavioral factors. Observational and cohort studies have shown that excessive gestational weight gain substantially increases the risk of weight retention at 1 year and future long-term weight gain at 15–21 years postpartum.[26–28] Weight retention is particularly more evident for women who are obese prior to pregnancy. Based on the existing literature, the Institute of Medicine published revised recommendations on appropriate weight gain during pregnancy. For underweight women the recommended total weight gain is 12.5–18 kg; for normal weight women, 11.5–16 kg; for overweight women, 7–11.5 kg; and for obese women, 5–9 kg.

Among patients who have undergone bariatric surgery, counseling about pregnancy is essential, as almost half of all bariatric procedures are performed on women of reproductive age. Bariatric surgery is thought to improve fertility based on normalization of sex hormones, menstrual irregularities, and improvement in polycystic ovarian syndrome. Most authorities urge patients to delay conception for at least 1 year post-bariatric surgery to minimize complications from nutritional deficiencies and optimize weight loss.

Maternal weight gain after bariatric surgery has not been well studied. In a prospective study of 79 consecutive first pregnancies following AGB, mean maternal weight gain was 9.6 ± 9.0 kg compared to 15.5 ± 9.0 kg among 79 obese subjects

matched for parity and maternal age.[29] The incidence of postpartum weight retention was not reported. Neonatal outcomes such as incidence of stillbirths, preterm
deliveries, and birth weight have been shown to be consistent with community values.[29,30] In one retrospective study, patients who conceived during the first postoperative year ($n = 104$) had short-term perinatal outcomes comparable to those of
patients who conceived after the first postoperative year ($n = 385$).[30] No significant
differences were noted regarding hypertensive disorders, diabetes mellitus, or bariatric complications.

The years surrounding menopause are linked to weight gain. Simkin-Silverman
and Wing[31] were among the first to observe this pattern in the Healthy Women's
Study, a longitudinal investigation of biobehavioral factors during menopause in a
cohort of 541 healthy and initially premenopausal women. Data published after the
first 3 years of this study showed that the women gained on average 2.25 kg, and
about 20% of subjects gained 4.5 kg.[31] Body composition studies demonstrate an
increase in total body fat and visceral adipose tissue.[32] Change in weight and body
fat is primarily due to decreased energy expenditure and physical activity along with
loss of estrogen. Menopausal weight gain is associated with development of hyperlipidemia, hypertension, and insulin resistance. Literature on menopausal weight
gain in patients who have undergone bariatric procedures is limited. However, it can
be postulated that the same factors that contribute to weight gain in a nonsurgical
menopausal woman can also affect a postsurgical menopausal patient.

Medication-induced weight gain can occur in individuals who have undergone
bariatric procedures. However, currently there are no studies that have identified
the effects of weight gaining medications in this population. It is, however, well
documented that many types of medications are associated with weight gain; these
include antipsychotics, mood stabilizers, antidepressants, antidiabetics, and glucocorticoids. The degree of medication-induced weight gain varies by medication.
Prescribed psychotropics may cause 2–17 kg of weight gain over the course of clinical treatment. In an analysis of four prospective trials of glucocorticoids in rheumatoid arthritis, the use of 5–10 mg/day of prednisone over 2 years was associated with
an increase of mean body weight of 4–8%.[33]

Although uncommon, medical causes of weight gain include Cushing's syndrome,
acquired hypothalamic obesity syndromes, and myxedema from hypothyroidism. In
a single center study of 783 consecutive patients who were evaluated for endocrine
disorders before bariatric surgery, Cushing's syndrome was diagnosed in six patients
and adrenocorticotropic hormone (ACTH)-dependent hypercortisolism in an additional five.[34] Diagnosis of Cushing's syndrome can be challenging since obesity and
hypercortisolism share many clinical features: central obesity, facial plethora, dorso-
cervical hump, and viloaceous stria. A thorough clinical examination and biochemical workup, along with a heightened suspicion, are necessary for diagnosis.

Tobacco use is a significant health behavior to assess in bariatric candidates.
One study found that 67% of bariatric surgery candidates have a lifetime history
of smoking and 27% are current smokers.[35] Since current guidelines recommend
smoking cessation at least 8 weeks prior to bariatric surgery, the effect of cigarette
smoking on body weight may be an important factor. Longitudinal cohort data of
1885 smokers from national surveys showed that mean weight gain after cessation

of smoking was 2.8 kg in men and 3.8 kg in women; 9.8% of men and 13.4% of women gained more than 13 kg.[36] The etiology of weight gain is thought to be attributed to a reduction in energy expenditure and increased caloric intake. Smoking and smoking cessations rates have not been well characterized in the post-bariatric surgical population.

Patients presenting with loss of restraint or reduced restriction of food volume may require an evaluation of the surgical procedure to rule out surgical failure as a factor in weight regain. An upper GI x-ray is a reasonable first step to assess pouch enlargement, anastomotic dilation, or formation of a gastrogastric fistula among patients who underwent a RYGB, and for inadequate band restriction for patients who had a LAGB performed. Depending on initial results, an esophagogastroduodoscopy (EGD) will provide a more accurate delineation of the anatomy and intraluminal measurements.

15.3.2 Psychological

Data suggest that patients with postoperative depression experience poorer weight loss than those who are not depressed. Similarly, postoperative patients who exhibit disordered eating patterns, such as grazing and loss of control over eating, have poorer weight loss and greater weight regain.[37,38] Patients who are found to have mood disorders, disordered eating behavior, or substance abuse after bariatric surgery should be offered professional psychological counseling and support. It is not known, however, whether such treatment improves weight loss or other outcomes.

In epidemiologic studies, attendance at postoperative support groups is associated with improved weight loss outcomes.[22,39] There is a lack of data regarding the effects of other types of postoperative psychological support, such as group or individual therapy, on weight loss and other outcomes.

Currently there are no well-established clinical tools to help guide health care providers in assessing postoperative behaviors. In response, the WATCH has been recently proposed as a tool to help health care providers assess suboptimal outcome or maladaptive eating behaviors and cognitions in post-bariatric surgical patients.[40] This screening tool is comprised of five questions: (1) Have you lost more or less weight than medically expected? (2) Are you having a hard time consistently adhering to the recommendations of your surgery team? (3) Are you spending an excessive amount of time thinking about your weight, shape, or food? (4) Are you feeling a sense of loss of control while eating? (5) Are you engaging in any harmful behaviors to lose weight? The intention of the WATCH is to make routine behavioral screening a standard component of the postoperative care of bariatric surgery patients and encourage future research on its empirical validation.[40]

15.3.3 Dietary

Clinical practice guidelines for significant weight regain emphasize timely evaluation for decreased adherence to lifestyle modification and development of maladaptive eating behaviors. Interdisciplinary approaches should be implemented with an emphasis on dietary change, physical activity, behavioral modification with frequent follow-up, and if necessary, pharmacological or surgical revision.[23] Strategies to improve dietary intake and eating behavior to reduce weight regain include nutritional counseling and follow-up, with emphasis on following a calorie-restricted diet, self-monitoring of eating and lifestyle behaviors, and increasing physical activity.

Regular contact between the patient and the provider, especially for nutrition counseling, may promote long-term weight control and help prevent weight regain. Follow-up after bariatric surgery not only is crucial to assess outcomes, weight loss, and resolution of comorbidities, but also is necessary for the patient to receive continual accountability regarding diet, lifestyle modification, and ongoing nutrition education. Madan and Tichansky report that most patients forget their preoperative dietary counseling at least 1 year following surgery, making it vital that follow-up with a dietitian occur at regular intervals.[41]

In their study, 63 patients who underwent RYGB surgery were provided comprehensive preoperative surgery education, including informed consent, a true/false quiz, a CD-ROM video, preoperative appointments, support group meetings, and a 130-page educational booklet. The researchers wanted to assess how well patients recall information they are given preoperatively. All patients were given a true/false quiz prior to receiving RYGB surgery and were given the same test at least 1 month postoperatively. Patients greater than 1 year postoperatively were compared to patients less than 1 year postoperatively. Every subject was required to take the test until a score of 100% was reached before receiving surgery. When the test was administered again postoperatively, 46% of the subjects did not get all the questions correct and the mean passing score was 95%. Patients who were greater than 1 year out of surgery had a greater failure rate, 80%, as opposed to those who were less than 1 year out of surgery, 36% ($p < .01$). Madan and Tichansky stated that despite efforts to educate patients prior to surgery, patients will forget basic and critical preoperative education following bariatric surgery. Therefore, it is imperative that continual patient education is mandatory for successful long-term outcomes following bariatric surgery.[41]

Freire et al.[42] conducted a cross-sectional study of 100 post-RYGB patients to determine lifestyle habits and food patterns to identify predictive factors of weight loss or weight regain. Most patients reported following up with a nutritional counselor or registered dietitian postsurgery; however, as the years progressed, follow-up visits progressively decreased. During the first 2 postoperative years, 85.3% of patients were following up on a regular basis with their nutrition provider. From years 2 to 5, only 69% of the subjects reported nutritional follow-up visits, and by year 5, only 3% of subjects were still engaged in regular follow-up. Following surgery, 53 subjects received nutritional counseling and 47 subjects did not. Of the 47 subjects who did not receive nutritional counseling following bariatric surgery, 37 subjects experienced weight regain ($p < .01$, odds ratio (OR) 6.6). Freire et al. states that lack of nutrition counseling is significantly associated with weight regain ($p < .01$).[42] Additionally, the AACE/TOS/ASMBS guidelines recommend that all patients should be encouraged to participate in ongoing support groups after bariatric surgery.[23]

Follow-up visits with a registered dietitian are an essential factor for the prevention of weight regain following bariatric surgery. Clinical assessment of weight

TABLE 15.2

Suggested Postoperative Nutrition Follow-up Visit with a Registered Dietitian or Nutrition Counselor

Recommended	Anthropometric Data	Activity
	Current height/weight/BMI	Amount, type, intensity, and frequency of activity
	Weight loss to date	**Medications**
	Percentage of excess body weight or body fat	Encourage patients to follow-up with PCP regarding medications to treat comorbidities such as hypertension or diabetes mellitus
	Biochemical	**Vitamin/mineral supplements**
	Review laboratory results if available	Adherence to protocol
Dietary Intake	Usual or actual daily food intake	Address individual patient complaints or questions
	Protein intake	Address lifestyle and educational needs for long-term weight loss maintenance
	Fiber intake	
	Fluid intake	Estimated calorie intake (usual or actual intake)
	Food texture compliance or advancement	Reinforce intuitive eating style to improve food tolerance
	Food tolerance issues (nausea, vomiting, dumping)	Appropriate meal planning
Other Considerations	**Promote anti-obesity foods containing:**	**Discourage pre-obesity processed foods containing:**
	Omega-3 fatty acids	Refined carbohydrates
	High fiber	Trans and saturated fatty acids
	Lean quality protein sources	**Psychological**
	Whole fruits and vegetables	Changing relationship with food
	Foods rich in phytochemicals and antioxidants	Changes in support system
	Low-fat dairy (calcium)	Stress management
		Body image

Source: Adapted from Aills, L. et al., *Surgery for Obesity and Related Diseases*, 4, 2008, S73–S108.

regain involves evaluation of current eating practices, including increased caloric intake or increased consumption of calorically dense foods.[14] Table 15.2 displays a recommended outline of a post-bariatric surgery follow-up visit with a registered dietitian or nutrition counselor.[43] Frequent follow-up visits and continued patient-provider contact has been reported to improve weight maintenance and reduce the risk of weight regain. Sarwer et al.[16] emphasizes that obesity is a chronic disease, and behaviors that may contribute to obesity, such as lack of physical activity or inattention to diet, require continuous treatment.

To investigate whether postoperative dietary counseling from a registered dietitian may lead to greater weight loss and more positive changes in dietary intake and eating behaviors, Sarwer et al.[16] conducted a pilot study of 84 bariatric surgery patients who were randomly assigned to receive dietary counseling or standard pre-operative care for 4 months following surgery. Patients completed measures of mac-ronutrient intake and eating behaviors at baseline 2, 4, 6, 12, 18, and 24 months following surgery. Patients in the dietary counseling group were either seen in per-son or followed up with via telephone by the bariatric surgery program's registered dietitian. Patients who received dietary counseling had lower mean consumption of calories, sweets, and fats and a higher mean consumption of protein than those who did not have standard care. Although these differences were not significant ($p > .13$), dietary counseling produced a positive effect on patient's behaviors. Patients in the dietary arm reported changes in multiple eating behaviors that may be important to successful long-term weight loss and maintenance, including consuming fewer total calories, less consumption of sweets and fats and greater consumption of proteins, and fewer episodes of nausea, vomiting, and gastric dumping (in patients who under-went Roux-en-Y gastric bypass).

Follow-up visits with patients should reiterate the postsurgical dietary require-ments: protein, calories, vitamins, minerals, supplements, and fluid intake. For patients who have gained weight following surgery, it is advised that they decrease the overall calorie intake. The Academy of Nutrition and Dietetics suggests that the ultimate goal of weight management is to be achieved through sensible lifestyle mod-ifications including, but not limited to, improvements in caloric intake and exercise behaviors.[44] In patients who have experienced weight regain, dietary interventions should include a calorie-restricted diet, decreasing overall calorie intake, or decreas-ing intake of high-calorie dense foods. Low-calorie diets with an emphasis on portion control can also be modified to fit into the post-bariatric surgery nutrition param-eters of a high-protein and low-carbohydrate diet. Physical activity is also encouraged to promote a negative energy balance. AACE/TOS/ASMBS guidelines for exercise include a minimum of 150 min/week, with at least 2–3 days of strength training.[23]

In a behavior modification treatment program for weight loss, self-monitoring of food and beverage intake is imperative. This tactic helps patients identify suspect food choices and eating behaviors that can affect their long-term weight mainte-nance or contribute to weight regain. Targeting these problematic areas through documentation can provide the patient with feedback, such as daily calorie intake, and can give the patient an opportunity to self-regulate his or her food choices and eating behaviors.

Patients have many options available for self-monitoring. Over the past years, patients have mostly been reliant on manual methods such as keeping a written food diary or looking up calorie content in books to calculate total calorie intake. However, access to multiple online tools and applications for smart phones and tablets has made it easier for patients to keep track of their food intake and energy expenditure. These advantages may promote greater adherence to self-monitoring, and therefore dietary compliance.[16] The National Weight Control Registry has provided support-ing data regarding the importance and impact of self-monitoring. Individuals in the registry reported eating a reduced-calorie diet (average 1400 kcal/day), limiting fat intake, and regularly engaging in many self-monitoring behaviors such as diet track-ing and regularly weighing on scales.[45]

15.4 CONCLUSION

In conclusion, bariatric surgery is the most effective treatment for obesity and generally is safe and well tolerated. However, some patients respond suboptimally and experience weight regain postoperatively. Currently the incidence of weight regain following bariatric surgery is not well defined. The current literature suggests that a significant percentage of patients will experience regain beginning several years following surgery. There are multiple determinants of weight regain that include biological, surgical, behavioral, social, and psychological factors. However, the extent and significance of these factors remain uncertain. Patients who present with significant weight regain following bariatric surgery should undergo a comprehensive evaluation for determination of corrective factors. Additional clinical research is needed to further define this long-term postoperative problem.

REFERENCES

1. Prachand VN. The evolution of minimally invasive bariatric surgery. *World J Surg* 2011; 35: 1464–1468.
2. Buchwald H, et al. Bariatric surgery: a systematic review and meta-analysis. *JAMA* 2004; 292: 1724–1737.
3. O'Brien PE, McPhail T, Chaston TB, Dixon JB. Systematic review of medium-term weight loss after bariatric operations. *Obes Surg* 2006; 16: 1032–1040.
4. Shah M, Simha V, Garg A. Long-term impact of bariatric surgery on body weight, comorbidities, and nutritional status. *J Clin Endocrinol Metab* 2006; 91(11): 4223–4231.
5. Heber D, Greenway FL, Kaplan LM, Livingston E, Salvador J, Still C. Endocrine and nutritional management of the post-bariatric surgery patient: an Endocrine Society clinical practice guideline. *J Clin Endocrinol Metab* 2010; 95: 4823–4843.
6. Sjöström L, Narbro K, Sjöström CD, Karason K, Larsson B, Wedel H, et al. Swedish Obese Subjects study: effects of bariatric surgery on mortality in Swedish obese subjects. *N Engl J Med* 2007; 357: 741–752.
7. Sjöström L, Lindroos AK, Peltonen M, Torgerson J, Bouchard C, Carlsson B, et al. Lifestyle, diabetes, and cardiovascular risk factors 10 years after bariatric surgery. *N Engl J Med* 2004; 351: 2683–2693.
8. Synder B, Nguyen A, Scarbourough T, Yu S, Wilson E. Comparison of those who succeed in losing significant excessive weight after bariatric surgery and those who fail. *Surg Endosc* 2009; 23(10): 2302–2306.
9. Melton GB, Steele KE, Schweitzer MA, Lidor AO, Magnuson TH. Suboptimal weight loss after gastric bypass surgery; correlation of demographics, comorbidities, and insurance status with outcomes. *J Gastrointest Surg* 2008; 12(2): 250–255.
10. Kruseman M, Leimgruber A, Zumbach F, Golay A. Dietary, weight, and psychological changes among patients with obesity, 8 years after gastric bypass. *J Am Diet Assoc* 2010; 110(4): 527–534.
11. Patel S, Szomstein S, Rosenthal RJ. Reasons and outcomes of reoperative bariatric surgery for failed and complicated procedures (excluding adjustable and gastric banding). *Obes Surg* 2011; 21: 1209–1219.
12. Deylgat B, D'Hondt M, Pottel H, Vansteenkiste F, VanRooy F, Devriendt D. Indications, safety, and feasibility of conversion of failed bariatric surgery to Roux-en-Y gastric bypass: a retrospective comparative study with primary laparoscopic Roux-en Y gastric bypass. *Surg Endosc* 2012; 26: 1997–2002.

13. Scott WR, Batterham RL. Roux-en-Y-gastric bypass and laparoscopic sleeve gastrectomy; understanding weight loss and improvements in type 2 diabetes after bariatric surgery. *Am J Physiol Regul Integr Comp Physiol* 2011; 301: R15–R27.

14. Mechanick JI, Kushner RF, Sugarman JM, Gonzalez-Campoy M, Collazo-Clavell M, Guven S, Spitz AF, Apovian CM, Livingston EH, Brolin R, Sarwer DB, Anderson WA, Dixon J. American Association of Clinical Endocrinologists, The Obesity Society, and American Society for Metabolic and Bariatric Surgery medical guidelines for clinical practice for the perioperative nutritional, metabolic and nonsurgical support of the bariatric patient. *Obesity* 2009; 17(Suppl 1): S1–S70.

15. Sarwer DB, Dilks RJ, West-Smith L. Dietary intake and eating behavior after bariatric surgery: threats to weight loss maintenance and strategies for success. *Surg Obes Relat Dis* 2011; 7: 644–651.

16. Sarwer DB, Moore RH, Spitzer JC, Wadden TA, Raper SE, Williams NN. A pilot study investigating the efficacy of postoperative dietary counseling to improve outcomes after bariatric surgery. *Surg Obes Relat Dis* 2012; 8: 561–568.

17. Sarwer DB, Wadden TA, Moore RH, Baker AW, Gibbons LM, Raper SE, Williams NN. Preoperative eating behavior, postoperative dietary adherence, and weight loss after gastric bypass surgery. *Surg Obes Relat Dis* 2008; 4: 640–646.

18. Banjerjee A, Ding Y, Mikami DJ. The role of dumping syndrome in weight loss after gastric bypass surgery. *Surg Endosc* 2013; 27: 1573–1578.

19. Conason A, Teixeira J, Hsu CH, Puma L, Knafo D, Geliebter A. Substance use following bariatric weight loss surgery. *JAMA* 2013; 148(2): 145–150.

20. King WC, Chen JY, Mitchell JE, Kalarchian MA, et al. Prevalence of alcohol use disorders before and after bariatric surgery. *JAMA* 2012; 307(23): 2516–2525.

21. Odom J, Zalesin KC, Washington TL, Miller WW, Hakmeh B, Zaremba DL, Altattan M, Balasubramaniam M, Gibbs DS, Krause KR, Chengis DL, Franklin BA, McCullough PA. Behavioral predictors of weight regain after bariatric surgery. *Obes Surg* 2010; 20: 349–356.

22. Livhits M, Mercado C, Yermilov I, Parikh JA, Dutson E, Mehran A, Ko CK, Gibbons MM. Behavioral factors associated with successful weight loss after gastric bypass. *Am Surg* 2010; 76(10): 1139–1142.

23. Mechanik JI, Youdin A, Jones DB, Garvey T, Hurley DL, McMahon MM, Heinburg LJ, Kushner R, Adams TD, Shikora S, Dixon JB, Brethauer S. Clinical practice guidelines for the perioperative nutritional, metabolic and nonsurgical support of the bariatric surgery patient—2013 update: cosponsored by American Association of Clinical Endocrinologists, The Obesity Society, and American Society for Metabolic and Bariatric Surgery. *Obesity* 2013; 21(S1): S1–S26.

24. Bond DS, Evans RK, Wolfe LG, et al. Impact of self-reported physical activity participation on proportion of excess weight loss and BMI among gastric bypass surgery patients. *Am Surg* 2004; 70: 811–814.

25. American College of Sports Medicine. ACSM issues new recommendations on quantity and quality of exercise. 2013. Retrieved from http://www.ascm.org.

26. Vesco, K, Dietz PM, Rizzo J, Stevens VJ, Perrin NA, Bachman DJ, et al. Excessive gestational weight gain and postpartum weight retention among obese women. *Obstet Gynecol* 2009; 114: 1069–1075.

27. Amorim A, Rossner S, Neovius M, Lourenco PM, Linne Y. Does excess pregnancy weight gain constitute a major risk for increasing long-term BMI? *Obesity* 2007; 15: 1278–1286.

28. Manum AA, Kinarivala M, O'Callaghan MJ, Williams GM, Najman JM, Callaway LK. Associations of excess weight gain during pregnancy with long-term maternal overweight and obesity: evidence from 21 y postpartum follow-up. *Am J Clin Nutr* 2010; 91: 1336–1341.

29. Dixon JB, Dixon ME, O'Brien PE. Birth outcomes in obese women after laparoscopic adjustable gastric banding. *Obstet Gynecol* 2005; 106(Part 1): 965–972.
30. Sheiner E, Edri A, Balaban E, Levi I, Aricha-Tamir B. Pregnancy outcome of patients who conceive during or after the first year following bariatric surgery. *Am J Obstet Gynecol* 2011; 204: 50.e1–6.
31. Simkin-Silverman LR, Wing RR. Weight gain during menopause. Is it inevitable or can it be prevented? *Postgrad Med* 2000; 108(3): 47–50, 53–56.
32. Lovejoy JC, Champagne CM, de Jonge L, Xie H, Smith SR. Increased visceral fat and decreased energy expenditure during the menopausal transition. *Int J Obes* 2008; 32: 949–958.
33. DaSilva JA, Jacobs JW, Kirwan JR, Boers M, Saag KG, Inês LB, et al. Safety of low dose glucocorticoid treatment in rheumatoid arthritis: published evidence and prospective trial data. *Ann Rheum Dis* 2006; 65(3): 285.
34. Fierabracci P, Pinchera A, Martinelli S, Scartabelli G, Salvetti G, Giannetti M, et al. Prevalence of endocrine diseases in morbidly obese patients scheduled for bariatric surgery; beyond diabetes. *Obes Surg* 2011; 21: 54–60.
35. Levine MD, Kalarchian MA, Courcoulas AP, Wisinski MS, Marcus MD. History of smoking and post cessation weight gain among weight loss surgery candidates. *Addict Behav* 2007; 32: 2365–2371.
36. Williamsom DF, Madans J, Anda RF, Kleinman JC, Giovino GA, Byers T. Smoking cessation and severity of weight gain in a national cohort. *N Engl J Med* 1991; 324: 739–745.
37. Kofman MD, Lent MR, Swencionis C. Maladpative eating patterns, quality of life, and weight outcomes following gastric bypass: results of an Internet survey. *Obesity* 2010; 18(10): 1938–1943.
38. Colles SL, Dixon JB, O'Brien PE. Grazing and loss of control related to eating: two high risk factors following bariatric surgery. *Obesity* 2008; 16(3): 615–622.
39. Sogg S. Alcohol misuse after bariatric surgery: epiphenomenon or "Oprah" phenomenon? *Surg Obes Relat Dis* 2008; 3(3): 366–368.
40. Coughlin JW, et al. A screening tool to assess and manage behavioral risk in the postoperative bariatric surgery patient: the WATCH. *J Clin Psychol Med Settings* 2013. DOI 10.1007/s10880-012-9358-4.
41. Madan AK, Tichansky DS. Patients postoperatively forget aspects of preoperative patient education. *Obes Surg* 2005; 15: 1066–1069.
42. Freire RH, Borges MC, Alvarwez-Leite JI, Correia MITD. Food quality, physical activity, and nutritional follow-up as determinant of weight regain after Roux-en-Y gastric bypass. *Nutrition* 2012; 28: 53–58.
43. Allied Health Sciences Section Ad Hoc Nutrition Committee, Aills L, Blankenship J, Buffington C, Furtado M, Parrott J. ASMBS Allied Health nutritional guidelines for the surgical weight loss patient. *Surg Obes Relat Dis* 2008; 4(5): S73–108.
44. American Dietetics Association. Position of the American Dietetic Association: weight management. *J Am Diet Assoc* 2002; 1145–1155.
45. Kelm ML, Wing RR, McGuire MT, Seagle HM, Hill JO. A descriptive study of individuals successful at long-term maintenance of substantial weight loss. *Am J Clin Nutr* 1997; 66(2): 239–246.

Index

A

ABW, *see* Actual body weight
ACTH, *see* Adrenocorticotropic hormone
Actual body weight (ABW), 260
Addiction transfer, 235, 270
Ad hoc stomach BPD (AHS BPD), 183
Adjustable gastric band (AGB), 266
ADMA, *see* Asymmetric dimethyl arginine
Adolescents, *see* Special populations, adolescents
Adrenocorticotropic hormone (ACTH), 272
AGB, *see* Adjustable gastric band
Agouti-related peptide, 4
AHS BPD, *see* Ad hoc stomach BPD
Alcohol use disorder (AUD), 235, 270
Alendronate, 167
Alimentary hypoglycemia, 202
Amikacin, 162
Amino acid deficiency, 247
Anastomotic ulcer, 95
Anemia
    iron deficiency, 217
    menstrual changes and, 203
Anemia, bariatric surgery and, 61–75
    anatomic and physiologic mechanisms for
        post-bariatric surgery anemia, 62
    causes of anemia in immediate postoperative
        setting, 64–65
        disseminated intravascular coagulation,
            64
        most significant cause of acute anemia, 64
        thrombotic thrombocytopenic purpura,
            64–65
        uncommon causes of postoperative
            anemia, 64
    copper deficiency, 69
        myeloneuropathic syndrome, 69
        neutrophil production, 69
    iron deficiency, 65–67
        ferrous gluconate, 66
        hemachromotosis, 66
        heme iron, 66
        hypersegmented neutrophils, 66
        iron overload state, 66
        macrocytosis, 66
        nonanemia symptoms, 65
        proton pump inhibitor, 66
    late-onset anemia following bariatric surgery,
        65
    niacin deficiency, 70
        nicotinamide adenine dinucleotide, 70

pellagra, 70
    riboflavin deficiency, 70
        flavin adenine dinucleotide, 70
        flavin mononucleotide, 70
        galactoflavin, 70
    small bowel, 63–64
        blind-pouch syndrome, 64
        bone marrow biopsy, 63
        jejunum, 63
        trace element absorption in, 63
    specific causes of anemia following bariatric
        surgery, 65–72
        ascorbic acid deficiency, 71
        copper deficiency, 69
        folate deficiency, 67
        iron deficiency, 65–67
        niacin deficiency, 70
        protein deficiency, 71–72
        pyridoxine deficiency, 70–71
        riboflavin deficiency, 70
        thiamine deficiency, 69
        vitamin B_{12} deficiency, 67–68
    stomach, 62–63
        intrinsic factor, 62
        iron deficiency anemia, 62
        overgrowth of nonresident flora, 63
    thiamine deficiency, 69
        ketoacids, 69
        Wernicke encephalopathy syndrome, 69
    vitamin B_{12} deficiency, 67–68
        blind-pouch syndrome, 68
        lactate dehydrogenase, 68
        macrocytic anemia, 68
        neuropathy, 68
        parasthesias, 68
Anorexia nervosa, 178
APACHE II scores, 258
Arachidonic acid generation, 261
Arginine, 247
Ascorbic acid deficiency, 71, 249
Asthma, 24, 270
Asymmetric dimethyl arginine (ADMA), 261
AUD, *see* Alcohol use disorder
Autoimmune disorders, 257

B

Bacterial overgrowth syndrome, 180
Barbiturates, 142
Bariatric beriberi, 103
BED, *see* Binge eating disorder